Medical Physics Monograph No. 25

PRACTICAL DIGITAL IMAGING AND PACS

D1276251

Edited by

J. Anthony Seibert, Ph.D.
Larry J. Filipow, D.Phil.
Katherine P. Andriole, Ph.D.

American Association of Physicists in Medicine
1999 Summer School Proceedings
Sonoma State University
Rohnert Park, California

Published for the
American Association of Physicists in Medicine
by Medical Physics Publishing

To order American Association of Physicists in Medicine publications, contact:

Medical Physics Publishing
Phone: 1-800-442-5778
or (608) 262-4021
Fax: (608) 265-2121
E-mail: mpp@medicalphysics.org
Order on-line: www.medicalphysics.org

Published by:
Medical Physics Publishing
Madison, WI

Published for:
American Association of Physicists in Medicine
One Physics Ellipse
College Park, MD 20740-3846
(301) 209-3350
Fax: (301) 209-0862

Library of Congress Catalog Card Number: 99-62806
ISBN: 0-944838-20-0 (hardcover)
ISBN: 0-944838-92-8 (softcover)

Printed in the United States of America

CONTENTS

Preface

This book is a compendium of 25 papers presented at the 1999 American Association of Physicists in Medicine Summer School at Sonoma State University in Rohnert Park, California during the week of June 26 through July 1. At the direction of the summer school subcommittee of the Continuing Education Committee, the topic of Digital Imaging and PACS was selected. Certainly the timeliness of the topic and the recognized need for the medical physicist to play a key role in the implementation of these systems in diagnostic imaging are the major reasons. With this in mind, the scientific committee has designed the program with an emphasis on new advances in imaging technology, covering all of the inherently digital imaging modalities such as Computed Radiography, CT, MRI, Ultrasound, and Nuclear Medicine. Digital Imaging and Communications in Medicine (DICOM) standards provide the path to integration of an electronic network and PACS comprised of digital imaging modalities, image workstations, and image archive. Knowledge of these standards to ensure a successful PACS implementation, for which the medical physicist takes a primary responsibility, is essential. Therefore, the focus of this summer school is to provide the medical physicist and other interested individuals with tools and information to become conversant with the details of DICOM, and to enable the verification of optimal image acquisition, display, archiving, and quality control of PACS in the clinical environment.

These proceedings represent the work of truly dedicated professionals who have volunteered their time and effort to provide an educational experience that is much greater than the printed words in this monograph. The scientific program committee would like to thank the entire faculty for their timely manuscript submittals to allow the publication of the proceedings prior to the summer school. This book was produced and copy-edited by Betsey Phelps of Medical Physics Publishing under very tight deadlines and many long hours. We, the scientific program directors, are very grateful for her patience and diligence.

Steve Thompson has masterfully directed local arrangements in conjunction with members of the local arrangements committee, including Virgil Cooper, Kali Mather, Bob Miller of the San Francisco Bay Area Chapter of the AAPM, and Jeanne Levesque of Argus Software. Sherry Connors, our summer school expert, Bruce Thomadsen, Herb Mower and other members of the AAPM summer school subcommittee participating in the event are gratefully acknowledged for their support. All of the members of the Local Arrangements Committee are responsible for the support around the campus and many wonderful opportunities and extracurricular activities that are offered throughout the week for the attendees and their families. Fred Jorgensen and Sandy Bond of Sonoma State University summer conferences deserve much credit and recognition for their help.

Acknowledgments and thanks go to AAPM headquarters personnel, including Angela Keyser, Lisa Rose Sullivan, and Nancy Vazquez for tremendous assistance in negotiations, registration, assistance to the local arrangements committee, CAMPEP application, and Medical Physics Continuing Education Credits. Lee Goldman, chairman of the AAPM Summer School Subcommittee of the Continuing Education Committee, and Don Frey, Chairman of the Education Council have provided solid support and assistance to insure the success of this endeavor.

Finally, we wish to thank the attendees of the 1999 Summer School—your support allows the Education Committee to continue offering opportunities such as these year after year. Hopefully you will find this experience well worth your time and attention.

Tony Seibert, Larry Filipow, Kathy Andriole

American Association of Physicists in Medicine 1999 Summer School
Sonoma State University
Rohnert Park, California

Picture Archiving and Communication Systems—an Overview

Larry J. Filipow, D.Phil.
Department of Radiology
University of Alberta
Edmonton, Alberta, Canada

Introduction

As computers became more prevalent in the early 1980's and suggestions of a paper-less office were first being presented, the idea of eliminating film from radiology departments started to be discussed. Modalities such as Computed Tomography (CT) and Nuclear Medicine (NM) were already producing image data in a digital form, only to have the images sent to a high resolution video printer for subsequent display on film. Subtraction angiography was poised to become digital, and with the ability to transform the signal from an image intensifier into a digital one by using analog to digital converters, the possibility of general radiography becoming a digital modality seemed to be just around the corner.

Almost 20 years later, in 1999, we still do not have a paperless office system; in fact, we use more paper now than ever before in history. In diagnostic imaging, we have two new modalities producing copious digital images: ultrasound (US) and MRI (Magnetic Resonance Imaging). Yet, we also do not have a truly filmless department. And, it could be argued, we print more film now than ever before in history. So what happened?

Early estimates of the capability of digital imaging were extremely overly optimistic. 1980's digital technology was simply not capable of providing the quality, speed, and cost effectiveness necessary to replace film in the radiology department. In my simple terms, it was not better, faster, nor cheaper. Faced with a product that:

- provided inferior diagnostic quality on early computer displays,

- was considerably slower in transmitting image data across fledgling networks, and

- cost prohibitively more,

radiologists and administrators quite appropriately said "no thanks"!

However, once again, over the last few years, the concept of filmless, digital radiology departments has become a popular idea. But this time, discussions are far more realistic and focused on rational decisions regarding quality, performance, and cost-benefit. The reason? Only very recently, since approximately 1997, the technology in regard to:

1

- image quality of the displays (high resolution and high intensity);

- the power of the computers (fast CPUs, large amounts of RAM);

- the speed of the networks (100+ Mbit/sec copper, 600+ Mbit/sec fiber optics);

- the intelligence of the file management software (databases, archive servers);

- the size of the storage devices [RAIDs, (redundant array of independent disks) Jukeboxes];

- the engineered quality of all the components (reliability, accuracy);

- the standardization of the communications formats (DICOM); and, importantly, the overall cost of all the above;

have all come together to make a filmless department a very realistic, reasonable, achievable goal. It's even cost beneficial.

And the hospitals are starting to line up to convert.

Since the discovery of x-rays by W.C. Roentgen in 1896, radiology images have been provided to physicians on an emulsion coated plastic base, popularly known as "film."

Film has many basic advantages:

- It is easy to move from place to place.

- It yields spatial resolution better than the human eye can detect.

- It can be "viewed" using straightforward light boxes.

- It is relatively inexpensive, compared to the imaging equipment used to produce the image.

Film, however, also has some glaring disadvantages, made even more glaring by the distributed, regional or HMO manner in which healthcare is provided these days.

The main disadvantages are:

- Flm can only exist in a single place at any given time.

- Once printed, no further image manipulation or enhancement is possible.

- Processing of film requires harmful chemicals to be released into the environment.

- Film is relatively expensive, costing on the order of a dollar or two per sheet, the total cost of which can accumulate very rapidly for busy departments.

- Storage and retrieval (handling) of exams requires significant space and much manpower.

- Films get lost.

The advantages of Picture Archiving and Communication System (PACS) are:

- A digital image can exist in many places (e.g. Trauma, O.R., Radiology, Referring physician's office) simultaneously.

- A digital image can be extensively manipulated (brightness, contrast, smoothing, measurements) and its diagnostic information enhanced to provide better, more accurate assessment.

- A digital image costs nothing to display or copy.

- No environmental effects because no processing chemicals required.

- Retrieval of older exams (for comparison purposes) is very easy if not automatic and instantaneous.

- The quality of images for certain digital modalities surpasses that of film.

In summary, in simple terms, PACS <u>is</u> better, faster, and, in most cases, cheaper than film dependent radiology:

- Better quality of images improve diagnostic capability and hence patient care.

- Faster access and retrieval of patient images anywhere, anytime.

- (Proven) lower operating costs for most modalities than using a consumable resource such as film.

Definition of PACS

PACS is the popular term used to describe a filmless situation in diagnostic imaging where images are produced, analyzed, distributed, and stored in electronic form. I personally do not like the term—filmless radiology is more than simple pictures, and we do not only archive and communicate them. A more appropriate and descriptive term, I believe, is IMACS (Image Management and Communication System). Being two syllables, however, it will (and already has to some extent) lose to the term "PACS."

PACS can be described as an amalgam of five fundamental processes/components:

1. Production of digital images (CT, MRI, US, NM, Film Digitization, Computed Radiography (CR), Direct radiography).

2. Communication/networking infrastructure (telephone lines, ethernet lines, fiber optic cable, digital switches, hubs, modems).

3. File and image management (patient and exam demographics, database of images, pre-fetching of old exams, auto-routing of images around the network).

4. Analysis and Display (computer workstations, radiologist reporting stations, clinical review stations, PC review stations).

5. Storage [RAIDs, digital archives, archive servers, WEB servers)].

Implementation of PACS

PACS/Film Comparisons

Is PACS for everyone? Not quite yet. At the world congress of Medical Physics held in 1991 in Kyoto, Japan, a whole day mini-symposium on PACS concluded with the following two main criteria only, for a radiology department to embark on the digital journey:

- A big problem managing film
- A friendly banker

Eight years later, these two main reasons for implementing a PACS still are relevant. PACS can solve some big problems with respect to film management, and still at large capital cost. But PACS has now matured to the point where it provides its own advantages, and does not need to be installed solely to solve problems.

So why is PACS not for everyone just yet? Because it cannot yet be cost-justified for smaller departments, where savings from reduction of film use and reduction in clerical staffing do not exist or are insufficient to offset the capital costs, even after a number of years of operation. Nevertheless, the size requirement for departments to be suitable candidates for PACS is shrinking.

Process and Operational Review of a Department

PACS will <u>not</u> cure an inherently bad process. Those hoping to purchase technology to correct a poor operational situation are in for an unpleasant surprise. PACS in its worst implementation can easily stand for "Picture a Chaotic Scene." Even in a benign form, it can simply stand for "Purchase Ample Computer Systems."

Careful scrutiny and analysis of a department's operations can clearly point out deficiencies in the process that a PACS cannot overcome, and those it can. Realistic objectives, before spending large amounts of cash, can produce user satisfaction and support of a PACS initiative, rather than frustration and enmity towards the system.

The operational review of a department should firstly consider the diagnostic imaging modalities present, which would typically be:

- CT
- Ultrasound
- Nuclear Medicine
- MRI
- Angiography
- General Radiography
- General Fluoroscopy

A thorough analysis of workload, volumes, exam recalls, distribution of images, and medico-legal storage requirements needs to be completed for each of these modalities.

The next step would be to assess the radiology "clients" needs, and their processes of interaction with radiology. These are the attending medical disciplines that use radiology resources. They would include:

- Emergency
- Neurosurgery
- Critical care
- Neurology
- Pediatrics
- Outpatient Clinics
- Inpatient Wards

Again, a thorough analysis of exam volumes, exam recalls, distribution of images, and numbers of users and user groups (physicians, interns, residents, nursing staff) needs to be completed for each of these areas.

The operational review needs to account for regional and local linkages, i.e., requirements for the images/exams to move around a region, or a city, or a multi-facility organization. Here, network issues become important because high-speed communication line rental costs across a city or region can be prohibitive, and can significantly impact operational budgets.

The operational review must closely scrutinize staffing levels. The four areas of staffing affected by PACS would be in:

- Clerical (Film and File Management)
  Displaying/Communicating
  Archiving
  Retrieving
  Report Gathering

- Technologist
  Total time for Examination

- Radiologist
  Reporting Efficiency

- Referring Physician
  Film retrieval efficiency

Benchmarking at this point is a useful exercise. Comparisons of Exams per FTE, Cost per Exam, Exams per bed, type of exams provided, and Workload units; with respect to inter-hospital, inter-state, or national standards can highlight areas of excellence or problem areas.

Growth should be factored into any PACS initiative. An accurate estimate of anticipated exam volumes and demands for diagnostic imaging services will be extremely helpful in appropriately sizing the PACS and establishing an initial infrastructure (both physical and economic) that will be able to cope with future expansion.

In summary, a thorough and well-conducted Process and Operational Review of the diagnostic imaging services and service demands before implementation of a PACS will go a long way to help address current and future needs. The conflicting issues of ever increasing service demands but ever decreasing funding can be resolved to some extent with PACS. It can (and will) do this by increasing overall efficiency of the radiology service by the judicious and careful application of digital technology.

PACS/IMACS Requirements

When designing and installing a PACS, the five distinct components mentioned earlier need to be considered:

- Production of Images
- Network Infrastructure
- Image Management
- Display and Analysis

- Storage of Images

Production of Images

Before any image can be digitally manipulated, analyzed, communicated or stored, it of course must be first created. In most departments there are four modalities that produce images inherently in a digital format. This would be a good place to start a PACS initiative— no significant extra expense needs to be accrued to provide these images to a PACS (it will be seen that the equipment required to produce digital images is the most costly aspect of a PACS).

The four modalities that are inherently digital are:

- Computed Tomography
- Ultrasound
- Nuclear Medicine
- Magnetic Resonance Imaging

In most departments, these modalities are probably already operating in a "mini-PACS" environment. The CT scanner will have a vendor specific workstation connected to do multi-planar reformatting and other reconstruction tasks. A similar configuration will be found in the MRI area. A lot of large ultrasound departments will already be connected to a small local network that provides images to large monitors for soft copy reporting. And most nuclear medicine departments will likely have a home-built network to move images between acquisition units and workstations. In most cases, communications will probably be vendor-proprietary. Standardization of the formats to DICOM (Digital Imaging and Communications in Medicine) will be required, usually achievable without major cost. An addition of an archive, and archive and file server starts the inevitable evolution of a PACS.

Subsequent additions to the PACS would follow logically:

- Angiography (new equipment all digital)
- Fluoroscopy (new equipment all digital)

At this point, all images in the department would be digital, except for general radiography. This is the final challenge or hurdle to a virtually filmless department. And it is the largest one.

General radiography probably accounts for 70% of diagnostic imaging workloads, and the image resolution required to provide accurate diagnoses for chest images is the greatest of all modalities. So general radiography creates the largest exam volumes and demands the highest resolution. This places the greatest demands on network speed, database management, display quality, display size, and storage volumes.

There are currently three ways to produce digital data from general radiography:

- Film Digitizers
- Computed Radiography
- Direct Radiography

Film digitizers are at a level of maturity and engineering design that enables them to provide very good digital analogs of plain film x-rays. The only problem is that filming is still required, so there can be no savings realized from reduction of film use. Nevertheless, for remote clinics where there is no access to radiologist resources, film digitization and subsequent transmission of the data to a central facility is a practical, relatively inexpensive way to get connected.

Computed Radiography (CR) is currently the most common method of "digitizing" general radiography. Film cassettes are replaced by cassettes containing photostimulable imaging plates, which capture the latent image and are subsequently read by a laser reader. The processes of acquiring the image are unchanged from those of plain film radiography, so there is no change to the technologist's function. The digital images are of very good quality, and are subsequently provided to the PACS, for reporting and analysis.

The main drawback to CR is the large capital cost of the laser readers, which are 5 to 10 fold more expensive than chemical film processors, and the increased cost and reduced durability of the phosphor plates, as compared with film cassettes. The durability problems are being addressed, and the cost of the plates is coming more in to line with film cassettes. CR will enjoy a long future in general radiography.

Direct Radiography (DR) is a term used to describe a very recent technology, one which is still largely in the development stages. DR uses large plates (43×43 cm) of thin film transistor (TFT) arrays to either directly convert incident x-ray photons into electrical signals sent directly to a PACS, or to convert incident x-ray photons into light photons via a scintillator painted on a TFT array, which then converts the scintillation photons into electrical signals sent directly to a PACS.

Image quality with respect to both spatial resolution and contrast resolution is excellent, better than film. The direct connection to a PACS eliminates the timely process of reading the phosphor plate required in CR. DR is definitely the direction filmless imaging will go. The problem? DR is, at this point, prohibitively expensive, and cannot address the needs of portable radiography. Also, the engineering requirements of durability and consistency in the field have really not been assessed. As well, a single DR image can occupy 12 Mbytes or more of digital space, and managing such large images around a network places great demands on all components of a PACS.

Network Infrastructure

The network is a very integral part of the PACS. A well-designed, sufficiently fast network will do much to provide satisfaction with the PACS, while a poorly designed network that is too slow, or shares bandwidth with other applications, can easily produce sufficient frustration to retard or reverse PACS evolution.

Network design should be done with the full cooperation of the Information Systems (IS) or Information Technology (IT) departments. Their expertise and resources will be invaluable in designing and implementing the network, and in some cases there may already be adequate spare bandwidth available in buildings or across campuses to reduce additional costs for PACS network infrastructure. However, having involved IS/IT people in the PACS network design, it is imperative for the Diagnostic Imaging (DI) people to ensure that they (IS/IT) fully understand the unique requirements for PACS communications. Usually they do not, and will attempt to assign shared lines for the PACS. This will benefit nobody. DI is not like Lab Medicine, or Admitting, or Finance, or other network users. PACS will move <u>large</u> files around a network, and will usually need to move them <u>quickly</u>. The best configuration for a PACS network is to be physically isolated (typically by means of switches) from the hospital backbone.

"Pipes," which, in my definition, consist of both the conduit and the wire, (either copper or fiber optic) need to be appropriately sized in terms of bandwidth. Between facilities, the rental cost of these lines, usually supplied by telcos, can be a major drain on a PACS operating budget. Appropriateness of bandwidth can only be determined by a careful study of digital traffic rates and volumes. As an example: a very expensive, high-speed connection between two hospitals may not be necessary if it is found that only 10 patient files a day are sent between the institutions, and physician requests for images are not *ad hoc*, but rather after the patient arrives from the other institution (which perhaps takes 30 minutes for travel). Thus a "push" can be initiated from the first institution, and the images will arrive electronically long before the patient does, even across a slow, inexpensive POTS (plain old telephone system) line.

Image Management

The management of image data around a busy, large network is anything but a trivial task. A good file management system is the "guts" of a well-functioning PACS, and comprises database and file management software. It includes the functionality of the archive server and archive, although these will be discussed later under "storage."

Good image management is optimized with the presence of a Radiology Information System (RIS) or Hospital Information System (HIS), which will provide the PACS with order/entry, patient demographic, and scheduling information. This will enable the PACS file manager to compare new and old patient data and rationalize it in case of errors, hunt for and pre-fetch prior exams done on a patient, and auto-route the prior and current exams to the relevant reporting stations or physicians. The file management software should also allow systemwide configurability for a number of housekeeping tasks:

- Purging rules—removal of old images/exams from hard drives after certain criteria have been met (for example—exam reported + exam archived + exam older than 3 weeks).

- Load balancing—distribution of reporting workload between stations and/or radiologists.

- User access privileges and security of information.

- Configurability of GUIs (graphical user interfaces) and FUIs (functional user interfaces).

- Redundancy of data repositories (i.e., no single point of failure or irretrievable data loss).

A good file management system needs to be scalable, and should incorporate comprehensive management statistics to allow for effective decision making regarding its own evolution.

Display and Analysis

There are, I believe, currently six different generic types of display and analysis systems/stations that can be identified. The distinctions separating these devices are dependent on the functionality, the connection, or simply the use. Near-future technology evolution will reduce these six types to two, or perhaps ultimately only one type.

- Radiologist Work Station

  This term is usually misapplied and can lead to confusion. In my opinion, it should only be applied to a (usually) vendor-specific computing station, which provides reformatting or 3D display and analysis capabilities. These are typically used to work the raw data from CT, MRI, NM to produce a variety of displays: maximum intensity projections, minimum intensity projections, 3D surface rendering, 3D volume rendering, multi-planar reformatting, angiographic images, curve processing, disarticulation images, cardiac analysis, etc. These are the very highest performance computers, usually with vector processors/array processors, and would not normally be used for routine reporting duties.

- Radiologist Reporting Station

This is the device that replaces film view boxes for radiologists. It will typically be a two monitor station, incorporating medium to high resolution, 1600×1600 pixel, high intensity, 100+ Foot Lambert, monochrome monitors. The monitors will be either in landscape or portrait layout, and there can be up to four of them, depending on use. They can also have resolutions of $2K \times 2K$ pixels or even more, although the expense for these increases exponentially.

These reporting stations will typically be PC based (apologies to Apple), running Windows NT, although the majority of current devices are SUN-based, running Unix. The stations have full analysis and functionality software:

> Multi-modality
> Multi-exam
> Region of interest (ROI)
> Window/level
> Roaming zoom
> Pixel read-out
> Edge enhance
> Smooth
> Distance
> Angle
> Multi-display
> "Page format save"
> Image format conversion (i.e., "save as")
> Print

They will be "loaded" with RAM, of the order of 256 Mbytes or more, and they will have a substantial local hard drive, of the order of 6 to 9 Gbytes. They will possess full query/retrieve access to the archive, and will possibly be directly linked to the reporting/dictating system.

- Clinical View Station

The clinical view station provides straightforward image review capabilities for attending or referring staff. Older stations are Unix- based systems, whereas current ones can be simple PCs, running Windows NT. The view station will be directly interfaced to the network, and will typically be found in the hospital, on the wards, and in the care units. The single monitor will be a standard 17" or 19" color monitor. The local hard drive needs to be sized appropriately for a minimum of 24 hours of storage capacity of estimated film volumes. In most cases, images will be pulled from the image server and reside only in RAM during the duration of the viewing, and then be deleted. The clinical view station will contain very simple, <u>intuitive</u> software:

File directory
Fetch, Display
Brightness/Contrast
Roaming zoom
Image collage
Image format conversion (i.e., "save as")

- PC Review Station

Identical to the clinical view station, running Windows 95,98, or NT. It will have a network interface card, and run the same PACS software as the clinical view station, but may also run other hospital applications. It will be a multi-purpose device, not used exclusively for PACS.

- Home/Office Review Station

Identical to the PC review station, but situated at home or in a physician's office. It will be connected to the PACS network via telephone modem, ADSL (asynchronous digital subscriber link), or cable modem. It may run the PACS software, or a third-party version. It may not have the privilege of querying the archive, but instead, have images pushed to it.

- Intranet/Internet Web Browser

This is a standard, found-in-the-home PC or MAC, that has minimal hardware requirements, and no additional or proprietary software other than a Web browser such as Netscape Navigator or Internet Explorer. This device will access the image/exam archive through a Web server that the hospital needs to install. Software viewing applications will be downloaded with the images/exams, most likely as Java applets. This device will (and is already starting to) supplant Clinical View Stations, PC Review Stations, and Home Review Stations. Connections will be as before, depending on location (hospital care unit, physician's office, home), but the attraction of no additional software requirements will be the primary reason for expansion of this technology. Advantages include the fact that through a Web server, the hospital can provide images to all relevant persons—attending and referring staff, care unit staff, clinics, offices, and homes. Expansion is easy, and will not be costly. There is even some indication that radiologist reporting stations may ultimately be connected to the Web server.

In summary, therefore, the display and analysis required for a PACS will eventually involve only two types of computer stations. The first will be for reporting by radiologists—multi-monochrome monitor, RAM heavy, full functionality, high-end CPU platforms. The second will be for everybody else—single color monitor, basic functionality, standard PC based platforms.

Storage

Images/exams in a well-designed PACS will, at any point in time, be stored at several locations. This is to provide quick response to viewing requests, and to ensure no single point of catastrophic data loss. Images/exams will be first stored in the local hard drive of the modality by which they are produced. They will also be immediately sent to the PACS image server, where they will be stored on the system RAID (redundant array of independent discs) for a preset period of time, usually a few weeks or months. The file manager will also auto-route the images/exams to the appropriate reporting and review stations, to reside on their local hard drives for a period of a few days to a week, depending on disc size and exam volumes. Once reported, the exam will be stored on the long term archive. This will typically be a "jukebox" with robotic arms to select from an array of discs or tapes that are used to store anywhere from one to more years of image/exam data.

A careful assessment of total volumes of exams, exam sizes (in Mbytes), recall rates, specific routing requirements, user requirements, and long-term archiving requirements needs to be done. This will enable the appropriate sizing of fairly expensive local hard drives and RAIDs, as well as the less expensive long-term archive. Long-term archiving can be further subdivided into on-line or off-line. Off-line means the storage discs or tapes can be stored on a bookshelf, to be remounted when an old exam is requested. While this requires human intervention, if the recall rate for images that are more than 5 years old is only one per day on average, this may be more cost effective than buying a larger archive to keep them on-line.

Archive media choices are currently many, and there are advantages and disadvantages for each. A general rule of thumb is that, the faster the access and download speed for a given media, the more costly it will be. The graph below provides a comparison of costs and transfer speeds for current archive media. The costs are relative—they were correct in early 1998, but prices for storage continue to drop.

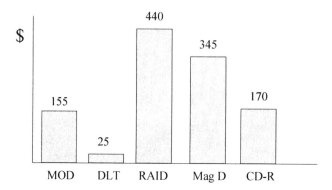

MOD: magneto-optical disc   DLT: digital linear tape
RAID: Redundant array of independent discs
Mag D: Magnetic disc   CD-R: compact disc-recordable

The next graph shows the transfer speeds for the various media to read/download a 40 Mbyte file.

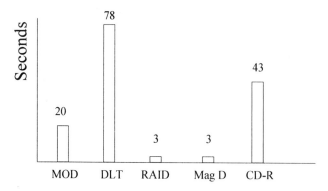

The access and read speeds may not be relevant if the archive has an appropriately sized front-end RAID, and images from the jukebox are moved to the RAID in the "dead of night" or other quiet network periods to be available for quicker recall when required. The assumption here is that the archive would store prior images that can be called up several days or weeks in advance. Current (last 3 months) images would reside on the system RAID.

Physical Logistics

An often overlooked area—siting of the stations—is very important, and can go a long way in ensuring success of the PACS. A radiologist reporting station should be located with a thought to the following:

- Accessibility (optimized process flow)

- Ambient light (as low as possible and adjustable)

- Consult environment (adequate space for referring staff to stand around the station)

- Monitor configuration (number, orientation)

- Proximity of lightboxes (for the odd film, and for the transition period between film and PACS)

- Outlets (power, network, dictation, telephone)

- RIS terminal

Similar consideration should be given to locating the clinical view stations.

Connectivity

PACS implementation needs to account for connectivity issues between components. Existing equipment in the department must be assessed as to the compatibility/connectivity it offers to a new PACS. Existing radiographic equipment that can handle CR cassettes needs no additional connectivity, whereas an older CT scanner may need a DICOM gateway to connect directly to a PACS. Other connectivity issues include compatibility with a hospital RIS or HIS, as well as vendor functionality within DICOM.

The current standard for text data exchange is HL-7, while for image data exchange it is DICOM 3.0. HL-7 information includes data from a RIS/HIS, which will empower a PACS file manager:

- Patient demographics
- Patient admitted/discharged
- Patient merge/change
- Exam scheduled
- Exam completed
- Exam reported
- Report verified

The DICOM 3.0 standard is more complicated, and considers the following:

- Information object:
    CT, X-ray, MRI, NM, US, CR

- Application entity:
    Workstation, Reporting station, Archive, Film Digitizer, Printer, CR, Modality

- Service class:
    Store, study content notification, patient management, query/retrieve, study management, print management, verification, results management

Patient management within DICOM includes ADT (admitting/discharge/transfer) information, demographics, and event/visit information. Study management includes creation, scheduling, performance, and tracking of studies. Results management includes creation, dispersion, and tracking of results.

DICOM links an information object with a service class to create a SOP (service-object pair). This SOP will be used to ensure that disparate types of equipment from different vendors will work together in pre-defined ways. "DICOM compatible" does not mean "plug and play," nor does it guarantee full functionality.

PACS/RIS compatibility will provide the following necessary communications:

- Matching of demographic information

- Provide scheduling and order information to PACS to enable prefetching of previous exams

- Provide procedure code information to PACS to enable auto-routing of images (organ systems, reporting station locations, presets)

- Provide PACS with previous reports

- Provide RIS with exam status (type, images completed)

- Provide PACS with study status (view, reported, verified)

Implementation Plan

A well-thought-out implementation plan is essential to provide a clear path toward a clear goal. PACS is not a device, or a bunch of devices, but is instead a process, with concomitant process changes that will affect many people. All stakeholders should be consulted in developing the plan, or, at the very least, informed of the plan once developed. An effective PACS implementation plan will include the following:

- A review of current processes and operating costs

- A detailed description of the required PACS/IMACS system

- A multi-phase, logical, reasonable implementation timeline

- Comprehensive cost-benefit analysis which considers:
  Capital, operating, maintenance, consumables, upgrades Intangibles (productivity, eficiency)

- PACS Goals

PACS Goals

The PACS goals are straightforward: Better, faster, cheaper.

- Better:
  Reduce patient stay (improve care).
  Increase referring physician satisfaction.
  Increase attending physician satisfaction.
  More access to previous exams.
  More analysis capability for the radiologist.

- Faster:
  > Reduce report turnaround time.
  > Reduce access time to images for attending physicians.
  > Reduce access time to images for referring physicians.
  > Quicker access to previous exams.
  > Current/previous exam synchronized viewing.

- Cheaper:
  > Lower the cost per exam.
  > Increase productivity to meet future increases in service demands with same staff levels.
  > Increase productivity to meet service demands with reduced staff levels.
  > Save money through elimination of consumables (film, chemicals).

Process Changes

As stated earlier, PACS is a process, and its implementation affects process(es) in the radiology environment. I have broken up the radiology "event" into three distinct processes: (1) Patient booking, (2) Examination, (3) Exam reporting and distribution. They are shown in the following figures.

Process A - Booking

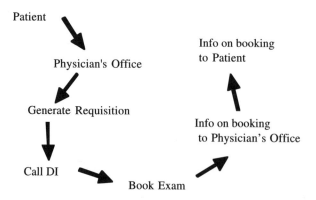

PACS will not impact nor affect any of the process steps in the Booking process (but an RIS will).

Process B - Examination

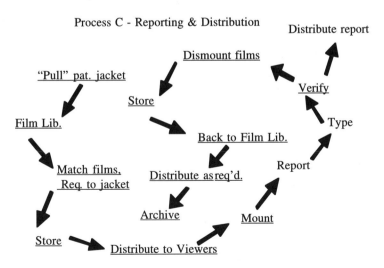

PACS will affect three process steps (underlined) in the Examination procedure: Process the images, Find the radiologist, and Audit. The images will be created digitally, and distributed within the PACS, which will negate the need to find a radiologist, assuming there is one somewhere on the PACS who can audit the images and authorize the release of the patient.

Process C - Reporting & Distribution

PACS will affect all processes underlined in Process C—Examination Reporting & Distribution. In fact, the majority of processes will be eliminated. It can be readily seen that PACS will have its major impact in this phase of the radiology "event." This is largely a clerical area, and so clerical functions will be the most changed after PACS.

Cost-Benefit Analysis

The cost-benefit approaches one would use in attempting to cost-justify a PACS would include:

- Reduce the use of film for reporting and viewing.

- Reduce/eliminate clerical need to retrieve previous exams from film library.

- Reduce/eliminate clerical need to mount previous exams on viewers.

- Reduce/eliminate clerical need to mount current exams on viewers.

- Reduce/eliminate clerical need to transport patient film jackets around department or between hospitals.

- Reduce/eliminate clerical need to find lost films (e.g., ER, OR).

- Reduce time required to find radiologist to audit images and release patient (especially in CT).

- Reduce time required to find films in ER, OR, so radiologist can report and reduce patient wait/length to stay.

The cost-benefit analysis should include both capital and operating costs. Operating costs should include PACS maintenance, network maintenance, staff training costs, software and hardware upgrade costs. A simple table that summarizes the components would look like the following:

Cost-Benefit Analysis

	Capital	
Net Savings:		Net Costs:
Camera/Processor Replacement		PACS
		Network Infrastructure

	Operating	
Net Savings:		Net Costs:
Film		PACS Maintenance
Chemistry		Network Maintenance
FTE Savings		Training

Evaluation of these items will provide a "pay-back" point in the future, where the accumulated cost savings from film elimination will balance the capital and operating costs of a PACS initiative. The graph of a CT/MRI/US PACS initiative will look something like the following:

Cost-Benefit Analysis
(MRI, CT, US)

Phase X

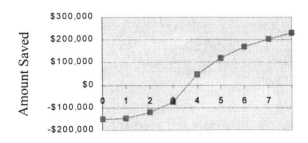

Year

Tangible items such as film savings and equipment capital costs are easy to incorporate into a costing evaluation. What is harder to do is to include the benefits of intangibles. Attempts, however, can be made to at least get a reasonable idea of the savings associated with these. Two examples of "intangibles" analysis follow.

Cost-Benefit Analysis

Intangibles:
FTE Savings from Elimination of Previous Exam "Pulls"

Total # of Exams	10,000
Total # of patients	8,000
% requiring previous exam pulls	75 %
--> Previous Exam Pulls	6,000
<Time> to pull Previous Exam	5 min
Total time for pulling P.E.'s	500 hrs
% FTE equivalent	25 %
FTE yearly pay	$25,000
Total annual saving	$ 6,182

Cost-Benefit Analysis

Intangibles:
Physician Savings from Elimination of Requirement to Access Film
library

Average # of Film Lib. Visits/week*	3.9
Average time / visit *	12.8 min
--> Average visit time/week	45 min
--> Average visit time/year	37.5 hrs
Physician hourly cost *	$ 250.00
Total cost for Film library visits/physician	$9,375.00

*University of Washington study
SPIE Med.Img. IV: PACS Sys.Dsgn. & Eval.

Conclusion

In summarizing, it must be understood that PACS will create a major culture change with respect to the manner in which a department of diagnostic imaging operates. PACS will also significantly change the way outside staff will interact with the diagnostic imaging department. Not only will images be available wherever there is a view station or PC, but even the process of consults will change considerably. PACS will absolutely separate the need to have the radiologist, referring physician, and film at the same physical location at the same time.

This last point is an important one. The push for PACS should and will eventually come from outside radiology—it is the clients of radiology services that will benefit most from a PACS.

In conclusion, therefore, the four following main statements accurately reflect the impact and the implementation of a PACS:

1. PACS is not primarily for Radiology, it's for Radiology clients.

2. PACS is not a bunch of devices, it's a process.

3. PACS is not a single purchase or endeavor, it's a continuum.

4. PACS is not static, but will continually evolve, and at a very rapid pace.

The following chapters and manuscripts in this book will deal with the issues discussed in this overview in a detailed, comprehensive manner.

References

Barnes, G.T., Lauro, K. "Image processing in digital radiography: basic concepts and applications." *Journal of Digital Imaging* 2: 132-146, 1989.

Bidgood, W.D. Jr., Horii, S.C. "Introduction to the ACR-NEMA DICOM Standard." *Radiographics* 12: 345-355, 1992.

Cleary, S., Cormier, L., Gilpin, D., Hunter, T., Lui, T., Mao, G., McMahon, C. An Analysis of the Viability of a Filmless MRI/CT Department. London Health Sciences Centre, Richard Ivey School of Business Entrepreneurship Project; Report 96/04/24, 1996.

Drew, P.G. "Cost Analysis of Image Management and Communications Systems (IMACS)." AAPM Monograph 22; *Digital Imaging.* Medical Physics Publishing; 569-588, 1993.

Glass, J.M. "The Economics of Information Technology." Agfa Division, Bayer Corporation Report 6, 21 pages, 1998.

Hendee, W.R. Digital Imaging Imperatives and Responsibilities. AAPM Monograph 22; *Digital Imaging.* Medical Physics Publishing, 2-21, 1993.

Honeyman, J.C., Frost, M.M., Huda, W., Loeffler, W., Ott, M., Staab, E.V. "Picture Archiving and Communications Systems (PACS)." *Current Problems in Diagnostic Radiology* 23(4): 101-160, 1994.

Imation Corporation Publication. Customer Migration—A Six Phased Approach to PACS. 1997.

Lindhardt, F.E. "Viborg Sygehus: routine digital operation with SIENET—a user reports." *Electromedica* 63(1): 13-17, 1995.

Offenmuller, W. "Managed Workflow between HIS, RIS, Modalities and PACS: Now—with DICOM—or beyond?" SPIE Proceedings: *PACS Design and Evaluation: Engineering and Clinical Issues,* Vol. 2711: 144-155, 1996.

Orth, A. "Phasing in a clinical network." *Medical Imaging* 10: 41-42, 1996.

PACS. Digest of the World Congress on Medical Physics and Biomedical Engineering—XVI International Conference on Medical and Biological Engineering. *Medical and Biological Engineering and Computing* 29(1): 300-311; 1991.

Nuclear Medicine Imaging Technology

David A. Weber, Ph.D. and Marijana Ivanovic, Ph.D.
Department of Radiology
University of California Davis Medical Center
Sacramento, CA 95817

Introduction

Nuclear medicine is the medical specialty that involves the administration of radio-pharmceuticals for use in diagnosis and therapy. Gamma and/or x-rays emitted from administered radiopharmaceuticals serve as molecular probes when imaged to diagnose and stage disease, monitor the effects of therapy, measure function, evaluate physiology, and investigate mechanisms underlying disease processes. Larger doses of radiopharmaceuticals are used for nuclear medicine therapy to treat disease.

Approximately 16 million diagnostic nuclear medicine imaging procedures are performed in the United States each year. Greater than 95% of these procedures involve single photon emission computed tomography (SPECT) and planar imaging. Although the number of positron emission tomography (PET) procedures is gradually beginning to increase, these currently account for far less than 5% of all imaging procedures performed in nuclear medicine. We will provide here a survey of the current imaging equipment used in nuclear medicine, the types of procedures conducted on this equipment, the types of image processing routines performed on different procedures, and the types and format of imaging data provided for display, networking, and archiving within a nuclear medicine unit and with an enterprise Picture Archiving and Communication System (PACS). This will include consideration of the diversity in nuclear medicine acquisition protocols and the use of proprietary image processing routines that can result in unconventional image formats for storage, transmission, and display.

Imaging Instrumentation

The primary imaging systems used for planar and tomographic procedures for diagnostic studies include: 1) scintillation cameras, 2) single and multiple detector (scintillation camera) single photon emission computed tomography (SPECT) imaging systems, 3) dedicated positron emission tomography (PET) imaging systems, and 4) camera coincidence PET and collimated 511 keV photon SPECT imaging systems.

Scintillation Camera Technology

The scintillation camera (also referred to as Anger or gamma camera) was first introduced by H. Anger (Anger 1958). It very quickly replaced the rectilinear scanner as the primary imaging technology and became the major instrument for nuclear medicine imaging. The camera provided an imaging system that could be used to image the 2-D distribution properties of radiopharmaceuticals in organs and regions of the body without requiring detector motion. The scintillation camera was the first instrument to allow simultaneous measurement of localization and turnover properties for imaging changing activity patterns of radiopharmaceuticals in organs and tissues in the human body. Subsequent changes in the camera technology and camera gantry design have extended the functionality of these systems to now include: 1) whole body imaging with a scanning scintillation camera, 2) physiologic gated imaging such as implemented in R-wave gated cardiac studies for planar and tomographic myocardial imaging, 3) SPECT, adding the capacity to image radiopharmaceuticals in 3-D by mounting one or more scintillation camera detectors on a rotating gantry so that complete sets of projection images can be collected for tomographic image reconstruction, 4) collimated 511 keV photon SPECT to provide tomographic images of positron emitting radionuclides imaged in the SPECT acquisition mode using high energy (511 keV) collimators and substituting thicker NaI(Tl) crystals (5/8" or 3/4") to improve the counting efficiency for 511 keV annihilation photons, and 5) annihilation photon PET camera imaging accommodated by the use of slit or axial collimation or no collimation of co-linearly opposed scintillation camera detectors employing 5/8" or 3/4" thick crystal detectors and adding coincidence circuitry and higher count rate capability options.

In addition to the recent changes in technology that have made camera PET more practical and feasible, other approaches to further extend the performance properties of a dual-purpose instrument are being investigated. The potential advantage of having dual PET/SPECT functionality in a single instrument has led to work in progress on developing a new phoswich detector camera PET (Dahlbom et al. 1997). This system uses scintillation camera signal decoding to define the position of events, taking advantage of the combined physical properties of two different scintillators. Small blocks of cerium doped lutetium orthosilicate (LSO) and yttrium orthosilicate (YSO) are sandwiched together to make small area detectors. Arrays of these scintillator blocks are assembled to form a single large area, modular detector for imaging annihilation photons. Characterized as scintillators with short scintillation decay times and having a much higher effective density than NaI(Tl), the phoswich sandwich detector is expected to offer major improvements in counting sensitivity and count rate capacity for coincidence PET imaging. Despite considerable ongoing research on other detector technology for providing more efficient and higher resolution systems, scintillation camera technology continues to dominate the approach to imaging in nuclear medicine.

Dedicated PET Technology

Dedicated PET imaging systems use several different detector designs to achieve adequate counting efficiencies for imaging the 511 keV annihilation photons accompanying positron decay. This range from the use of co-linearly opposed cylindrical NaI(Tl) detectors operated in the coincidence mode to current generation systems that use multiple ring or cylinder systems (Budinger 1998). Since the overall number of dedicated PET units being used for clinical nuclear medicine is limited and of several different designs, we will not attempt to detail the types of instruments that are currently being used. There are fewer than 100 units actively used for clinical imaging in the United States. Interest in dedicated PET systems has centered recently on systems which employ rings or cylinders of multiple small detectors or arrays of small or large detectors made of bismuth germinate (BGO) or NaI(Tl) to achieve adequate sensitivity, resolution, and scan volume. Multiple ring detectors now offer in excess of 40 transverse sections over an axial distance of 15 cm. Greater scan areas are achieved by moving the patient through the ring detector and collecting multiple sets of tomographic sections. BGO has been used in preference to NaI(Tl) as the scintillation detector of choice in many of the newer systems to gain higher efficiency for imaging the 511 keV annihilation photons. Multiple rings or larger surface area modular detectors have been used to maximize the scanning volume with these systems. Image resolution achieved with the highest resolution systems has been of the order of 2.6 mm; however, conventional state-of-the-art systems offer spatial resolution of the order of the order of 4 to 6 mm. Currently dedicated PET units provide much better spatial resolution, of the order of a factor of two, than can be achieved with camera PET. With enthusiasm building for using coincidence camera PET, we expect that this technology will undergo many changes, and performance properties could dramatically change as new detector materials and detector designs are introduced.

Imaging Equipment Specifications and Performance Properties

Scintillation Camera

With camera technology playing such an important role in nuclear medicine imaging and accounting for more than 95% of the imaging procedures performed in nuclear medicine, we briefly detail selective specifications and performance properties that influence image matrix size, spatial resolution, image quality, and related imaging variables. Each of these variables directly influences clinical interpretation and imaging archiving for subsequent review or referral.

The scintillation camera employs a rectangular or circular NaI(Tl) scintillation crystal detector which is backed by an array of photomultiplier tubes (PMTs) that detect the position and energy of γ- or x-photons absorbed in the collimated NaI(Tl) crystal (Figure 1).

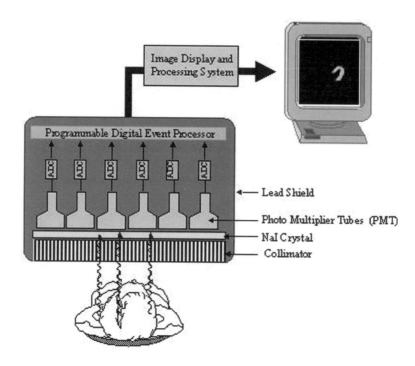

Figure 1. Detector housing of a scintillation camera includes a shielded, large area NaI(Tl) scintillation crystal, collimator, PMTs, and signal processing electronics that are connected to an image display and processing system.

Gamma and x-ray photons pass through the camera's collimator holes perpendicular to the face of the detector and absorbed in the scintillation crystal. Light is released which is detected by one or more PMTs mounted on the back of the NaI(Tl) detector. With the position of each absorption event determined by the detector electronics, large area, circular fields of view of the order of 10"-22" or rectangular fields of the order of ~6.7" × 12.6" to 16.5" × 22.3" can be imaged continuously without moving the detector. Position signals from analog to digital converters (ADCs) on each PMT are processed to obtain the centroids of absorption events and the Z signal from the PMTs are processed to determine the energy of an event for the camera's pulse height analyzer to accept or exclude from the image.

SPECT

Most new purchases of imaging equipment for nuclear medicine imaging involves the purchase of SPECT systems. These systems provide the advantage of supplying the acquisition and processing hardware and software for both planar (with equivalent of scintillation camera performance) and SPECT imaging. The majority of SPECT systems used in nuclear medicine typically employ one to three detectors (1-3 cameras) which are mounted on a rotating gantry. The systems are usually available as open or closed gantry systems and as fixed or variable angle imaging systems (Figure 2). Most of the initial dual and triple camera detector SPECT imaging systems were manufactured with the closed gantry design.

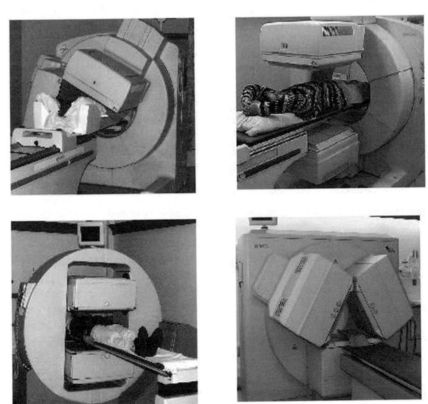

Figure 2. Upper: Example of open gantry, variable angle dual camera detector imaging systems (Picker Axis) with detectors separated by 102 degrees for cardiac SPECT (left) and by 180 degrees for SPECT, whole body scans, or coincidence PET imaging (right). Lower: Closed gantry, fixed angle dual camera detector SPECT imaging system (Picker Prism 2000) positioned for SPECT or whole body scans (left) and fixed angle, triple camera SPECT imaging system (Picker Prism 3000, right).

Although the closed gantry, fixed-angle system can be used efficiently for whole body scan procedures and body SPECT, the greater versatility offered by the variable angle, open gantry SPECT systems has led to its preferred use for general purpose SPECT imaging. The open gantry design typically facilitates better patient positioning, especially for those attached to physiologic monitors, respiratory support, and/or other life-support systems. The variable angle gantry SPECT provides for optimum positioning of detectors for regional body imaging; it facilitates more efficient, limited angle projections acquisition such as used in 180 degree cardiac SPECT. Here, a 90-degree rotation of the gantry assembly with the heads offset 90 or 102 degrees can facilitate closer positioning of the camera detectors to the patient for better spatial resolution images. The offset positioning further facilitates each of the detectors to only image over 90 degrees. This decreases the imaging time needed to complete cardiac SPECT by approximately a factor of two compared with that required by a fixed 180-degree opposed, dual-detector SPECT system.

In the simplest form, a single gamma camera is mounted on a slip ring or other type gantry that rotates the camera in a 360-degree circular or body contour orbit about a patient. Figures 2 show photographs of closed gantry, fixed angle, and open gantry, variable angle dual detector camera SPECT imaging systems. The open gantry, variable angle imaging system in Figure 2 shows a system that can be used for conventional SPECT, collimated annihilation photon SPECT, and coincidence PET imaging.

In SPECT acquisition a series of planar images, called projections, are collected at selectable equal angular increments about the subject, e.g., 60 projections collected at 6-degree increments or 120 projections collected at 3-degree increments. Image processing typically includes an attenuation correction applied to the projections before image reconstruction. Tomographic slices are then processed using image reconstruction software to obtain 3-D images of the structures imaged. The most commonly used image reconstruction software for SPECT is based on the filtered back projection reconstruction algorithm. Additional image filtering is typically performed to enhance, smooth, or suppress image data and to improve image quality. Images are stored and viewed as sets of transaxial, sagittal, and coronal slices. Additional oblique reconstructions are frequently used in other studies such as cardiac perfusion. Projection images are sometimes viewed cinematically to provide the viewer a 3-D presentation of the organ or structures that were imaged. Viewing these images along with the more conventional transaxial, sagittal, and coronal slices is often found useful in visualizing and isolating sites of abnormality from adjacent normal structures. A schematic representation of the gantry rotation and examples of SPECT projections and reconstructed tomographic slices are shown in Figure 3.

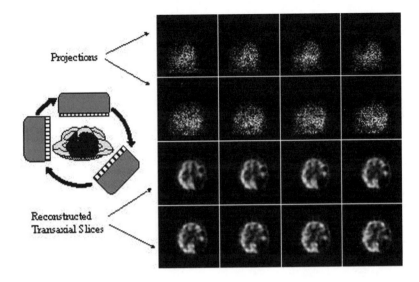

Figure 3. Left: One or more scintillation camera detectors on SPECT imaging system rotates about patient following circular or elliptical orbit to collect projections. Upper right: series of eight consecutive projections taken from 120 projection set shows localization of a 99m-Tc labelled radiopharmaceutical used to image cerebral perfusion. Lower right: series of transaxial slices of the brain reconstructed from SPECT projections.

Typical performance properties and specifications of current generation SPECT systems are listed in Table 1. Depending upon the type collimator selected and the tissue structures imaged, the best spatial resolution is of the order of 6 to 8 mm FWHM. The thicker NaI(Tl) scintillation crystals used to achieve a greater efficiency for coincidence imaging will degrade the spatial resolution by approximately 1 mm at 511 keV accompanied by a gain of almost a factor of two in efficiency for photons of this energy. Whereas in SPECT acquisition, one or more collimated cameras are required to collect projection data for image reconstruction, coincidence detection of annihilation photons requires at least two opposed detectors with limited or no collimation to perform coincidence imaging (Figure 4). Projection data is collected in list mode for on-line or post acquisition processing to provide line of projection or line of coincidence data suitable for subsequent reformatting to frame mode projections for image reconstruction.

Table 1. Typical SPECT Detector Specifications and Performance Properties

Specifications

Detector FOV	
Rectangular	6.7" × 12.6" to 16.5" × 22.3"
Circular	10" to 22" diam.
NaI (Tl) thickness	
SPECT mode	0.375"-0.5"
Coincidence mode	0.625"-0.750"
# PMTs/detector	37-95
Energy Range	55-170 keV to 40-960 keV
Pulse intergration time	
SPECT mode	850 ns
Coincidence mode	225 ns
Coincidence pulse pair resolution	15 ns
Number of detectors	1-4

Performance Properties

Spatial Resolution (UFOV)	
Intrinsic:	2.7-4.5 mm FWHM 5.2-9.0 mm FWTM
System (LEHR):	7.4-9.8 mm FWHM 13.8-18.0 mm
FWTM	
Uniformity	
System Integral:	± 2.5%-± 5.0%
System Differential:	± 1.2%-± 3.0%
Energy Resolution	9.5-10.6%
Maximum Count Rate	
SPECT mode	> 150 kcps
HCR Coincidence mode	> 350 kcps
System sensitivity (LEGP)	230-350 c/m/mCi

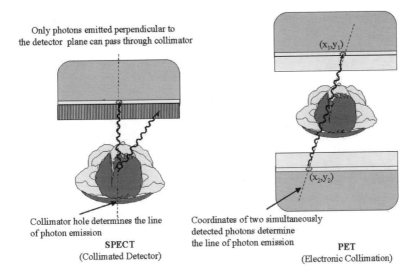

Only photons emitted perpendicular to
the detector plane can pass through collimator

(x_1, y_1)

Collimator hole determines the line
of photon emission

SPECT
(Collimated Detector)

(x_2, y_2)

Coordinates of two simultaneously
detected photons determine
the line of photon emission

PET
(Electronic Collimation)

Figure 4. Diagram (left) shows the principle of camera detector SPECT image acquisition involves the collection of a series of projection frames acquired from the collimated scintillation camera field of view. Diagram (right) shows dual-camera PET image acquisition involves uncollimated detectors imaging geometry in which the coordinates of lines of projection or coincidence are stored in list mode for subsequent processing and reformatting to frame mode data for image reconstruction.

Images and Image Formats

Imaging procedures performed on scintillation cameras include a wide variety of planar imaging studies with options for frame and list mode static and dynamic gated or ungated procedures. SPECT imaging systems provide similar frame mode options for projection acquisition and reconstructed tomographic slices. Although systems vary, a state-of-the-art scintillation camera or SPECT imaging system will use image acquisition modes that include all or most of the image acquisition modes listed below.

Acquisition Mode	Image Matrix (pixels)
Planar static	64×64, 128×128, 256×256, 512×512, 1024×1024 (16 bit)
Planar Dynamic*	64×64, 128×128, 256×256 (8 and/or 16 bit)
Physiologic Gated*	64×64, 128×128, 256×256 (16 bit)

SPECT Projections	64×64, 128×128, 256×256 (16 bit)
Camera PET	list mode acquisition of line of projections, reformat to 64/128 frame
Whole Body	256×512 or 1024

* List mode data acquisition may be offered as an option with operator selected frame mode conversion.

In practice, with the exception of routine whole body images, the majority of image files are acquired and stored in 64×64 or 128×128 pixel matrices. Most images are stored in 16-bit word pixels; however, some systems offer 8-bit byte pixels for dynamic studies to limit storage requirements. As such, these image formats place minimal demand on conventional PACS used in radiology. The number of pixels per image is in general substantially less than found in most radiological images. The large number of different image acquisition protocols used for nuclear medicine procedures, however, does interfere with the standardization of nuclear medicine images for PACS considerations.

Variables such as static vs. dynamic image sets, list vs. frame mode images, gated dynamic vs. dynamic images, and a wide variety of image formats with a variable number of frames per study make it difficult to systematically standardize and classify image sets. This is further complicated by imaging procedures that involve more than one radiopharmaceutical. Here this can involve the storage of one to four data sets for different photopeaks on each detector of a SPECT system.

Proprietary image processing is involved in most SPECT, camera PET, cardiac, and many other procedures involving dynamic physiologically gated and ungated studies. Some processed image data sets can only be viewed on the monitor and photographed without provision for archiving or image transfer. Others can be saved and stored in a standard image format; however, there are many processed images that provide displays consisting of graphs, tables, and dynamic and/or static activity maps of the processed images.

An example of a processed image set for quantitative gated SPECT (QGS) myocardial perfusion imaging is shown in Figure 5. Manufacturer's proprietary QGS software creates several results review screens that can not be stored in standard image format and require the QGS software for viewing.

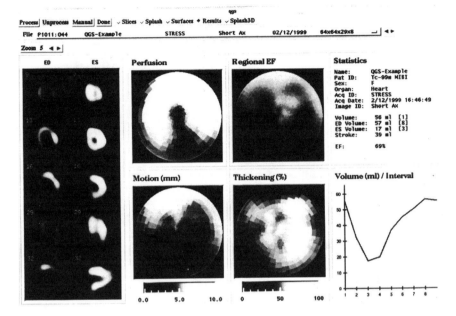

Figure 5. An example of one of results review screens from QGS analysis application for gated myocardial perfusion imaging. The results review screen displays summaries of regional and global left ventricular function and analysis via polar plots, statistics, images, and graphs.

Here we will review the special needs of the various nuclear medicine image formats and other variables that affect the archiving, transfer, and display of nuclear medicine images. We will review how an intermediate file format called interfile was developed and introduced to assist in translating proprietary processed images through the use of a data dictionary driven format (Todd-Pokropek 1994). Providing a means to develop file format specifications, this was not a transfer protocol, but provided a means of communication with interfile objects using more conventional means of file transfer. We will then look at how the DICOM standard administers medical image communication and review how the various nuclear medicine image formats and data sets are addressed by this standard. Studies of this type present a challenge to the investigator, the nuclear medicine physician, and the PACS manager when a comprehensive enterprise wide PACS is to be used for imaging data communication.

References

Anger, H.O. "Scintillation Camera." *Rev. Sci. Instrum.* 29:27-33, 1958.

Budinger, T.F. "PET instrumentation: what are the limits?" *Semin. Nucl. Med.* 28:247-267; 1998.

Dahlbom, M., MacDonald, L.R., Eriksson, L., et al. "Performance of a YSO/LSO phoswich detector for use in a PET/SPECT system." *IEEE Trans. Nucl. Sci.* 44:1114-1119, 1997.

Todd-Pokropek, A. "Interfile conformance claim." *Nucl. Med. Comm.* 15:659-663, 1994.

Computed Tomography: Technology Update on Multiple Detector Array Scanners and PACS Considerations

John M. Boone, Ph.D.
Department of Radiology
University of California, Davis
UC Davis Medical Center
Sacramento, California 95817

Introduction

Computed Tomography (CT) remains a steadfast clinical tool, capable of delivering cross sectional anatomical images with excellent image quality and rapid acquisition. While Magnetic Resonance Imaging (MRI) technology has enjoyed a vast amount of technological change and improvement in recent years, CT scanner technology has been relatively static until recently. With the advent of multiple detector array technology, however, CT scanners are back on the technological cutting edge, and these systems now offer unique features with significantly enhanced clinical utility.

In this chapter, it is assumed that the reader is already familiar with the basics of CT, both from the theoretical and clinical perspectives. For those who may require some basic background information on CT scanner systems, there are many fine texts which discuss CT (Marshall 1982, Hendee and Ritenour, 1992). The focus here is to introduce multiple detector array CT technology, and discuss the ramifications of how this technology will impact the medical physicist in terms of acceptance testing and quality assurance. Furthermore, with Picture Archiving and Communication System (PACS) becoming increasingly viable, the issues related to PACS specific to CT are also discussed.

The discussion in this chapter is intended to be generic with respect to the different CT manufacturers, however our institution has recently acquired a General Electric multiple detector array scanner ("Lightspeed"), and some of our experiences with that system are reported. There is, however, no intention to endorse a particular vendor's product over another. Effort is taken to describe features of other manufacturers' products, where this information is known.

What are Multiple Detector Arrays?

A conventional, single detector array CT scanner of course has many detectors. There are approximately 1000 individual detectors on a single detector array on a third generation (rotate/rotate) scanner. The individual detectors span the length of the detector array, and they simultaneously detect x-rays across the entire fan angle of the scanner during acquisition. Figure 1A illustrates the detector array for a third generation scanner design.

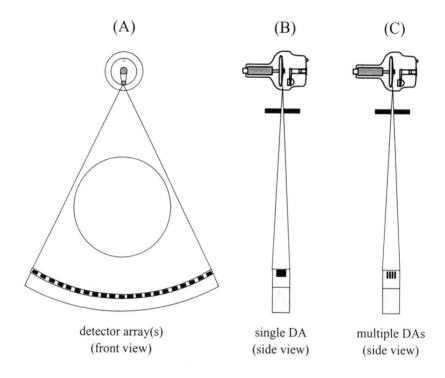

(A)   (B)   (C)

detector array(s)   single DA   multiple DAs
(front view)   (side view)   (side view)

Figure 1. All modern CT scanners use multiple detectors; for example, third generation scanners use about 1000 detectors to cover the fan angle (A). The side view of a single detector array scanner is shown in (B). Multiple detector array CT scanners have many different detectors *arrays* along the z-axis of the scanner (C).

In the case of a conventional, single detector array (DA) system, each detector along the array represents a single, wide (~25 mm) detector element, as shown in Figure 1B. For a single detector array scanner, the slice thickness is completely governed by the mechanical collimation of the x-ray beam (and other less significant factors which impact the slice sensitivity profile, such as focal spot size). A multiple detector array scanner employs a series of detector elements along the z-axis of the scanner, as shown in Figure 1C. The multiple detector array scanner uses pre-patient collimation, but the slice thickness is dictated by the width of the individual detector elements.

The Big Picture: Why Multiple Detector Arrays?

CT has evolved substantially since its initial clinical introduction three decades ago, and the "generations" of CT scanners are familiar to most medical physicists (Bushberg et al. 1993). The driving force for multiple detector array CT scanners (seventh generation?) is the same that drove earlier innovations: Reduced patient scan time, increasing patient throughput, and expanded clinical applications.

Prior to the introduction of helical scanners, individual slice acquisition time was limited by gantry rotation speed (the x-ray tube had to be accelerated to constant velocity from a stopped position), and total scan time was limited by the need to stop the x-ray tube, move the patient table, then start up the x-ray tube rotation again. The stop/start cycles were necessary between each slice acquisition because the x-ray tube was tethered by its high tension cables to a cable spool which let out (odd-numbered slices) or took up (even-numbered slices) the cables as the gantry rotated. This technology was adequate in the late 1980's, because modest computer power and limited x-ray tube output were also factors which prohibited major reductions in CT scan time.

As greater computer power led to reduced reconstruction times, and as CT x-ray tubes became significantly more powerful (with higher mA for extended duration), the inertial gantry start/stop cycle became the rate-limiting step of CT acquisition. Slip ring scanners, which use sliding electrical contacts instead of cables, eliminated the need for the start/stop cycle of the gantry. Slip ring technology allowed the gantry to rotate continuously in one direction, and consequently rotation times decreased from several seconds to less than one second per rotation. Immediately, the start/stop motion of the patient table became the rate limiting step, and slip ring scanners addressed this by simply keeping the patient table moving at constant velocity during the scan, leading to helical acquisition techniques. Even with these improvements, typical scan times in the abdomen and thorax of 30 seconds or more required that the patient be given an opportunity to breathe between scan sequences.

Helical CT scanners have no inertial limitations during the scan cycle since both the gantry and table move at constant velocity during the scan. Computer horsepower continues to increase; however CT x-ray tube technology development has probably reached asymptotic growth given the constraints of physics and cost. Given this state of the technology, the next most obvious way to decrease total scan time is to make more efficient use of the x-rays that are produced by the tube, and this is done by increasing the collimated slice thickness. For example, scanning with 5-mm collimation for a 30 cm extent of the patient using conventional parameters (1 second gantry rotation, pitch = 1.0) requires 60 seconds. Using a multiple DA system employing four 5-mm detectors and opening up the mechanical collimation to 20 mm, the scan time is reduced to 15 seconds. Importantly, for many patients this means that the entire scan can be performed within a single breath-hold.

Helical Pitch Redefined

With conventional single DA scanners, the concept of helical pitch is straightforward. Referring to Figure 2A, with the collimated beam width given by C (in mm) and the table travel per gantry rotation defined as T (in mm), "pitch" and more specifically *collimator pitch* is defined as:

$$\text{collimator pitch} = \frac{T}{C}.$$

With the introduction of multiple DA scanners, ambiguity arises in terms of the definition of pitch. Consequently, collimator pitch (which is consistent with the conventional notion of pitch) needs to be distinguished from *detector pitch* (see Figure 2B), which is defined as:

$$\text{detector pitch} = \frac{T}{D}.$$

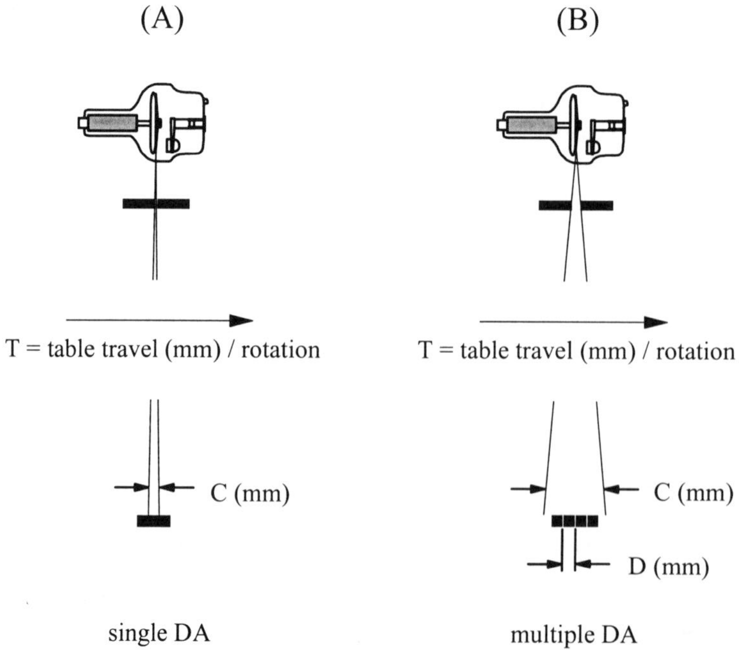

(A)   (B)

T = table travel (mm) / rotation   T = table travel (mm) / rotation

C (mm)   C (mm)

D (mm)

single DA   multiple DA

Figure 2. (A) The concept of *collimator pitch* is illustrated, where collimator pitch = T/C. Collimator pitch is consistent with previous notions of pitch in a helical scanner. (B) With multiple detector array scanners, pitch needs to be defined more precisely. The *detector pitch* is defined as D/T, while the definition of collimator pitch still holds as well.

One manufacturer in the quad detector CT market, General Electric, quotes pitch values of 3 and 6. A pitch of 3 refers to a *detector pitch* of 3, and this is roughly comparable to a collimator pitch of 0.75, whereas the detector pitch of 6 corresponds to a collimator pitch of 1.5. If the x-ray beam is collimated to N active detectors in a multiple DA system, the relationship between collimator and detector pitch is:

$$\text{collimator pitch} = \frac{\text{detector pitch}}{N}.$$

Image Generation with Multiple Detector Array CT Scanners

In helical acquisition mode with a collimator pitch of approximately 1 (a detector pitch of 4 for a four DA scanner), a small point in the patient's anatomy (or a BB as illustrated in Figure 3) casts its x-ray shadow across all four detector arrays during one 360° rotation of the gantry. The top of Figure 3 shows the translation of the shadow of a BB placed on the patient table. While the x-ray shadow of the BB translates from detector array to detector array (side view), it does not necessarily strike the same detector number (front view). The bottom of Figure 3 illustrates a front view of the BB in the scanner, and during the 360° scan the shadow of the BB cycles back and forth across the detectors in sinusoidal manner. The time points shown (1-4) are just four points along the many view angles that produce the CT sinogram.

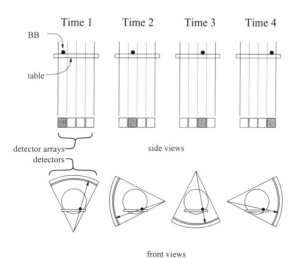

Figure 3. The position of a BB placed on the patient table is shown at four different time points during a scan. In the side view, the BB moves at constant velocity laterally, and its shadow progresses from one detector array to the next. In the front view (bottom of figure), the shadow BB is cast onto the individual detectors. As the scanner rotates, the shadow of the BB follows a sinusoidal path on the detectors (resulting in the CT *sinogram*) (in the front view only).

Each detector array detects the shadow of the BB for a limited range of angles. For example, for a 360° CT image reconstruction and a detector pitch of 4, each detector array will primarily contribute to the image for about 90° of acquisition, or about 25% of the projection data for the scan. If the slice sensitivity profile of one of the detector arrays was (for example) much wider than the other 3, then the data from that detector array may include shadows of objects that were not included in the other 3 detector arrays. For about 90° of the CT reconstruction, a slightly different set of data would be backprojected, and this would cause streak artifacts in the image.

The Small Picture: Multiple Detector Array Details

The impact of multiple detector arrays is most obvious when looking at the slice thickness dimension of CT acquisition, that is the dimension parallel to the long axis (cranial-caudal) of the patient laying on the CT table. Here the long axis is referred to as the z-axis, while the x- and y-axes are defined in the plane of the CT image. Figure 4 compares single and multiple detectors.

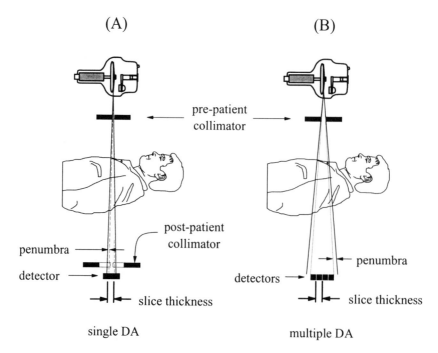

Figure 4. (A) With conventional signal detector array scanners, the pre-patient collimator determines the slice thickness. For the thinnest slices, some single DA scanners make use of post-patient collimators to improve the slice sensitivity profile (and the z-axis resolution). (B) With multiple detector array scanners, the detectors themselves determine the slice thicknesses. To avoid a mis-match between the slice sensitivity profiles between the four detectors shown, the system is aligned so the x-ray focal spot penumbra strikes outside the edge detectors in the array.

With conventional (single detector array) scanners, the collimated slice thickness is always smaller than the width of the detector. Pre-patient collimators define the slice thickness in single detector array systems; however, some CT systems make use of additional post-patient collimators for the smallest slice thicknesses (e.g., 1 mm slice thickness) to improve the slice sensitivity profile. Whenever post-patient collimation is used, some amount of the primary x-ray beam that has already passed through the patient is attenuated (usually in the penumbra), reducing the dose efficiency of the scanner.

In multiple detector array scanners, the pre-patient collimation determines the overall beam width, but it does not determine the slice thickness. Slice thickness is determined by the width of the individual, active detector elements along the z-axis, as illustrated in Figure 4B. Consequently, the collimated slice thickness is always *greater* than the dimensions of an individual detector in multiple detector array systems. Most manufacturers of multiple detector array CT systems are employing four active detector arrays for acquisition, and for convenience a four detector system will be assumed. The reader should keep in mind that other numbers are possible.

The use of discrete detector elements along the z-axis (Figure 4B) is similar to post-patient collimation, since x-rays that do not strike the active surface of a detector are not detected. During helical acquisition with a multiple detector array scanner, the data from all four detector arrays are used to reconstruct every CT slice, and thus the slice sensitivity profile (z-axis resolution) of each of the four detector arrays needs to be similar, otherwise artifacts might occur. The slice sensitivity profile for the two center detector arrays is governed primarily by the detector aperture since they are near the center of the radiation beam, and are away from the penumbra induced by the focal spot and pre-patient collimation (Figure 4B). The relative placement of the edge of the x-ray beam with respect to the outside edges of the two edge detectors, however, will have a significant effect on the slice sensitivity profile. To circumvent potential problems, manufacturers of multiple detector array CT scanners adjust the collimation such that the penumbra falls *outside* the sensitive area of the edge detectors, and thus the outer detectors have similar slice sensitivity profiles as the two inner detectors. The downfall of this is that the x-ray beam is under-collimated, such that primary x-rays that pass through the patient go undetected in the penumbra region, and dose efficiency suffers.

Slice Thickness Options in Multiple Detector Array Scanners

With conventional single detector array scanners, the desired slice thickness is adjusted by moving the collimators, a simple mechanical operation. With multiple detector array scanners, however, since the width of the detector arrays defines the slice thickness, the effective detector array width needs to be selectable. Changing the width of four contiguous detector arrays by mechanical means is unfeasible (although Elscint used this approach with a two detector array system), and therefore most manufacturers have adopted an electronic strategy as illustrated in Figure 5.

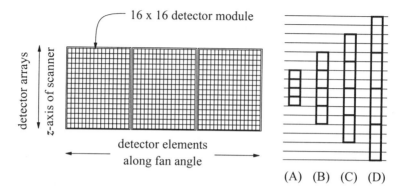

Figure 5. (A) Multiple detector array scanners make use of modular detector systems, small area arrays of detector elements. The CT gantry is lined along the fan direction with a series of modules. In the orthogonal dimension (parallel to the *z*-axis), the individual detector elements comprise the different detector arrays. (B) Slice thickness is determined by how many individual detector elements are binned together to form an active detector. (a) with only one detector element as the active detector, the slice thickness is at a minimum. (d) with four detector elements binned into one active detector, the slice thickness is four times the *z*-axis dimension of the detector element. The electronic signal from the four active detector elements shown for different slice thicknesses (a, b, c, and d) is sent to the four-channel data acquisition system on the scanner.

The detector modules allow the detector configuration to be adjusted by electronically combining the signals emanating from adjacent individual detector elements. For example, the General Electric system uses a 16 x 16 detector module. Along the z-axis of the scanner, the 16 detector elements measure ~2.15 mm, and projected back to the isocenter of the scanner, each detector's width is 1.25 mm. The scanner has four data acquisition channels. By changing the way that the 16 detector elements report their signals to the four acquisition channels, different slice thicknesses are possible. Four binning strategies are used, with 1, 2, 3 or 4 adjacent detectors combined (corresponding to labels A, B, C, and D in Figure 5) to provide slice thicknesses of 1.25, 2.50, 3.75, and 5.0 mm, as measured at isocenter. The Toshiba detector array uses a similar approach as General Electric, except that in the center of the detector array, the detector elements are thinner than at the periphery. This allows a thinner minimum slice thickness (0.5 mm) on the Toshiba scanner. Four 0.5-mm detectors are at the center of the detector, sandwiched by 15 1.0-mm detectors on both the top and bottom. This design results in 34 individual detector arrays spanning 32 mm. Picker has built (but not sold) a multiple detector array CT scanner based on the fourth generation design. Picker and Siemens will rely on the Elscint multiple DA scanner currently under development. The Elscint (and therefore Picker and Siemens) detector module has 8 detector arrays spanning 20 mm. Going from the center toward the edge (in both directions), the detector array widths are 1.0 mm, 1.5 mm, 2.5 mm, and 5.0 mm.

Scattered Radiation

Opening up the collimation to accommodate four detectors makes better use of the x-rays emitted by the tube, but an increase in scattered radiation will result. A Monte Carlo simulation (Boone and Seibert 1988) was performed to assess the scatter to primary ratio for various CT beam collimation widths. The scatter/primary ratio is plotted versus the z-axis position at the detector plane in Figure 6A. The geometry simulated in the Monte Carlo experiment is shown in Figure 6B. Water was used as the scattering medium, an 80 keV (monoenergetic) x-ray beam was simulated, and complete energy absorption at the detector was assumed. The geometry of Figure 6B is consistent with a 32 cm thick patient placed at the isocenter of a commercially available multiple detector array scanner (dimensions of the GE scanner were used). Notice that in CT, in addition to a much narrower beam than in radiography, the air gap (25 cm) is quite large by comparison as well.

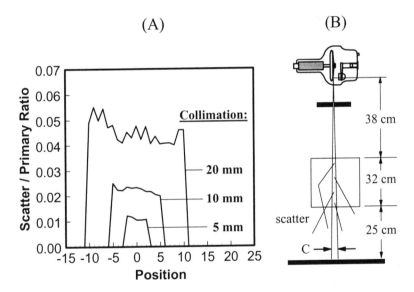

Figure 6. (A) The results of Monte Carlo simulations are shown, indicating that the S/P ratio (measured at the detector) for a 5-mm collimated x-ray beam is ~0.01, increases to 0.02 for a 10-mm collimated beam, and to 0.05 for a 20-mm x-ray beam width. (B) The geometry used in the Monte Carlo simulations is illustrated.

The S/P ratio increases from about 1% at 5 mm collimation, to 2% with 10 mm collimation, and then increases to 5% with a 20 mm collimated aperture. Comparing the 5-mm collimated beam width of a single detector array scanner with the 20-mm beam width of a quad detector array scanner (in four × 5 mm mode), the S/P increases approximately five-fold for the 5-mm CT slice thickness. While a five-fold increase in scattered radiation is substantial, the overall magnitude of scatter is still quite low at 5%. The influence that this additional scatter has on clinical image quality is not completely understood; however, if there is an effect, it is likely to be small.

Acceptance Testing Multiple Detector Array CT Scanners

A complete discussion of acceptance testing CT scanners is provided elsewhere (Fullerton and Zagzebski 1980, Gould 1994, Mattson 1994, Loo 1994, and Rothenberg 1994). The acceptance testing procedures for multiple detector array scanners are very similar to those for a conventional single detector array scanner. Because the x-ray beam collimation and detector configuration is fundamentally different with multiple detector array scanners, however, additional focus during acceptance testing should be made in these areas.

The collimated x-ray beam widths can be measured on the image using film placed on the patient table. A ready-pack type of film such as therapy verification film (e.g., Kodak X -Omat Type V) works well and has the proper sensitivity. Type TL film is too sensitive and might cause overestimation of the beam width. The physically measured beam width should be compared with the slice thickness as set on the console, recognizing that on a four detector array scanner, the beam width should be approximately four times the set slice thickness. The x-ray beam width can be simply measured with a ruler or reticule with the film on a light box.

The slice sensitivity profile width should be measured off the image for each slice thickness, using a thin wire scanned at a known angle. Commercially available CT phantoms provide angled-wire sections. The Catphan CTP401 module (23° wire) was used in our measurements. To determine the width of the slice sensitivity profile, software for measuring distances must be available on the scanner. The GE measurement software rounds off to the nearest millimeter, so to get better accuracy we transferred the images to a workstation for analysis.

Figure 7 illustrates the beam thickness and slice sensitivity width measurements for the GE Lightspeed scanner recently installed at our institution. The collimated x-ray beam is 200% wider than the slice sensitivity profile for the thinnest slice (1.25 mm nominal), but for the thickest slice (5 mm nominal) the beam width is only about 10% wider than the slice sensitivity profile. These measurements are qualitatively consistent with the fact that the collimation was designed so that the penumbra is outside the detector field (Figure 4B) for this scanner. As mentioned previously, many single detector array scanners use post-patient collimation to exclude detection of some of the x-ray beam for the thinnest slices (to achieve a narrow slice sensitivity profile, Figure 4A), so conventional scanners also suffer from poor dose efficiency at the thinnest slices.

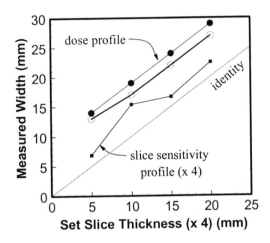

Figure 7. The width of the x-ray beam (measured using film) is illustrated as a function of the slice thickness set on the scanner. The filled circles represent measurements made at UC Davis, and the open circles were data acquired at MD Anderson Cancer Center (thanks to Donna Moxley for providing this data). The collimator width should be four times the slice thickness, and that correction is made on the figure. The width of the slice sensitivity profiles was determined off reconstructed images of an angled wire, and these are plotted as filled squares. The collimated x-ray beam width is substantially wider, and the slice sensitivity profiles are somewhat wider than the nominal slice thickness.

In addition to the thickness of the slice sensitivity profile, it is very useful to quantitatively assess the slice sensitivity profile itself. Figure 8 illustrates isometric plots of a patch of the CT image corresponding to the angled wire. Height on these plots is the CT number. Isometric plots are shown for all four slice thicknesses, acquired in *axial* (non-helical) mode. The small dead zone between individual detectors causes a reduction in the slice sensitivity profile between detectors, causing a saw-tooth appearance in the isometric plot. When N detectors are used, there are N-1 dead zones between the detectors, and this is clearly evident in Figure 8.

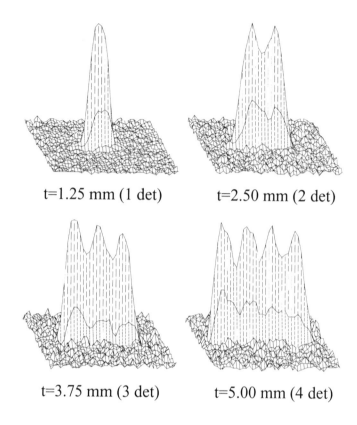

t=1.25 mm (1 det)   t=2.50 mm (2 det)

t=3.75 mm (3 det)   t=5.00 mm (4 det)

Figure 8. Isometric plots of the slice sensitivity profile are illustrated, for the slice thickness as indicated. The saw tooth pattern is a consequence of the small dead space between the individual detector elements.

The saw-tooth slice sensitivity profile is only apparent in axial (non-helical) mode acquisition, because in helical acquisition the slice sensitivity profile is blurred along the z-axis due to the table motion. When the highly angled wire was imaged in helical mode with the multiple DA scanner, it produced an interesting artifact. Figure 9 illustrates a scalloping artifact emanating from the angled wires. Because these artifacts are not seen in the axial acquisition, it is thought that they are a consequence of the data interpolation between detector arrays in the helical acquisition, combined with the highly angled wire. It is suspected that the wire caused the signal to experience a detector phase shift between detector arrays because of its angled orientation (something that the interpolation algorithm cannot generally anticipate), and thus the backprojected data from a given projection angle will not precisely compensate for the backprojected data acquired from the opposite (180°) projection angle. This would cause both positive (overshoot) and negative (undershoot) components in the reconstruction, both of which are visible in Figure 9.

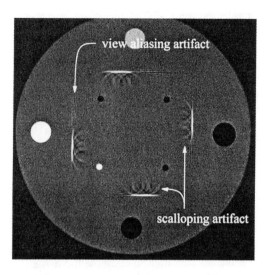

Figure 9. A helical CT scan through the angled wires shows a scalloping artifact. View aliasing artifacts are also seen radiating off parallel the ends of the wire. It is suspected that the high angulation of the wire in the slice plane causes the scalloping artifact.

Dose Measurement—CTDI

As part of acceptance testing a new scanner, the computed tomography dose index (CTDI) should be measured. Multiple detector array scanners require a slight adjustment in the measurement technique for the CDTI. There are several definitions of CTDI (Rothenberg 1994). The CTDI defined in 21 CFR subchapter I 1020.33 is given by:

$$\text{CTDI} = \frac{1}{nT} \int_{-7T}^{+7T} D(z) \ dz$$

where:

n = number of tomographic images produced
T = nominal slice thickness
D(z) = dose profile along the z-axis

We approximated the measurement of the CTDI by using a ~100 mm pencil chamber placed at various positions in the large (32 cm diameter) and small (16 cm diameter) Lucite CDRH Dose Phantoms. For the 5 mm nominal slice thickness (T=5 mm) placed in the center of the ~100 mm chamber, the limits of integration are really from –10 T to +10 T rather than from –7 T to +7 T as in the above equation. Since the dose distributed so far laterally, between ±7 T (3.5 cm) and ±10 T (5.0 cm) is very small, this difference in the CTDI is small. Furthermore, by measuring more of the integrated dose the results error toward being conservative.

Axial (non-helical) acquisition mode was used, and four (n=4) 5 mm simultaneous slices were acquired. Letting the electrometer reading be E, the correction factor for the CT pencil chamber be C (the units of the product CE should be in roentgen), the f-factor for Lucite be f, the length of the pencil chamber be L (L=10 cm) and the nominal slice thickness (as before) be T (T = 0.5 cm), the number of slices acquired be n (n=4), the CTDI is calculated as:

$$CTDI = f \times C \times E \times \frac{L}{nT}$$

This CTDI measurement is very close, as discussed by Rothenberg (1994) and Shope et al., (1981) to the Multiple Scan Average Dose (MSAD). CTDI values are often computed in plastic, but it is also important to compute the tissue (or water-equivalent) dose, since these values will be used to estimate patient dose. While the f-factor of 0.78 is often used for Lucite, there is an energy dependence in this value that should be taken into account for nonconventional CT beam energies such as 80 kVp or 140 kVp. Toward this end, computer simulated tungsten anode x-ray spectra (Boone and Seibert 1997) were filtered with various thicknesses of copper (0-1.2 mm), and the average beam energy and half value layer (HVL) in aluminum was computed. The x-ray spectra were then filtered by an additional layer of Lucite, corresponding to the radius of the Lucite CT dose phantoms in common usage, the radius being 8 cm for the head phantom and 16 cm for the body phantom. This corrects the primary spectrum to that actually incident upon the pencil chamber in the center position of the dose phantom. This x-ray beam will be approximately equivalent to that striking the pencil chamber at the peripheral positions. Using this technique, spectrum ($\Phi(E)$) weighted f-factors specific to each beam energy and dose phantom were calculated as:

$$f = 0.873 \frac{\int_{E=0}^{E_{max}} \Phi(E) \frac{\left(\frac{\mu(E)}{\rho}\right)_{med}}{\left(\frac{\mu(E)}{\rho}\right)_{air}} dE}{\int_{E=0}^{E_{max}} \Phi(E) \ dE}$$

The results of these computations are given in the appendix in Table A1 for the head phantom values, and in Table A2 for the body phantom values. The f-factors for both Lucite and water are given, and the ratio of the two are tabulated as well.

After confirming mAs linearity of the CT scanner ($r^2 > 0.9999$), the CTDI dose measurements were normalized to 100 mAs, and were computed for both Lucite and water-equivalent tissue. The f-factors listed in the appendix (Tables A1 and A2) were used, appropriate for the kV and HVLs measured on the scanner. The HVL at 80 kV was measured as 5.7 mm Al, and at 120 kV the HVL was 8.2 mm Al. With the aid of the GE service engineer, the HVLs were measured with the x-ray tube in the parked position and with the detector arrays covered with a lead apron. Representative CTDI values are listed in Table 1.

Table 1: Sample CTDI values, normalized to 100 mAs, measured on the GE LightSpeed multiple DA scanner (5 mm slice x 4 slices). The body phantom was 32 cm in diameter, the head phantom was 16 cm in diameter. No teflon collar was used on the head phantom.

kVp	Phantom	Position	Lucite CTDI Rad/100 mAs	Tissue CTDI Rad/100 mAs
80	Body	center	0.16	0.21
80	Body	6 o'clock	0.32	0.42
80	Head	center	0.56	0.76
80	Head	12 o'clock	0.74	0.99
80	Head	3 o'clock	0.65	0.87
80	Head	6 o'clock	0.59	0.79
80	Head	9 o'clock	0.68	1.00
120	Body	center	0.63	0.76
120	Body	12 o'clock	1.33	1.60
120	Body	3 o'clock	1.26	1.53
120	Body	6 o'clock	0.74	0.90
120	Body	9 o'clock	1.26	1.53
120	Head	center	1.93	2.39
120	Head	12 o'clock	2.35	2.90
120	Head	3 o'clock	2.12	2.61
120	Head	6 o'clock	1.91	2.36
120	Head	9 o'clock	2.20	2.71

Image Count and Multiple Detector Array CT

Most institutions installing multiple detector array scanners report an increase in the overall number of CT images generated, compared to single detector array scanner systems. While there is no fundamental reason why multiple detector array scanners should produce more CT images than conventional single slice scanners, the thickest slice that the GE multiple detector array scanner allows in helical acquisition is 5 mm (giving better z-axis resolution). Adjacent 5 mm slices can be added together to produce a 10 mm thick CT slice (the only reason for this would be to reduce noise by compromising z-axis resolution); however, this requires additional steps on the part of the technologist. With single detector array scanners, most institutions use scan protocols using 7 and 10 mm slice thicknesses. With multiple detector array scanners producing 5 mm thick CT images as their normal "thick slice" images, a 40% (7/5) to 100% (10/5) increase in the number of images can be expected for most clinical protocols. This has implications on many practical aspects of clinical CT, including the number of images sent to the PACS and the number of images that the radiologist ends up having to interpret. Initial experience with our multiple DA scanner based on film utilization indicates about a 40% increase in images.

Picture Archiving and Communication Systems (PACS) and CT

Perhaps the most difficult thing to a medical physicist about PACS is that it is not physics: There are few equations that do not include dollar signs, and there are few "first principles" to provide rational guidance towards making a PACS work. To a medical physicist used to working on a strong scientific footing, the pursuit of PACs is a long walk on thin ice—and the ice is constantly moving. Because the ice *is* still moving, many observations made below involve speculation, initial impressions, and subjective interpretation. Please keep this in mind.

Proceed with Caution

The PACS implementation at a medical institution needs to match the specific needs of that institution. Despite the similarity in the physical topology of most hospitals, the specific needs of an institution related to PACS really depend upon many factors beyond topology, including the economic strength of the institution, the local patient referral network dynamics, the strength of the information technology (IT) resources, the status of interdepartmental politics, the amount of trauma seen, and the chutzpa of the responsible hospital and radiology administrators, among many other factors. The development of a PACS is an expensive undertaking, and its cost effectiveness will only truly be known after implementation. The mandate that a PACS be budget neutral (pay for itself) may be unrealistic at the current state of the technology, and other more noble goals such as improved patient throughput, better patient care, increased referring physician satisfaction, and more rapid dissemination of the radiologist's report should underlay the justification for CT PACS. Efforts which begin with shoestring budgets and only modest commitment from top administrators should be avoided.

The medical physicist should become involved in defining the specific goals and requirements of a PACS, working with the Information Technology (IT) department, radiologists, and other physicians and administrators involved in the project. Be fore-warned, however, that if the medical physicist is placed in the role of managing the PACS effort, this will likely consume virtually all of his or her time for several years, and perhaps beyond.

CT PACS

The production of film copies of CT images is the conventional approach to CT inter-pretation. While many institutions will make the transition between interpreting CT studies off film to reading CT images off the computer monitors gradually (to build the previous study archives), for the purposes of the following discussion, a CT PACS is considered to be a principally soft-copy read environment, where producing a film hardcopy is the exception and not the rule. Interfacing a CT system to a PACS while still depending upon film-based interpretation combines the worst attributes of both approaches: the high cost of PACS, with the low efficiency of handling film (cost of film, film library personnel costs, the need to manually load films onto alternators, etc.). Except for a transition period designed to build a database of serial studies and for radiologist training and migration to soft copy readout, a CT PACS system predi-cated on printing film for interpretation is not recommended.

Due to the enormity of the task, it makes sense to implement a PACS in a phased approach. For many institutions, starting the PACS implementation with CT (and MR), instead of digital radiography, makes good sense for the following reasons:

(1) CT images are 512×512, ½ Megabyte (MB) each, and a busy scanner might put out an average of 60 images per patient for 18 patients per day, totaling only around ½ Gigabyte of data (uncompressed) each day.

(2) The matrix size of the CT image, 512×512, makes it possible to use computer monitors (with typically 1000×1500 display capability or better) for accurate visualization. High resolution chest radiographs, with 4000×5000 or even 2000×2500 matrices challenge current computer monitors both in terms of cost and performance.

(3) Radiologists are very familiar with having to window and level CT images, and preset window and level values for CT images (possible because of the intrinsic normalization of CT grayscale) are well-defined at most institutions. The proper window and level settings for digital radiography is a less-explored territory.

(4) CT images are backed-up in digital format at most institutions without PACS, *anyway*. When implemented, the PACS becomes the primary image archive, and in some instances it replaces the back up at the CT modality, saving the cost of media, technologist time, and managing the separate archive.

Many other reasons can be added to the above list. One possible permutation of starting with a CT PACS, is to start with a neuroradiology PACS, combining image data from CT, MRI, and neuroangiography (digital subtraction angiography, DSA). Because of the low reliance on the interpretation of plain films in neuroradiology, a neuroradiology PACS can ramp up to a full digital soft copy read implementation somewhat quickly. Because neuroradiologists comprise a small fraction of the entire radiologist group (or faculty), fewer primary diagnostic workstations are needed initially and fewer radiologists need to be trained for soft copy interpretation at the beginning. Because large matrix plain films are the exception in neuroradiology, the monitors do not need to be ultra-resolution (2k+), and so workstation costs can be kept to reasonable levels.

The CT Workstation

The *primary diagnostic workstation* is where the radiologists do their work in a networked soft-copy image-interpretation environment. It is important that the medical physicist realize that details of image display are of paramount importance to the radiologist. Some physicists tend to dismiss the reluctance of radiologists to embrace soft copy displays as some flaw in radiologists' character, but such attitudes are counterproductive. For a radiologist to read off of a monitor requires a *major* adjustment in his/her daily professional life, and represents a huge shift away from training experience. It is analogous to putting a Cessna pilot at the controls of a Lear Jet, *in flight*. The first step in migrating to a PACS system for CT, long before money is spent, is to assure that the radiologists see the need—professionally, financially, and logistically. The radiologists need to be an intrinsic part of this decision if a PACS is to be implemented smoothly and successfully.

One way of getting the emotional commitment on the part of radiologists for PACS is to demonstrate to them what the brave new world will entail. Toward this end, the various primary diagnostic (PD) workstation options that exist in the marketplace need to be fully evaluated, by both technical individuals (the medical physicist in some instances) and the radiologist. Invite a number of vendors in to show off their workstations, and make sure they have an area where ambient light can be turned down low. It is important to realize that if a PD workstation is placed in a reading area with conventional alternators, glare and ambient lighting conditions may cause major problems in the clinical performance and radiologist acceptance of the workstation.

There are many hardware considerations concerning primary diagnostic workstations, importantly the resolution capabilities and numbers of image monitors that each workstation will have. Typical primary diagnostic workstations have either two or four monitors for a CT reading area. Active matrix flat panel monitors are currently ready to challenge cathode ray tube (CRT) monitors in the role of image display, albeit at higher cost, but with perhaps longer lifespan. Monitor brightness is also an issue that needs attention. Software is probably the biggest distinguishing factor between different workstation designs. General hardware and software considerations for workstations are discussed elsewhere in this proceedings. Here, the workstation details specific to CT are addressed.

A general purpose alternator (two over four) can simultaneously display 8 14" × 17" films with 20 CT images on each film, for 160 CT images at full 512×512 resolution. Even if a CT workstation employed four 2048×2048 monitors, it could only display 64 CT images at full resolution (40% of the image display at 400% of the cost!). Workstations with more than four monitors get bulky and very expensive, and so competing with conventional display technology in traditional terms is not realistic. Rather than simply replicating the display paradigm of the past (parallel image display with little interactivity), a CT workstation should provide the interactive display functionality that only a computer can offer (some parallel image display with a lot of interactivity). The number of displayed images can be reduced substantially if the window and level presets can be toggled in real time, and this is a must for any CT workstation. A reasonable selection of window and level presets should be instantly available on the keyboard (without having to go through layers of software menus), implemented for example as the function keys.

Radiologists spend a great deal of time orienting themselves in front of a set of CT images. They follow anatomical structures from slice to slice (and from film to film on the alternator), chasing down diagnostic clues and searching for pathology. Stack mode display on a workstation facilitates this diagnostic task, once a radiologist becomes familiar with the workstation software. Stack mode display is useful for studying a serial set of temporally- or spatially contiguous images, such as DSA, MRI, CT angiography, and CT. A typical method of operation for displaying CT images using stack mode is to display the scout view (or "scanogram"), and the CT slice that is displayed is indicated on the scout view (dotted line on Figure 10)). Moving the mouse selects the CT slice for display (it also moves the dotted line on the scout view). Rapid movement of the mouse should allow real-time fly-by's of the CT volume data set, and the workstation hardware should have enough processor speed and memory to assure real time performance in stack mode viewing. Figure 10 shows one possibility of stack mode display, where the single selected slice is displayed at two different window and level settings.

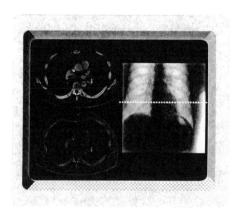

Figure 10. One rendition of "stack mode" display is shown. The CT image is displayed with two different window/level settings on the left side of the monitor, while the scout view is shown on the right and the dotted line indicates the position of the CT image shown. Movement of the mouse or trackball scrolls through the CT images in succession.

Once a radiologist becomes facile with stack mode interpretation of CT images, gains in interpretation efficiency may be achieved. Rather than having to change the spatial location of one's gaze and reorient on a different image (as on an alternator), the radiologist can concentrate on the same spatial location and move the anatomy underneath his/her gaze (by pushing or pulling the mouse). This mode of display permits tasks such as following vessels to be accomplished easier and with less physical motion of the head and eyes. The radiologist can then concentrate on the cognitive diagnostic issues surrounding the case, and not waste time having to spatially reacquire landmarks on each image.

As CT workstations become more sophisticated, it will be reasonable to expect that a lot of off-line image processing can be performed at the workstation, rather than at the CT scanner itself. For example, workstations have the capability of performing three dimensional rendering, maximum intensity projections, multi-planar reconstruction, and quantitative analysis of CT images. The benefits of performing these types of functions at the workstation instead of the scanner are many: software packages from CT vendors are very expensive and need to be replicated at each scanner (replicating the cost), local processing on the workstation gives more interactivity to the user (e.g., rotating a 3-D rendered vascular tree in real-time), and image analysis (evaluation of the CT number of a pulmonary nodule) by the radiologist at the time of interpretation is a more logical approach than having the technologists at the scanner do this.

Work Lists

In the traditional way of handling CT images (film), a film library technician is responsible for finding the CT cases for a particular radiologist to interpret, and then the technician hangs the films on the alternator. After the alternator has been loaded with many cases, the radiologist sits down and goes through the cases, dictating the diagnostic report for each case. For workstations to provide a similar functionality as alternators, the radiologist needs to sit down and be presented with a series of CT cases. In this case, however, the computer (instead of the film library technician) selects the cases to be read out by the radiologists working each area in the radiology department. The computer matches the clinical cases produced by the CT scanners to the various radiologist workstations using *work lists*. In a simple example of how a work list might be used, a cross sectional imaging PACS sends all the MRI images to the MR workstation, CT images to the CT workstation, and ultrasound images to the ultrasound workstation. Radiologists sitting at those respective workstations go through the images and interpret them—very simple. The real world isn't quite so straightforward, however. Most radiologists specialize by organ system (pulmonary, neuro, bone, genitourinary, etc.), and so the neuro CT images should be sent to the neuroradiology workstation, and the bone CT images should be sent to that workstation. But there is the pediatric radiologist, who should be reading the pediatric cases (bone, neuro, GU, etc.), so those CT cases need to be sent to the pediatric workstation. Perhaps there is an emergency room radiologist workstation, and the radiologist working in that area needs to be sent all the emergency CT scans, which could be neuro, bone, GU, or pediatric. Some trauma patients will have multiple CT studies, including neuro, bone, and pulmonary for example. Should these studies be split up and read individually by three different sub-specialist radiologists? Probably not. If not, who gets those cases?

Workstations are located spatially, but it may be more appropriate to have work lists associated with radiologists (who move around), not specific workstations. For example, a bone radiologist walking through the pediatric area of the hospital should be able to sit down at the pediatric diagnostic workstation, log on as a bone radiologist, and receive the bone cases she needs to interpret. Moreover, some radiologists cross-cover other areas (e.g., bone and pediatrics), and the PACS software should be able to seamlessly concatenate multiple work lists, when appropriate.

As the above examples demonstrate, the clinical reality of how a radiology department operates is actually quite complex in terms of work flow. In the opinion of many, a PACS absolutely has to have the ability to create and use work lists to orchestrate the flow of clinical studies from the acquisition sites to the appropriate workstation locations. How well the PACS software addresses work lists, and how flexible the work list assignment algorithm is, should be a major factor in the consideration of one PACS vendor over another.

How does the PACS system software, which is responsible for routing the images (work list control), know which CT case goes where? Each case has a set of parameters associated with it (e.g., medical record number, referring physician, date of birth of patient, type of study, name of patient, accession number, CPT code, etc.), and presumably from this multi-parametric data the PACS should be able to build an efficient work list. To exacerbate matters, however, the PACS software is just one part of the

PACS. An institution may have three CT scanners, each one from a different vendor, and the type and quality of DICOM data set from each scanner to the PACS may vary widely, depending on the age of the scanner and its manufacturer. While DICOM conformance has the promise of uniformity across vendors and across modalities, DICOM implementations can differ in their adherence to the standard. Furthermore, a system can be DICOM conformant yet not be DICOM compatible. The CT-PACS interface(s), however, need(s) to be robust enough to allow the accurate transfer of electronic data from different scanners and in some cases in different formats.

One robust approach to the work-list assignment dilemma is to allow the institution to construct its own algorithms for assigning individual studies to work lists. For example, Boolean logic can be applied to the parameters associated for each case (e.g., if [referring physician = Dr. Xia] **and** [age of patient <=18] **and** [study != head], then route to pediatric radiologist). Although the Boolean logic approach is brute force, if enough time is spent developing all possible permutations, the PACS will execute work lists with reasonable accuracy. Other artificial intelligence techniques such as neural networks could also address this same problem, once enough cases have been correctly sent so as to provide the training data set for the neural network. While work lists are straightforward in concept, the successful implementation of work lists is a challenge in the PACS environment. What is important when purchasing a PACS, however, is to make sure that the PACS can handle work flow issues in a manner appropriate for the institution.

The PACS should also keep track of whether cases have been read or not, so cases do not end up getting lost in the system. This functionality requires that the PACS be informed in some manner as each study proceeds through dictation, transcription, report editing, and report sign-off. The status of the clinical report is typically monitored by the radiology information system (RIS), and therefore for the PACS to locate delayed reports, communication needs to occur between the RIS and the PACS. Locating lost or delayed cases is a very important issue that impacts both patient care and clinical revenue.

CT PACS: Distribution Beyond Radiology

Referring physicians in many instances need to see representative CT images, in addition to the radiologist's written report. A representative set of images are those images which demonstrate the salient aspects of the diagnosis in a concise manner (as few images as practical). As part of the primary diagnostic workstation software, the radiologist should be able to flag representative images for reference in the report and to make available to the referring physicians if requested.

Referring physicians should then be able to access the representative image set via the PACS at a *physician's review workstation*. A physician's review workstation provides nonradiologist users a place to review the CT images and to evaluate the patient's diagnosis and the corresponding image data flagged by the radiologist. A physician's review workstation needs superior display capability, but not at the same level as a primary diagnostic workstation. For example, physician's review workstations may use monitor resolutions on the order of 1500×1000. Physician review workstations need to be provided around the medical center to provide realistic access to those referring physicians and others who need to see the images. In some cases, referring physicians and other professionals will need access to the entire CT image data base, for example for radiation treatment planning or for surgical planning. For CT scanner installations where radiation oncology patients will be scanned, it is a very good idea to communicate with the therapy physicists concerning the radiation treatment planning computer system used, prior to purchase. The CT vendor should be informed in the bid specifications that DICOM conformance to the radiation treatment planning computer system is required, and vice versa.

Not all individuals will be able to access the physician review workstations at the medical center, and so some hard-copy print capability is needed with a CT scanner. This requires that the CT software provide DICOM interfaces, which include targets for printing via application entity (AE) titles for printers on the PACS network. Hard copy films are also required to fulfill legal requests, for physicians outside the local network environment, and in some cases for the operating rooms (depending on whether a secondary review workstation is available there). The hard copy technology needs to suit the needs of the institution. High-end computer printer technology has become very image oriented, and in many cases CT images printed onto plain paper may be sufficient for the end user. Transparency CT images can also be produced using a conventional laser camera or a dry laser system. It is preferable that the printers used for making hard copy CT images be connected not directly to the CT scanner (in the traditional fashion), but to the PACS network. This allows the printer to be a shared resource across all networked modalities, but it also allows the production of hard copy directly from the archive through the primary diagnostic workstations and perhaps through secondary review workstations. Because of the need to produce the occasional hard copy image, the PACS needs to be able to adequately indicate onto the film the technical data related to the CT image acquisition—the slice thickness, the kV, mA, time, pitch, etc; the same information that is available with conventional CT hard-copy images.

Teleradiology

A PACS is designed principally to service medical care directly at the institution (on the local area network), however a successful PACS implementation provides the backbone for a teleradiology system. Teleradiology in the context of CT is useful for radiologists who take a lot of CT-related calls. In many cases, CT images can be downloaded to a computer workstation at the radiologist's home, and a late night trip to the hospital can be avoided. A teleradiology network really is just an extension of the PACS, which makes use of remote review workstations (usually a personal computer) and typically modem-based communication. Teleradiology may also be useful for transmitting CT images to remote referral centers or from remote radiology clinics. High bandwidth connections may be necessary for these applications.

HIS/RIS/PACS Integration

The hospital information system (HIS) and the RIS are well established entities at most health care institutions. These computer services have helped to create an information systems (IS) dynasty at many hospitals and medical centers. Fortunately, a strong IS department is a crucial component in the successful implementation of a PACS. The degree of involvement and cooperation between Radiology and IS varies between institutions, but in the best of environments there is a good relationship between key members of both departments. The potential for friction between radiology and IS is great, especially when implementing a PACS where the expertise of specialists from both departments is needed. It is important that the key individuals from both departments know what the overall institutional goal is with respect to a PACS implementation, and that each player has a good understanding of his/her responsibilities. A strong team leader with big biceps is an asset.

A broad view of the relative roles of the HIS, RIS, and PACS is beyond the scope of this chapter. CT scanners need to communicate directly to the PACS of course. Often the PACS is not integrated in any meaningful way to the RIS system, however, and so the CT scanner does not have direct digital access to the information in the RIS system. This information often includes the patient schedule for the scanner, but more importantly here, the RIS holds basic patient information such as the medical record number, patient name, accession number, date of birth, etc. In lieu of direct communication between the RIS and the CT scanner, the technologist has to hand-enter the patient demographics for each study.

The utility of the PACS depends on the accuracy of the data it contains, and multiple sessions of hand data entry associated with each patient should be avoided where possible. There is the occasional overt keyboard entry error; for instance, typing in the medical record number incorrectly. More insidious, however, are errors caused by human variability. A patient Jose Roberto Rodriguez can be entered into the CT console as J.R. Rodriguez, J. Rodriguez, Rodriguez, JR, Jose R. Rodriguez, and so on. Because of this, at our institution we have pursued connecting the CT scanners directly to the RIS system. With such an interface (which is typically custom since DICOM standards do not apply here), the RIS downloads the patient demographics electronically to the CT scanner console.

With connectivity between the RIS and the CT scanner, the technologist does not have to enter patient data and some minor improvement in CT throughput may be realized there. More importantly, however, the DICOM format images will contain the patient demographic data which came directly from the RIS; so when it comes time for the computer to match the radiologist report (on the RIS) with the images on the PACS system, the two systems have the same exact patient data fields and matching them becomes much easier. This may sound trivial, but at our institution about 25% of the studies do not get matched correctly—a feat which requires exactly matching the patient name, the accession number (a day number assigned by the department in the RIS), and the medical record number. Being a Level 1 trauma center, many of our ER patients get registered initially as Jane or John Doe. Once the patient is stabilized and his/her name is entered into the system, the imaging studies under the Doe alias needs to be merged with the real name, and with subsequent imaging studies performed under his/her real name.

DICOM Specifications for CT

The details of DICOM are discussed in other chapters in this proceedings. The goal here is to indicate what aspects of the DICOM standard are applicable to Computed Tomography. CT is a *storage service class*, but other *abstract classes* (a DICOM term) that are important include *Query and Retrieve, Print, HIS / RIS*, and *Work List*. The CT scanner console can act as either a *service class user* (SCU) or a *service class provider* (SCP), depending on the function. For example, if a remote workstation (acting as a SCU) queries the CT scanner, the CT acts as a SCP, but if it then sends requested images to the workstation (as a result of the query), the CT scanner console acts as a SCU and the workstation becomes the SCP while it receives the images.

Table 2 illustrates the DICOM functionality that a CT scanner should have (marked on the table as CT). Other *desirable* features are marked as CT*. When developing bid specifications for a CT scanner, it is recommended that those items indicated by the table be requested in the bid. The physicist is traditionally involved in developing the bid specifications for imaging equipment such as a CT scanner. It is important for the physicist to participate in developing the DICOM language in the bid as well, usually working with an IS technical person or the PACS manager at the institution. IS professionals know computers and computer networks, but they usually do not have a complete understanding of how a radiology department works from a patient flow or work-flow perspective.

Table 2: A matrix showing which DICOM features are necessary for CT (labeled as "CT") and those features which would be desirable (CT*).

Abstract Class	Service Class User	Service Class Provider
Storage Service Class	CT	CT*
Query & Retrieve	CT*	CT
Print	CT	
HIS / RIS		CT
Work List	CT	

After the CT scanner is purchased and installed, it will become necessary to verify the performance of the scanner. The more traditional CT acceptance testing procedures should be done, of course, as discussed elsewhere in this chapter. Once connected to the PACS, the CT scanner should then be tested for its ability to communicate with the PACS. These tests, which should be performed by the PACS network technical manager, should be explicitly scheduled and performed. It is likely that the PACS tests may take longer than the more traditional physics acceptance testing, and resolution of problems uncovered may require months.

Summary

The difference between the promise and the reality of PACS is substantial. A realistic understanding of what can and can't be done in the short term is necessary in making implementation plans and procurement decisions which match an institution's needs. Despite the shortcomings of PACS, the computer-savvy medical physicist should keep the pressure on the vendors—the CT manufacturers, PACS vendors, workstation companies, and the RIS vendors—to deliver an electronic imaging system that performs at the highest levels of expectation. There will invariably be disputes between vendors in a highly interconnected environment, each vendor insisting that the problems encountered are the fault of the other. This is where the conflict resolution skills of the medical physicist or PACS manager will be honed. It is also where a set of well-written bid specifications comes in handy.

PACS will become an increasingly important part of the radiology equipment armamentarium, and the diagnostic medical physicist should take steps sooner rather than later to prepare him or herself for this eventuality.

References

Boone, J.M. and Seibert, J.M., "An accurate method for computer-generating tungsten anode x ray spectra from 30 kV to 140 kV." *Medical Physics* 24: 1661-1670; 1997.

Boone, J.M. and Seibert, J.A., "Monte Carlo simulation of the scattered radiation distribution in diagnostic radiology." *Medical Physics* 15: 713-720; 1988.

Bushberg, J.T., Seibert, J.A., Leidholdt, E.M., Boone, J.M., *The Essential Physics of Medical Imaging*. Baltimore, Williams and Wilkins, 1993.

Fullerton, G.D., Zagzebski, J.A., "Medical Physics of CT and Ultrasound: Tissue Imaging and Characterization." AAPM Monograph 6, New York, American Institute of Physics, 1980.

Gould, R.G., "CT Overview and Basics" in: Seibert, J.A., Barnes, G.T., and Gould, R.G., "Specification, Acceptance Testing and Quality Control of Diagnostic X-ray Imaging Equipment." AAPM Monograph 20, New York, American Institute of Physics, 1994.

Hendee, W.R. and Ritenour, R. *Medical Imaging Physics*, 3rd Edition, St. Louis, Mosby Year Book, 1992.

Loo, L.-N. D., "CT Acceptance Testing" in: Seibert, J.A., Barnes, G.T., and Gould, R.G. "Specification, Acceptance Testing and Quality Control of Diagnostic X-ray Imaging Equipment." AAPM Monograph 20, New York, American Institute of Physics, 1994.

Marshall, C. *The Physical Basis of Computed Tomography,* St. Louis, Warren H. Green, Inc., 1982.

Mattson, R., "CT Design Considerations and Specifications" in: Seibert, J.A., Barnes, G.T., and Gould, R.G. "Specification, Acceptance Testing and Quality Control of Diagnostic X-ray Imaging Equipment." AAPM Monograph 20, New York, American Institute of Physics, 1994.

Rothenberg, L.N. "CT Dose Assessment" in: Seibert, J.A., Barnes, G.T., and Gould, R.G. "Specification, Acceptance Testing and Quality Control of Diagnostic X-ray Imaging Equipment." AAPM Monograph 20, New York, American Institute of Physics, 1994.

Shope, T.B., Gagne, R.M., and Johnson G.C. "A method for describing doses delivered by transmission x-ray computed tomography." *Medical Physics* 8: 488-495; 1981.

Table A1: f-factors for various beam qualities pertinent to CT. These data were calculated using a spectral model (Boone and Seibert 1997) with 10% voltage ripple, the kV, and added copper filtration as shown. The data in this table also include 8 cm of Lucite filtration, simulating the beam filtration path of x-rays reaching the pencil chamber on a 16 cm diameter Lucite head phantom. The average x-ray energy and HVL in mm of aluminum are given. The f factors were calculated for Lucite (f_L) and water (f_w) , and the ratio f_w/f_L is given as well.

Values for HEAD PHANTOM

kV	Cu (mm)	E (keV)	HVL (mm Al)	f_L Rad/R	f_w Rad/R	Ratio —
80	0.0	46.7	2.3	0.671	0.944	1.408
80	0.2	52.0	5.2	0.700	0.946	1.351
80	0.4	55.0	6.6	0.718	0.947	1.318
80	0.6	57.1	7.4	0.731	0.947	1.296
80	0.8	58.7	8.0	0.741	0.948	1.279
80	1.0	60.0	8.5	0.749	0.949	1.266
80	1.2	61.1	8.8	0.756	0.949	1.256
100	0.0	53.2	2.8	0.707	0.947	1.340
100	0.2	58.9	6.3	0.738	0.948	1.285
100	0.4	62.2	7.9	0.757	0.950	1.255
100	0.6	64.6	8.8	0.770	0.951	1.234
100	0.8	66.5	9.4	0.780	0.951	1.219
100	1.0	68.0	9.9	0.789	0.952	1.207
100	1.2	69.3	10.3	0.796	0.953	1.197
120	0.0	58.5	3.4	0.732	0.949	1.296
120	0.2	64.5	7.3	0.763	0.951	1.246
120	0.4	68.2	8.9	0.782	0.952	1.218
120	0.6	70.9	9.8	0.795	0.953	1.199
120	0.8	73.2	10.5	0.805	0.954	1.185
120	1.0	75.1	11.0	0.814	0.955	1.173
120	1.2	76.8	11.4	0.821	0.956	1.163
140	0.0	63.0	3.9	0.749	0.950	1.268
140	0.2	69.2	8.1	0.779	0.952	1.222
140	0.4	73.2	9.7	0.798	0.954	1.195
140	0.6	76.3	10.6	0.811	0.955	1.177
140	0.8	78.9	11.3	0.822	0.956	1.163
140	1.0	81.1	11.8	0.830	0.957	1.152
140	1.2	83.1	12.2	0.838	0.957	1.143

Table A2: f-factors for various beam qualities pertinent to CT. These data were calculated using a spectral model (Boone and Seibert 1997) with 10% voltage ripple, the kV, and added copper filtration as shown. The data in this table also includes 16 cm of Lucite filtration, simulating the beam filtration path of x-rays reaching the pencil chamber on a 32 cm diameter Lucite body phantom. The average x-ray energy and HVL in mm of aluminum are given. The f factors were calculated for Lucite (f$_L$) and water (f$_w$) , and the ratio f$_w$/f$_L$ is given as well.

Values for BODY PHANTOM

kV	Cu (mm)	E (keV)	HVL (mm Al)	f$_L$ Rad/R	f$_w$ Rad/R	Ratio —
80	0.0	50.1	2.3	0.689	0.945	1.371
80	0.2	53.9	5.2	0.712	0.946	1.329
80	0.4	56.4	6.6	0.727	0.947	1.303
80	0.6	58.2	7.4	0.738	0.948	1.284
80	0.8	59.6	8.0	0.747	0.948	1.270
80	1.0	60.8	8.5	0.754	0.949	1.259
80	1.2	61.8	8.8	0.760	0.949	1.250
100	0.0	57.1	2.8	0.728	0.948	1.302
100	0.2	61.3	6.3	0.751	0.949	1.263
100	0.4	64.0	7.9	0.767	0.950	1.240
100	0.6	66.1	8.8	0.778	0.951	1.223
100	0.8	67.7	9.4	0.787	0.952	1.209
100	1.0	69.2	9.9	0.795	0.953	1.199
100	1.2	70.4	10.3	0.801	0.953	1.190
120	0.0	63.0	3.4	0.754	0.950	1.260
120	0.2	67.5	7.3	0.777	0.952	1.224
120	0.4	70.5	8.9	0.793	0.953	1.202
120	0.6	73.0	9.8	0.804	0.954	1.186
120	0.8	75.0	10.5	0.813	0.955	1.174
120	1.0	76.8	11.0	0.821	0.956	1.164
120	1.2	78.4	11.4	0.828	0.956	1.155
140	0.0	68.0	3.9	0.772	0.952	1.232
140	0.2	72.8	8.1	0.795	0.953	1.200
140	0.4	76.2	9.7	0.810	0.955	1.179
140	0.6	79.0	10.6	0.821	0.956	1.164
140	0.8	81.3	11.3	0.830	0.957	1.152
140	1.0	83.4	11.8	0.838	0.958	1.143
140	1.2	85.3	12.2	0.845	0.958	1.134

Magnetic Resonance Imaging and PACS

John D. Hazle, Ph.D. and Edward F. Jackson, Ph.D.
UT M. D. Anderson Cancer Center
Houston, TX

The goal of this presentation is to introduce Picture Archiving and Communication System (PACS) issues specific to nuclear magnetic resonance imaging (MRI). A review of MRI fundamentals will precede an overview of some of the unique demands magnetic resonance (MR) has on PACS.

MRI is still an immature technology that continues to evolve at a rapid pace. Recent advances, particularly in fast-imaging, have resulted in MR scanners capable of acquiring large numbers of images (>1000) in a single examination. These data often undergo significant post-processing for efficient presentation to the reviewer. This impacts the PACS archive and bandwidth requirements and creates new issues related to image presentation. Consensus solutions are not available at this time for many of the image viewing issues. However, identifying the issues is the first step in defining the appropriate solutions at individual institutions.

MR Fundamentals

The basis for nuclear magnetic resonance (NMR) is the interaction of nuclei possessing non-zero magnetic moments with external magnetic fields. This moment-field interaction was first postulated by Pauli in the early 1920's. However, it was not demonstrated in bulk matter until 1946 when independent experiments performed by Bloch at Stanford (Bloch, Hansen et al. 1946) and Purcell at Harvard (Purcell, Torrey et al. 1946) demonstrated the effect. Since their experiments were based on a resonance phenomenon, the term "nuclear magnetic resonance" (NMR) was coined. Eventually, the marketing components of the major equipment manufacturers were able to "lose" the nuclear nomenclature when related to human imaging, resulting in the common MR or MRI terminology. The reader is referred to several good chapters on basic MR physics (Wehrli, Shaw et al. 1988; Cho, Jones et al. 1993).

Magnetic Moment and Nuclear Spin

The nuclear species of most interest in MRI is the proton. Protons exist in large quantities in most biological materials. The protons that make up water and fat (lipids) constitute more than 99% of the detectable protons in the human body. Therefore, this presentation will be limited to protons associated with water and lipids.

The proton, a "spin-1/2" magnetic moment, can be thought of as a small dipole magnet. This dipole will interact with an external magnetic field and will prefer to be aligned parallel or anti-parallel to the field. The torque resulting from the interaction of the magnetic moment and the external field causes the proton to precess about an axis parallel to the external field. The rate of precession is dependent on the magnetic field interaction, which is proportional to the external field. This relationship is given by the Larmor equation:

$$\omega_0 = \gamma B_0$$

where W_0 is the precessional frequency, γ is the gyromagnetic ratio, and B_0 is the applied field (this term describes the main static field of the MRI system). Therefore, the base operating frequency of the system is a characteristic of the static magnetic field strength. As will be seen, expansions of this equation form the fundamental basis for MRI spatial encoding and image formation.

Image Formation

As with other tomographic imaging modalities, such as x-ray CT (computed tomography), MRI is inherently a three-dimensional imaging modality. Similar to CT, one dimension is defined independently as the *slice* direction and the other two dimensions are derived from complex projection or encoded data. In CT the slice is defined by the x-ray tube collimators and is always *axial* relative to the patient (or within a few degrees of axial). Multiple projections of the patient from a slice limited by the collimators result in a data-space that can be back-projected to form a CT image (Herman 1980; Cho, Jones et al. 1993). In MRI the *slice* plane can be defined electronically to be in any orientation. The image is then formed by spatially encoding the other two dimensions using linear gradients.

The diagram in Figure 1 is a simplified MR *spin-echo* pulse sequence. Slice selection is achieved by applying a bandwidth limited excitation radiofrequency (rf) pulse in the presence of a linear magnetic field gradient. Spatial encoding of the other two directions is performed by applying a *frequency-encoding* gradient during signal detection and variable *phase-encoding* gradients during the spin evolution period.

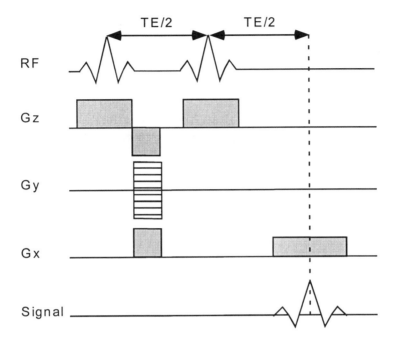

Figure 1. A simple spin-echo pulse sequence diagram showing the major rf pulses, gradients, and signal acquisition period.

Slice Selection

Slice selection in MRI is achieved by applying a bandwidth limited rf excitation pulse in the presence of linear magnetic gradient fields. This results in the selective excitation of a plane of protons orthogonal to the applied gradient axis (remember, this could be an axial, sagittal, coronal, or oblique gradient plane). Consider the diagram in Figure 2 where a linear gradient, G_z, is applied parallel to the static field.

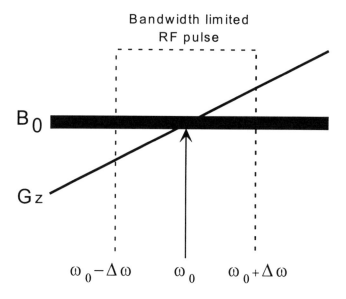

Figure 2. The mechanism of slice selection using a linear magnetic field gradient (G_z) and bandwidth limited rf pulse is demonstrated. The rf pulse only excites frequencies of $\pm\Delta\omega$ which are defined by B_0 and G_z.

The total magnetic field at any point, z, along the plane is given by

$$B_z = B_0 + \left(G_z \cdot z\right).$$

The magnetic resonance frequency at any location z is then:

$$\omega_z = \gamma B_z .$$

Therefore, the spins with frequencies $\Delta\omega_z$ can be selectively excited using bandwidth limited rf pulses to define a slice of width Δ_z.

Frequency Encoding

In conventional imaging sequences a second linear gradient, G_x, is applied during the acquisition of the MR signal. This results in a line (or view) of k-space data. Again, the linear magnetic field gradient serves to cause spins at different locations, in this case, in the x dimension, to resonate at different frequencies. When these data are Fourier transformed, the frequencies and amplitudes of the individual frequencies are extracted to serve as the image data.

Phase Encoding

The final direction is encoded by inducing small phase perturbations between successive lines of k-space data using a third linear gradient, G_y. This results in the sinusoidal modulation of the spins in the direction of the encoding gradient; here the y gradient. After phase-encoding we have now generated a dataset from a defined slice with the x and y directions encoded so that following a 2D FT a tomographic image is formed.

k-space and the 2D Fourier Transform

Following excitation of the spins in the prescribed plane, the spin system is manipulated to return an image with a particular contrast. A rigorous discussion of contrast mechanisms is beyond the scope of this article and the reader is referred to several thorough discussions of MR contrast mechanisms (Wehrli, Shaw et al. 1988). Regardless of the desired image contrast, a set of raw data must be acquired with sufficient density to achieve the desired spatial resolution. This set of raw data will be processed by 2D Fourier transform to convert *k-space* raw data into a spatially encoded image. The requirements of the 2D Fast Fourier Transformation (FFT) are that the raw image data have the same dimensions (matrix size) as the image space. "k-space" is the term for the raw data space that will be transformed to yield the MR image. Figure 3 is the raw k-space data and transformed image data from a T2-weighted image of a human brain. Note that the bulk of the image information or energy is located at the center of k-space which constitutes the low frequency components of the image. Figure 4 shows the conventional rectilinear sampling of k-space. The first time a pulse sequence is executed the protons in the defined slice are excited, a phase aberration is introduced, and a *line* of k-space is acquired during the readout period. A magnetization recovery period or repetition time, TR, is then allowed for the magnetization in the slice to return to equilibrium. The next line of k-space is acquired in the same manner, except that the phase aberration is changed. Therefore the total imaging time is n_y (number of phase-encoding lines) times TR (the repetition time).

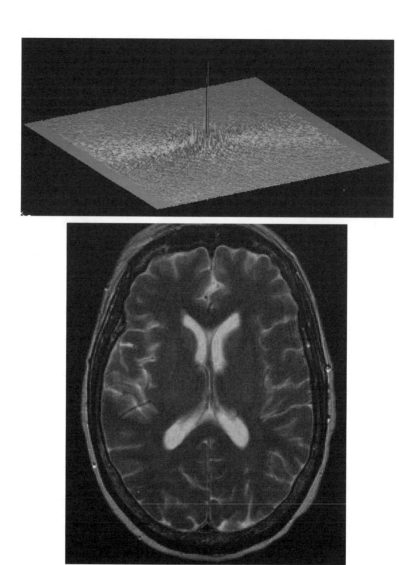

Figure 3. The top plot is the raw k-space data used to generate the T2-weighted image of a brain in the lower half of the figure. Note that most of the energy in k-space is located near the center or low frequencies.

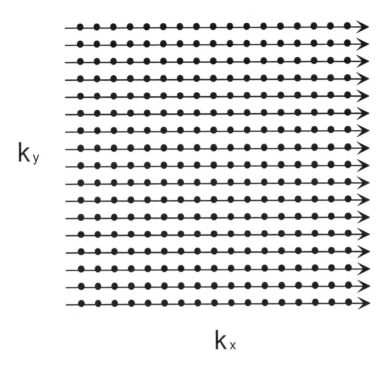

Figure 4. k-space is covered by conventional imaging sequences in a piecewise manner one line at a time. The time between each line acquisition is defined by TR. Therefore, the total acquisition time is TR times the number of lines acquired.

Signal-to-Noise

Signal-to-noise ratio (SNR) in MRI is a very complex parameter that depends on many object characteristics, scanner hardware specifications, and operator defined parameters (Sprawls 1988). There are a few parameters that are of global significance. Generally, higher static field strengths result in higher SNR (for the same imaging times and resolution). Using surface-coils will also usually increase signal and decrease noise, significantly raising SNR, but at the expense of restricted fields-of-view (FOVs) and often inhomogeneous sensitivities.

SNR, as you might intuitively guess, is linearly dependent on slice thickness. All things being equal, as we increase the slice thickness, we are linearly increasing the number of protons excited by the slice select pulse. Also, as the FOV is increased, the absolute number of protons observed in each voxel increases linearly with each dimension (i.e., increasing the FOV from 20 cm to 40 cm results in a factor of 4 improvement in SNR).

Density-weighted images typically have higher SNR than their T1 and T2 counterparts. This is because the relaxation effects that result in image contrast also result in signal loss. Also, spin-echo sequences have inherently better SNR than gradient-echo sequences. These are all described in excellent detail in (Wehrli, Shaw et al. 1988).

Contrast

Contrast in MR has a complex dependence on multiple independent tissue parameters (Hendrick 1988). This is significantly different from the singular dependence of tissue contrast on the linear attenuation coefficient parameter as in x-ray. The three fundamental MR contrast *weightings* are proton density, spin-lattice (T1) relaxation, and spin-spin (T2) relaxation. MR angiography (MRA) is gaining significant clinical acceptance and the ability to visualize flowing blood without the use of i.v. (intravenous) contrast materials is a distinct advantage for MRA. We will treat MRA separately since it is one of the first advanced MR imaging techniques to gain widespread clinical acceptance and which can put significantly greater demands on data archive capacity. MRA also requires more sophisticated post-processing and visualization. Other, newer contrast mechanisms that appear headed for routine clinical use will also be briefly discussed.

Proton Density, T1, and T2 Contrast

The following equation is a simplification of a universal contrast equation for MR describing the influence of proton density, T1, and T2 relaxation times on MR signal intensity:

$$S = k \cdot \rho \cdot \left(1 - e^{-T1/TR}\right) \cdot e^{-T2/TE}$$

where k is a constant, ρ is the proton density, TR is the repetition time, and TE is the echo time. Several good textbooks are available for more detailed descriptions of MR contrast (Wehrli, Shaw et al. 1988). The point here is that by adjusting TR and TE, the operator can manipulate the contrast in the image to enhance the differential diagnosis. Additionally, paramagnetic contrast agents are available which dramatically alter T1 and are used routinely for imaging tumors and other pathology. Figure 5 demonstrates the common contrast presentations of proton-density, T1, T2, and post-contrast T1-weighting for a case of glioblastoma multiforme.

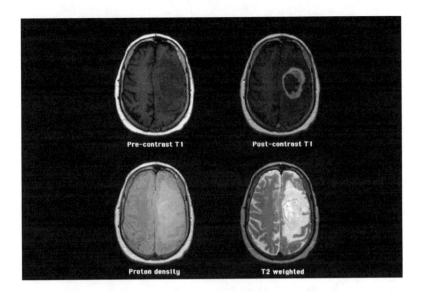

Pre-contrast T1 Post-contrast T1

Proton density T2 weighted

Figure 5. The most common MR contrasts are shown in this figure
(T1, T1+contrast, T2, and Proton density).

Volume Imaging

All tomographic imaging is inherently three-dimensional; that is to say that when we consider the contrast between two pixel elements, we in fact know the planar (2D) relationship from the image and the third dimension from slice selection. MR and CT are now capable of acquiring *isotropic* data—image data where the scale of the pixel dimensions are equal in all three planes. For example, consider a 24-cm FOV image with a resolution of 256 elements per side. This results in an in-plane pixel resolution of about 1 mm (240 mm ÷ 256). Using 3D gradient-echo imaging sequences it is possible to obtain 1.0-1.5 mm thick slices through most or all of the cranium. The significant point to be made for volume imaging is that reformatting or volume or surface rendering is enhanced by the fact that image planes can be created in any orientation from the dataset without a significant loss in resolution. Figure 6 is a volume rendering of a volume image set (top) and a shaded-surface rendering of the same data (bottom). Post-processing in this manner is a growing component of the radiology practice for surgical and radiotherapy planning (Siebert and Rosenbaum 1993).

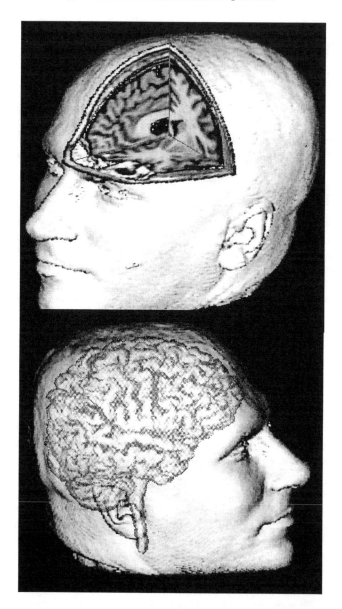

Figure 6. The upper half of the figure shows a volume rendering with a quadrant cut-out to expose inner surfaces. The lower half show a shaded surface rendering of the same data set with the skin being translucent, allowing visualization of the inner brain surface.

Volume imaging raises two issues: archive capacity and visualization. Archive bandwidth and storage depth will be affected by these higher resolution (more slices) studies. A typical whole-brain volume study will typically generate 124 images, a series larger than many conventional studies.

Visualization can be considered to have two components: diagnosis and post-processing. Diagnosis is impacted because now the radiologist has 124 images to consider rather than the 20-25 of a typical T1 series. This means that they either have to wade through all the images, the technologist selects *representative* slices (usually every nth image printed), or new paradigms of image viewing must be considered (i.e., cine viewing on soft-copy workstations). Finally, the image data may undergo significant post-processing for a rendered display. This brings up the thorny issue of quality control on the post-processed data and the issue of archiving *non-standard* data. These should all be addressed when considering incorporating MRI into PACS.

Other Contrast Mechanisms

Significant interest is now focused on functional or physiologic imaging techniques. These include dynamic contrast-enhanced, arterial spin-labeled, and diffusion-weighted MR imaging sequences. These techniques all rely on significant post-processing of the MR data. Off-line workstation capabilities, quality assurance procedures, and archiving strategies must be developed to include these as well.

Advanced Imaging Techniques

Echo-planar Imaging (EPI)

Currently, the fastest commercially available image acquisition technique is echo-planar imaging (EPI) (Jackson 1999). The basic idea behind the EPI sequence is that multiple phase- and frequency-encoding gradients are applied in a given TR interval, thereby reducing the time required to acquire a given number of lines of k-space. Figure 7 shows the k-space trajectory for a single-shot EPI sequence. In "snapshot" or "single-shot" SE EPI acquisitions, for example, *every* echo is obtained following a single 90°-180° pulse pair. This results in image acquisition times as short as 50-100 ms, and makes EPI ideal for imaging dynamic processes. The acquisition of snapshot EPI images, however, requires an MR scanner that has very fast acquisition rate capability, i.e., high bandwidth, and extremely good gradient field subsystems. Otherwise, high-quality snapshot EPI images are difficult to obtain reproducibly. To ease the requirements of single-shot EPI somewhat, multishot or "mosaic" EPI techniques have also been introduced. While not as fast as single-shot scans, multishot EPI scans demonstrate decreased geometric distortions and other artifacts. While clinical applications of EPI in routine oncological MRI are currently limited, EPI imaging techniques are commonly used for perfusion, diffusion, and functional MRI research (discussed below). Typically, EPI images are acquired with lower matrix sizes than, for example, routine clinical proton density-weighted images. Therefore, one might expect that the bandwidth and storage needs in terms of a PACS would be significantly reduced. However, when used to monitor dynamic processes with temporal resolutions on the order of 100 ms per image, the total number of images in a given EPI run can be quite large.

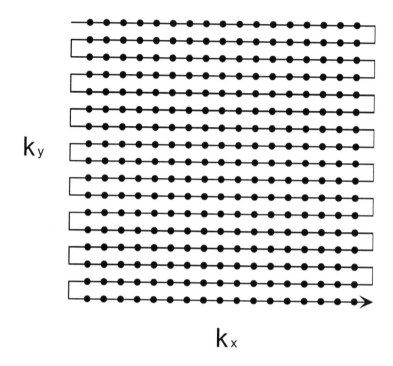

k_y

k_x

Figure 7. In echo-planar imaging k-space is traversed in a single shot or multiple shots. At the end of each line of k-space the magnetization vector is "wound" back into the other direction for continued data collection.

Spiral Acquisition

Although MR is dominated by rectilinear k-space acquisition strategies, non-linear strategies were proposed as a means to accelerate acquisition times in the early 1990's (Ra, Rim et al. 1991). However, it was not until gradient system performance improved to the point that these techniques gained significant interest (Sachs, Meyer et al. 1994). Since then many applications in vascular (Gatehouse, Firmin et al. 1994), cardiac (Hardy, Pearlman et al. 1991), functional neuro-imaging (Lee, Glover et al. 1995), and dynamic (Glover and Lee 1995; Liao, Sommer et al. 1995) imaging have been proposed.

Spiral imaging is similar to rectilinear in the sense that the same contrast mechanisms available to rectilinear sequences can be used in spiral sequences. Further, spin- or gradient-echoes can be formed. The most significant differences are that 1) rather than using *blipped* phase-encoding, gradients of x and y gradients are applied simultaneously during signal detection and 2) an additional post-processing step, *regridding,* is necessary to prepare the spiral k-space data for 2D FT. The k-space trajectory for a spiral acquisition is shown in Figure 8. The magnetization vector starts at the center of k-space and is spiraled out. While the use of spiral imaging is still largely a research endeavor, spiral imaging is likely to quickly become a clinical sequence for cardiac, dynamics and for functional neuroimaging (fMRI) applications.

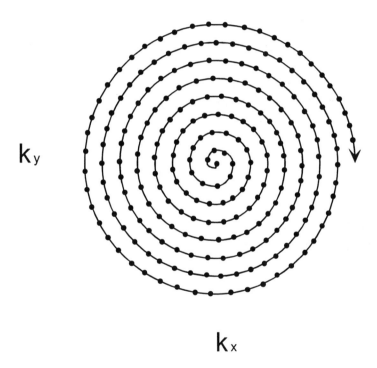

Figure 8. In spiral imaging the magnetization vector starts at the center of k-space and spirals out to achieve the desired field-of-view. Data sampling is linear in time, therefore the data points are not acquired in a rectilinear grid. Following data acquisition the k-space data is *regridded* for 2D fast-Fourier transformation.

Angiography

All current MRA techniques are based upon gradient-echo sequences and time-of-flight (TOF), phase contrast (PC), or bolus contrast agent-enhanced techniques.

Time-of-flight (TOF)

The physical basis for TOF MRA techniques is known as "flow-related enhancement" (Keller and Saloner 1993). In TOF MRA, T1-weighted images are acquired with very short TE and TR times. Since the images are being acquired from a volume or slice of tissue, the spins in that volume or slice become partially saturated due to the rapidly repeated RF pulses, i.e., the net magnetization never recovers completely during the TR. However, the signal from the volume of tissue being imaged is decreased due to this partial saturation. Blood flowing into the imaging volume, however, has not been partially saturated. Therefore, the signal from the blood is typically significantly larger than the signals from the surrounding tissues. As a result, the vessels appear bright relative to the surrounding stationary tissue. MRA data is usually presented in the form of a maximum intensity projection (MIP). Figure 9 is the MIP of a circle of Willis study with and without magnetization transfer normal tissue suppression (Parker and Haacke 1993).

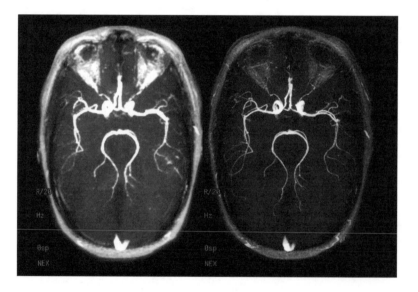

Figure 9. These two maximum intensity projection (MIP) cerebral angiograms demonstrate the ability of MR to accurately depict vessels in the brain. The image at left is using conventional TOF techniques, while the image on the right also uses magnetization transfer to reduce signals from brain tissue, improving vessel conspicuity.

The TOF technique works best for relatively rapid flow that is perpendicular to the slices in the imaging volume since this maximizes the flow-related enhancement. However, it is frequently necessary to spatially saturate the vessels flowing in the opposite direction to the vessels of interest in order to minimize contribution from these opposing vessels. In this case, "spatially saturate" means to apply a 90° pulse (outside of the imaging volume) to the blood in the vessels that are to be suppressed. If the saturated blood then flows into the imaging volume and receives a 90° pulse (or other large flip angle pulse), the resulting magnetization will primarily be in the longitudinal direction, i.e., parallel to the applied static field. As no signal is detected from magnetization that is parallel or antiparallel to the static field, the signal from the saturated blood will be suppressed. If such spatial saturation techniques are not employed, arterial and venous vessels may both appear in the resulting image and overlap of the two can cause confusion.

TOF techniques are the most commonly utilized sequences for MRA, particularly for studies of relatively fast flow. They work well with very short TE values, which minimize loss of signal secondary to dephasing of the spins by turbulent flow. Such dephasing can cause significant over-estimation of stenosis as the TE times increase. The same MR system improvements that have resulted in faster and faster imaging, especially the improved gradient subsystems, are also resulting in continuous improvement in the quality of MRA angiography by decreasing acquisition times (decreased patient motion artifacts, better contrast due to emphasized flow-related enhancement effects, and better throughput) and decreasing echo times (decreased dephasing and less overestimation of stenosis).

From a PACS standpoint, many of these "improvements" come at a price. For example, it is not uncommon these days to use "zero-interpolation" (ZIP) methods in MRA to improve the apparent in-plane resolution. In a 3D acquisition mode, "slice ZIP" methods also can provide two to four times the number of acquired slices to yield apparent overlap of the slices in order to improve the quality of the maximum intensity projections commonly used to display a pseudo 3D representation of the vasculature. Therefore, while one might acquire 64 slices with an acquisition matrix of 256×256, the resulting image dataset that must be transmitted and stored may be 128 images, each with a 512×512 matrix size.

Phase-Contrast (PC)

TOF techniques currently dominate the MRA scene. However, PC techniques have some particular benefits (Dumoulin, Souza et al. 1993). The basic mechanism behind PC MRA is quite different from TOF techniques. While TOF MRA relies upon flow-related enhancement and appropriate use of spatial saturation pulses, PC MRA capitalizes on the fact that the signal intensity from the nuclear spins can be made to depend upon the velocity of the spins. During a PC MRA pulse sequence, the moving spins accrue phase that is directly proportional to their velocity, and this phase can be measured. Therefore, PC MRA can depict the velocity (direction *and* speed) of the nuclear spins and, if the vessel diameter is also measured, the flow rate. Furthermore, such PC MRA acquisitions can be gated to the cardiac cycle to allow for the display of flow velocity as a function of cardiac cycle to examine multi-directional flow (biphasic or triphasic flow patterns).

Because of the way phase contrast images are formed, they have two main advantages compared to TOF MRA images. First, PC MRA is more useful when imaging slow flow. This is because the image contrast does not depend on flow-related enhancement, but rather on the actual velocity of the spins. Furthermore, careful placement of spatial saturation bands to suppress flow opposed to the direction of interest, and preferential placement of the scan plane perpendicular to the direction of the flow are not necessary. Second, quantitative measures of flow velocities and flow rates can be obtained using PC MRA. There are, of course, some disadvantages of PC MRA relative to TOF techniques. First, for the same spatial resolution, the image acquisition time for a PC MRA study is longer than is required for a TOF MRA study. Second, the user must specify the expected maximum flow velocity (the "VENC," or velocity *en*coding value) before the scan is initiated. If the actual flow velocity exceeds the specified VENC value, the flow will be "aliased" in the MRA images, typically resulting in the displayed flow velocity that underestimates the actual flow velocity. On the other hand, if the specified VENC is significantly greater than the actual flow velocity, the signal from the vessel will be small and the SNR in the resulting MRA will be poor.

Due to the increased acquisition time relative to TOF MRA, typically fewer slices are acquired, ZIP methods are not commonly used, and the maximum image matrix size is typically 256×256. Therefore, one's initial impression would be that the storage requirements and bandwidth necessary for accommodating PC MRA would appear to be much less than for TOF MRA. However, it is not uncommon to encode up to three spatial directions and to store images representing the magnitude of the flow velocity, as well as the individual flow-encoded images along each orthogonal direction. Therefore, the image storage requirements for PC MRA, like TOF MRA, can be very misleading if one only considers the number of slices and acquisition matrices of the acquired data; one must always consider the ultimate reconstructed data set characteristics.

Bolus Contrast Agent-enhanced MRA

With the recent boost in acquisition rates, a new type of MRA has become very prevalent in body MRA, and is becoming more common in MRA of the carotid arteries as well (Marchal, Bosmans et al. 1993). In the bolus contrast agent-enhanced MRA technique, rapid T1-weighted fast gradient echo images are obtained following (within a carefully chosen delay) the bolus infusion of paramagnetic contrast agent, such as Gd-DTPA. In this technique, the contrast is provided by the dramatic decrease in T1 relaxation times of blood relative to the surrounding stationary tissues (at least during the first pass of the contrast agent through the vasculature). With a rapid bolus, e.g., 5 cc/sec infusion of 0.2 mmol/kg Gd-DTPA, and rapid scanning, e.g., 28 images in ~20 sec, very high quality MRA of the descending aorta, renal arteries, etc., can be obtained in a single breath-hold in order to minimize motion due to respiration. As with TOF MRA, ZIP methods are commonly employed with bolus contrast agent-enhanced MRA, so the number of slices to be stored, as well as the image matrix, may be significantly larger than those used to acquire the data.

Functional Neuroimaging

Of the many other mechanisms for generating contrast in MRI, one that is likely to have significant impact on PACS is functional neuroimaging (fMRI) (Jackson 1999). fMRI is the generic term for one of many acquisition schemes that indirectly measure neuronal activity in response to a given task. These studies typically use ultra-fast pulse sequences (acquisition times on the order of several hundred milliseconds) repeated many times, typically for multiple slices, for an extended period of time.

Once again, archive and visualization become critical issues. In the case of fMRI it is not unusual to acquire thousands of images in a single *run*. In addition, in a single exam several such fMRI runs may be performed to map different areas of neuronal function, e.g., motor, sensory, and expressive speech activation tasks. Although these images may be acquired with reduced matrices relative to those used for anatomic imaging (64×64 or 128×128 instead of the usual 256×256 or 512×512), they may be reconstructed to the more typical resolution of 256×256.

Similarly, high speed imaging techniques for measuring perfusion and diffusion are becoming more widely used in the clinical environment, and potentially generate large numbers of images in relatively short scan times. For example, a typical 5 min. brain perfusion exam may easily generate 400 or more images.

Interventional MR

A relatively new area is that of interventional MR (iMRI). New system and magnet designs have been developed to allow for patient access during MR imaging. These systems typically use lower field magnets (<0.5 T) and may or may not have conventional body imaging coils. They are typically sited in semi-sterile (special procedures) to sterile (surgical suite) environments. The systems are used for guiding biopsies, minimally invasive surgery, and loaded orthopedic applications. The image management is typical of other MR scans. However, many of the applications are dynamic in nature and relatively large datasets can be expected. Display of the data may also be best performed in cine format on workstations, rather than in conventional film formatting.

PACS Issues Related to MR

Figure 10 lays out the components of PACS related to MRI and their interconnections. Image distribution strategies come in basically two flavors: store-&-forward and on-demand access. Deciding which approach you will take for your institution is perhaps the first question that should be addressed in selecting a PACS vendor. Store-&-forward system require that the images be moved from the archive to the workstation before viewing; they must be *prefetched*. While this approach significantly reduces the communication bandwidth demands, it has two distinct disadvantages. First, the "system" must know where to send the images (which workstation) for viewing. While this is not a major problem for diagnosis in radiology, it is a considerably more complex problem when all clinicians in a hospital are considered part of the PACS client base. The second drawback is related to the first in that images prefetched to a particular workstation are not available *on demand* at other workstations.

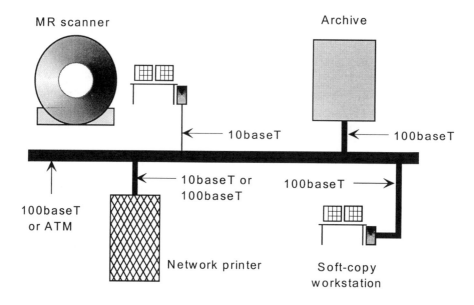

Figure 10. Typical configuration of an MR scanner integrated into a PACS network. The MR console is connected by conventional 10baseT (10 MB/s) ethernet. The hospital backbone is likely higher bandwidth 100baseT (100 Mb/s) ethernet or asynchronous transfer mode (ATM, 155 Mb/s). Printers and workstations are connected either using 10baseT or 100baseT depending on the bandwidth demands of the application.

We believe that the *on demand* configuration offers considerably more flexibility. First, images (or applications for that matter) are delivered from the archive to the workstation at the time they are requested. This means that the communication bandwidth must be adequate to move the images from the archive to the workstation in a matter of seconds. Radiologists and clinicians will not tolerate significant delays between requesting the images and viewing. However, the small image format size in MR (commonly $256 \times 256 \times 2$ byte = 135 kb file size) makes it relatively easy to maintain a short delay between study request and first image viewing.

While the institution or department communication backbone is typically high bandwidth, 100 Mb/s fast-ethernet or asynchronous transfer mode (ATM), other connections may be conventional 10 Mb/s ethernet. For example, the MR scanner generates images in a fairly continuous manner during the work day. Further, the output of those images is not an *on demand* service. Therefore, lower bandwidth 10 Mb/s ethernet is generally adequate for transferring images to the archive. Depending on the workload of the printer, this device may also be amenable to conventional ethernet transfer rates. However, if fast-ethernet is available it is probably wise to take advantage of the increased transfer speed for the operationally sensitive process.

Workstations, be they diagnostic or consultative, benefit from the additional bandwidth provided by fast-ethernet or ATM. Most Unix-based workstations and many Intel-based systems now offer fast-ethernet as an integated service. Certainly, the cost of fast-ethernet is now low enough to justify the incremental expense in the viewing workstations.

Printing

While soft-copy reading is hailed by many as the next revolution in medical imaging, the reality is that we will be printing MR images for several years to come. Printing in MR presents some unique challenges. First, it is not uncommon for an MR study to have 10 or more series, each with different tissue contrast requiring different window/level settings. This is complicated by the fact that unlike x-ray CT, the pixel intensity in the MR image has no absolute meaning. Therefore, preset window/level functions do not work as well. This all means that an extra burden is placed on the MR technologist to accurately adjust the window/level settings on each image to optimize and reproduce the desired contrast in the printed image. Strict quality control of printer, processor, and MR console display screens is required to make this process efficient and consistent.

Archiving

When specifying a PACS archive the impact of MR must be considered. Although the demands placed on the archive by MR usually pale relative to chest computed radiography and x-ray CT, it would be imprudent to plan a PACS installation without understanding the full scope of MR procedures that are currently performed, or perhaps more importantly, or are being considered. The very large data sets associated with volume MR, MRA, and advanced techniques like fMRI may place significant and unique demands on the image manager as well as the archive itself. In all cases Digital Imaging and Communications in Medicine (DICOM) compliance for MR image formats should be included in archive specifications.

Soft-copy Reading

It is likely that MR will move to soft-copy reading in the next few years. The contrast and resolution in MR is compatible with existing display hardware technology. The ever increasing number and different types of images acquired during an individual examination will make it increasingly difficult to manage the diagnostic workload using film as a display media. The ability to rapidly register and cine-loop large image series can be a significant enhancement to the visualization of volumetric, MRA, and post-processed data like fMRI. Figure 11 shows a neuroradiologist "cleaning" a board of filmed procedures with a cart of additional films to be read and the same radiologist reviewing films at a soft-copy reading workstation.

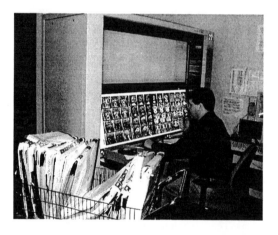

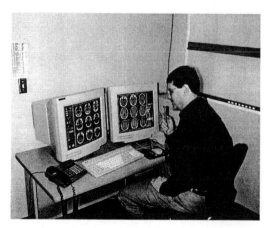

Figure 11. At top is a typical neuroradiology MR reading area with printed images loaded onto a multi-viewer and a cart of films to be read or compared against. At bottom is one potential solution for soft-copy read using only dual 1k × 1k color monitors. Note the smile on the radiologist's face when using the soft-copy workstation.

Off-line Processing

Many aspects of the MR clinic now rely on images that have been post-processed. This includes MIP for MR angiography, uptake kinetic analysis and parametric mapping for dynamic contrast enhanced studies, and cross-correlation analysis of functional neuroimaging studies. After processing you will typically want to print these on color printers, usually using opaque paper media, for documentation. It may also be desirable to store the processed images in the central archive. This will require that the post-processing workstation be capable of DICOM storage class functions. Many workstations today do support this capability, but the DICOM compliance statements of the workstation and archive vendors must be consistent in the types of image data they each support.

Transferring to Other Devices

With today's rapidly expanding image-guided surgery programs and products, there is an ever increasing demand for access to MR image data from outside diagnostic imaging. This can often be complicated by the fact that the surgical device vendors are not the MR scanner vendors, and so almost every connection must be nursed through the early stages of establishing DICOM compliance on both ends of the communication link.

Summary

While MR has not been considered a significant component of PACS to date, it is a modality that can easily be integrated into a filmless department, if appropriate considerations are made for the particular types of images in the MR study.

References

Bloch, R., W. W. Hansen, et al. "Nuclear induction." *Physical Review* 69: 127, 1946.

Cho, Z.-H., J. P. Jones, et al. *Magnetic Resonance Imaging. Foundations of Medical Imaging.* New York, NY, John Wiley & Sons, Inc.: 237-456, 1993.

Dumoulin, C. L., S. P. Souza, et al. "Phase-sensitvie flow imaging." *Magnetic Resonance Angiography: Concepts and Applications.* E. J. Potchen, E. M. Haacke, J. E. Siebert and A. Gottschalk (Eds.). St. Louis, MO, Mosby-Year Book, Inc., 1993.

Gatehouse, P. D., D. N. Firmin, et al. "Real time blood flow imaging by spiral scan phase velocity mapping." *Magn Reson Med* 31(5): 504-12, 1994.

Glover, G. H. and A. T. Lee "Motion artifacts in fMRI: comparison of 2DFT with PR and spiral scan methods." *Magn Reson Med* 33(5): 624-35, 1995.

Hardy, C. J., J. D. Pearlman, et al. "Rapid NMR cardiography with a half-echo M-mode method." *J Comput Assist Tomogr* 15(5): 868-74, 1991.

Hendrick, R. E. "Image contrast and noise." *Magnetic Resonance Imaging*. D. D. Stark and W. G. Bradley (Eds.). St. Louis, MO, C.V. Mosby, Co.: 66-83, 1988.

Herman, G. T. *Image Reconstruction From Projections*. Orlando, FL, Academic Press, Inc., 1980.

Jackson, E. F. "Magnetic resonance imaging: Physical principles to advanced applications." *Molecular Imaging in Oncology*. E. E. Kim and E. F. Jackson (Eds.). New York, Springer-Verlag: 17-46, 1999.

Keller, P. J. and D. Saloner. "Time-of-flight imaging." *Magnetic Resonance Angiography: Concepts and Applications*. E. J. Potchen, E. M. Haacke, J. E. Siebert and A. Gottschalk (Eds.). St. Louis, MO, Mosby-Year Book, Inc., 1993.

Lee, A. T., G. H. Glover, et al. "Discrimination of large venous vessels in time-course spiral blood- oxygen-level-dependent magnetic-resonance functional neuroimaging." *Magn Reson Med* 33(6): 745-54, 1995.

Liao, J. R., F. G. Sommer, et al. "Cine spiral imaging." *Magn Reson Med* 34(3): 490-3, 1995.

Marchal, G., H. Bosmans, et al. "Magnetopharmaceuticals as contrast agents." *Magnetic Resonance Angiography: Concepts and Applications*. E. J. Potchen, E. M. Haacke, J. E. Siebert and A. Gottschalk (Eds.). St. Louis, MO, Mosby-Year Book, Inc., 1993.

Parker, D. L. and E. M. Haacke "Signal-to-noise, contrast-to-noise, and resolution." *Magnetic Resonance Angiography: Concepts and Applications*. E. J. Potchen, E. M. Haacke, J. E. Siebert and A. Gottschalk (Eds.). St. Louis, MO, Mosby-Year Book, Inc., 1993.

Purcell, E. M., H. C. Torrey, et al. "Resonance absorption by nuclear magnetic moments in a solid." *Physical Review* 69: 37, 1946.

Ra, J. B., C. Y. Rim, et al. "Application of single-shot spiral scanning for volume localization." *Magn Reson Med* 17(2): 423-33, 1991.

Sachs, T. S., C. H. Meyer, et al. "Real-time motion detection in spiral MRI using navigators." *Magn Reson Med* 32(5): 639-45, 1994.

Siebert, J. E. and T. L. Rosenbaum "Image presentation and post-processing." *Magnetic Resonance Angiography: Concepts and Applications.* E. J. Potchen, E. M. Haacke, J. E. Siebert and A. Gottschalk (Eds.). St. Louis, MO, Mosby-Year Book, Inc., 1993.

Sprawls, P. "Spatial characteristics of the MR image." *Magnetic Resonance Imaging.* D. D. Stark and W. G. Bradley. (Eds.) St. Louis, MO, C.V. Mosby, Co.: 24-35, 1988.

Wehrli, F. W., D. Shaw, et al. *Biomedical Magnetic Resonance Imaging: Principles, Methodology, and Applications.* New York, NY, VCH Publishers, Inc., 1988.

Digital Angiography and Fluoroscopy: An Overview

Robert G. Gould, Sc.D.
Professor of Radiology and
Bioengineering
University of California
Department of Radiology
San Francisco, CA 94143

Introduction

Angiography is the predominate method for imaging vasculature and is used not only for imaging vessels in all body organs for disease detection but increasingly for interventional and therapeutic procedures. These procedures may involve changing blood flow (e.g., opening a vessel constricted by arteriosclerotic disease, correcting a vascular malformation, or placing coils in an aneurysm), or using the vessel as a conduit to a tumor for the purpose of drug delivery.

Angiography was significantly improved in the 1980's with the development of digital techniques for processing the video signal originating from the image intensifier/video camera system. Prior to this digital technique, angiography was done with film either 14" × 14" cut-film in film changes or cine film in 35 or 16 mm cameras. Current angiographic equipment is no longer designed to support film changes and cine cameras are rapidly being phased out.

This chapter will review the components of current angiographic systems including image intensifiers, video cameras, and digital signal processors. Image quality characteristics and patient dose and dose reduction techniques will be discussed. Challenges in integrating these systems into a Picture Archiving and Communication System (PACS) will be considered.

Angiographic System Components

Image Intensifier (II)

The principal difference between fluoroscopy and radiography is that fluoroscopy occurs at a greatly reduced x-ray fluence rate but over a much longer time. Fluoroscopy provides a continuous image allowing the observer to view dynamic changes within the patient such as organ motion or blood flow through a vessel. However, because of patient x-ray dose concerns, the fluence rate at the entrance to the detector as reflected by the x-ray tube current is several hundred times lower than the fluence rate used in radiography where an intense burst of radiation is used to record a static image. The consequence of the low x-ray fluence is that light levels from fluorescent detectors are very low and, if viewed directly, would limit acuity because of the performance of the human eye at low light levels.

The image intensifier was developed in the 1950's to electro-optically increase the available light level available for viewing during fluoroscopy. A cross-section of an II is shown in Figure 1. An II consists of an evacuated vessel containing an input phosphor and photoemissive layer, electron optics, and an output screen. The input phosphor absorbs x-rays and converts the absorbed energy into visible light. Since the late 1970's all image intensifiers have used CsI as the input phosphor material. A 300-600 μm layer of CsI is coated on a thin aluminum substrate but is formed in fine, needle-like crystals with the effect that emitted light is "channeled" through the phosphor layer with minimal spreading (Figure 2), greatly improving spatial resolution for a given layer thickness in comparison to settled phosphors. The thickness of the CsI layer affects the x-ray stopping power and thus patient dose. A 500 μm layer of CsI stops ~ 75% of 60 KeV photons.

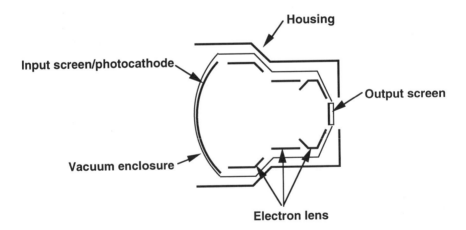

Figure 1. Cross-section of an image intensifier.

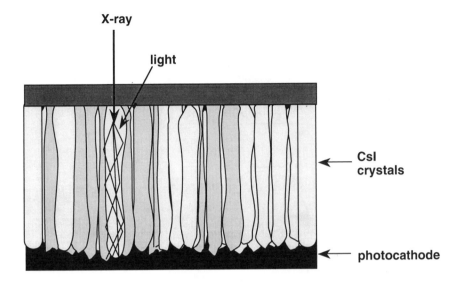

Figure 2. Cross-section through the input layer of an image intensifier showing how light is channeled perpendicular to the surface of the CsI layer. On the surface of the CSI, opposite the support substrate, a thin layer of antimony tri-sulfide (Sb_2S_3) is sputtered to form a photocathode. This material releases electrons in proportion to the light intensity emitted by the CsI. Thus, when x-rays strike the entrance surface of the image intensifier, a pattern of electrons is formed reflecting the x-ray intensity distribution.

The electrons are then accelerated along the axis of the image intensifier in coherent paths using a pentode electronic lens system. The electrons are focused onto an output phosphor screen and accelerated through a 25 KeV potential between the photocathode and the anode, located in the vicinity of the output screen. The settings of the electronic lens system can be changed so that input screen areas of different diameters are focused on the output screen which has a much smaller diameter than the input screen (Figure 3). These "magnification" modes cause a reduced patient area (the field-of-view, FOV) to be viewed but with improved spatial resolution.

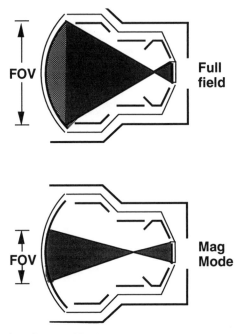

Figure 3. Illustration of a magnification mode of an image intensifier where a smaller area of the input phosphor is focused on the output phosphor, reducing the minification gain of the intensifier.

The output phosphor is usually P20, a zinc cadmium sulfide material. This phosphor converts the kinetic energy of the electrons back to visible light. Since electrons are easy to stop, this phosphor layer is very thin and made of small particles so that it has very high spatial resolution. Light emitted by the output screen is collected and focused onto the target surface of a video camera through a high quality lens system.

The brightness gain achieved by an image intensifier is due to two factors: a minification gain, resulting from the concentration of energy between the large input screen and the small output screen, and a flux gain, resulting from electron acceleration. The light per unit area given off by the input layer compared to that of the output area is proportional to the square of their diameters. Thus, for a 30 cm input area with a 2.5 cm output screen, the minification gain would be $(30/2.5)^2 = 144$. The flux gain is typically around 50 yielding a total brightness gain of ~7000. Because magnification modes alter the input area focused on the output screen, the brightness gain changes when magnification modes are used: smaller fields-of-view, although seen with better detail, have a reduced gain.

Image Intensifier Performance Characteristics: Spatial Resolution and Noise

As in any imaging system, spatial resolution and noise characteristics are determinates of image quality. In an image intensifier, spatial resolution depends primarily on the

characteristics of the input phosphor and on the diameter of the intensifier. The electronic lens system requires that the path length of the electrons between the
photocathode and output phosphor be nearly equal. While the small size of the output
screen allows it to be made flat, the large diameter of the input phosphor layer means
it must be curved (or the length of the II be unacceptably long) (Figure 1). This
curvature causes x-rays at the periphery of the FOV to strike the input phosphor at an
oblique angle, reducing spatial resolution at the edge of the image relative to the center.
The curvature also causes pincushion distortion in the image. Image intensifiers are
made with input diameters of up to 40 cm. These large diameter tubes are used in
clinical applications for imaging the belly and for leg run-offs, which are procedures
that image a bolus of iodinated contrast as it courses down the arteries of the legs.
Smaller diameter intensifiers (cm and often as small as 25 cm) are used for head and
cardiac angiography as both a smaller FOV and higher resolution are needed.

The thickness of the CsI input phosphor layer affects both the spatial resolution and
the detection efficiency and thus greatly affects the noise characteristics. CsI is an
excellent absorber of diagnostic x-rays having K edges at 36 KeV (Cs) and 33 KeV
(I) and a density of ~ 4 g/cm^3 can be achieved in the layer which is about 90% of the
bulk density of CsI. By comparison, for settled phosphor layers such as used in
intensifying screens in film imaging, the binder material reduces the layer density by
~ 50%. As discussed, the crystalline structure of CsI limits light spreading lateral to
the surface of the layer.

The electronic lens system and the output screen generally are not limiting components
in spatial resolution. However, image intensifiers are very sensitive to magnetic fields,
down to near the field strength of the earth (~0.5G), and should not be installed in locations where stray magnetic fields are present such as near some magnetic resonance
imaging (MRI) installations.

During fluoroscopy, image intensifiers are operated at low x-ray fluence rates and
photon noise is always present in the image. Typical exposure rates to the entrance surface of an II are 30-60 µR/s corresponding to ~10,000 photons mm^2/s (assuming 60
KeV x-rays). For 60 KeV photons, the absorption efficiency is 60-70% for a 400 µm
thick CsI layer. Thus, at the 30 µR/sec exposure rate, if a single video frame of the
fluoro image is digitized to 300 µm2 pixels (30 cm/1024), fewer than 20 x-ray photons
are used per pixel. The detective quantum efficiency is about 10% lower than
the absorption efficiency due to noise introduced by pulse height variations in the
scintillation process.

Contrast Ratio

The contrast ratio is a measure of the ability of an image intensifier to produce contrast
in the image of radio-opaque object, typically covering 10% of the input surface of
the image intensifier. Figure 4 illustrates how the contrast ratio is determined. In principle, the contrast ratio should be infinite since the object is completely absorbing of
x-rays. However, light scattering, primarily in the output window of the II, creates a

low level signal within the object. This light scattering is referred to as veiling glare and results in contrast ratios ranging from 20 to 30 for an object covering 10% of the II surface. The contrast ratio is significantly worse for small objects, such as an iodine-filled blood vessel.

A high contrast ratio is desired for intensifiers used in angiography. In effect, an angiographic run, wherein iodinated material is injected into the FOV while a rapid sequence of images is taken and a mask image subtracted from each image, reproduces the contrast ratio measurement. A low contrast ratio will result in poor contrast in the subtracted images of the vessels.

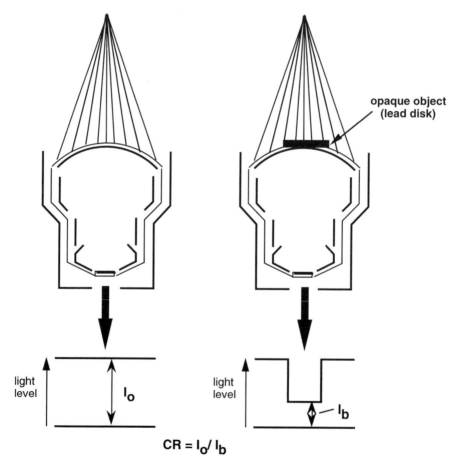

Figure 4. Illustration of the contrast ratio of an image intensifier. The contrast ratio decreases as the object size decreases.

Dynamic range

Image intensifiers have remarkable dynamic range and remain linear in their response over a 1000 fold increase in the instantaneous radiation exposure rate. While during fluoroscopy, the input exposure rate is around 30 μR/s, during angiographic runs where static images are being acquired, 1-2 μR are input to the intensifier in less than 10 msec. This exposure level is equivalent to that used for conventional screen-film imaging. Thus the image intensifier is not used as a dose sparing device but rather to achieve a high quality, high detail image. Consequently, the noise per pixel must be minimized so a significant dose level must be used. In addition, the response time of the intensifier must be fast: the CsI must have minimal afterglow. Dynamic range limitations in intensified images are the result of limitations in the video camera and not the intensifier. The aperture of the optical coupling (described below) is adjusted to a very small opening so that light levels to the video camera during angiographic runs do not cause camera saturation.

Optical Connection

The output screen of an image intensifier is optically coupled to a video pick-up tube. An infinite conjugate lens coupling is used between the output screen of the intensifier and the target of the video camera allowing an additional view port(s) as shown in Figure 5. However, most new angiographic and fluoroscopic systems are being sold with a single video camera as the output image capture device. The lens system is an important component of the imaging chain because it controls the amount of light emitted by the output of the II that reaches the camera. The speed of the imaging system can be changed by adjusting the aperture: as the aperture is opened, the speed increases, the radiation dose rate to the II and to the patient decreases, and the image noise due to photon statistical fluctuations increases. The aperture is set to assure that patient entrance exposure levels do not exceed state and federal regulations during fluoroscopy and adjusts to a small aperture when static images (e.g., those taken during an angiographic run) are acquired so that each image is obtained at a high dose without saturating the video camera.

Video Cameras

Two types of video camera systems are used in fluoroscopic systems: vidicons and charge coupled devices (CCDs). Vidicon systems in use may have one of several photoconductive targets including PbO (a plumbicon), CdZnTe (Newicon) antimony trisulfide ($Sb_2 S_3$), and SeAsTe (Saticon). The principle difference between these photoconductive materials is the amount of lag they exhibit, which affects the noise characteristics of the image and the ability to image rapidly moving objects. Lag describes the retention of signal in the photoconductor from frame-to-frame. Table 1 lists some vidicons and their characteristics. To some degree, in video tubes with low dark currents, lag can be adjusted by use of a bias light, which maintains a dark level current thus preventing lag induced by beam discharge.

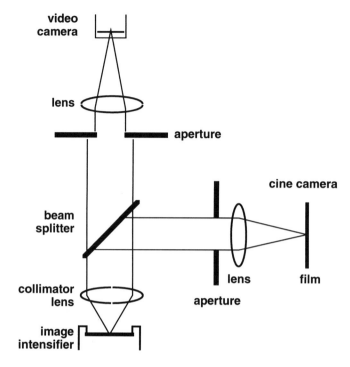

Figure 5. Optical coupling system between the output screen of an image intensifier and the video camera showing an auxiliary port. Rather than a cine camera, another video camera could be placed at this port optimized for angiographic applications as opposed to fluoroscopy.

The other type of video system used is a CCD. In a CCD, the target is pixellated into a large number of photosensitive regions. Signal readout occurs not by scanning the target with an electron beam as in a vidicon vacuum tube, but rather across the surface of the target using a series of registers into which the charge from each pixel is transferred at rates equaling the frame rate. CCD cameras have some advantages in comparison to vidicon vacuum tubes: they are smaller and more rugged; they are generally immune from local saturation effects bleeding into adjacent areas; they do not suffer "burns" from over exposure; and they do not degrade or "age" over time. However, a CCD has almost no lag and generally has a higher noise level than vidicons. Thus use of CCD camera in fluoroscopic systems usually requires some digital signal processing for noise reduction.

The video system also includes a camera control unit (CCU) for amplification of the video signal. The gain of this amplifier is adjusted so that regardless of the size of the pre-amplified signal from the pick-up, the full video signal range is used in the output video signal. This automatic gain control is important particularly when the image intensifier is being operated in magnification modes that limit the brightness gain of the image intensifier, lowering the light level from the output screen. The CCU also provides some γ correction and produces synchronization pulses in the video signal.

Table 1. Vacuum tube vidicons*

Type	Dark current (nA)	γ	Lag (fields)	Sensitivity (nA at 1 lux)	Burn resistance
Sb_2S_3	30	0.7	8	85-1	Low
Plumbicon	1	1	1	60-100	High
Saticon	1	1	2	80-120	High
Chalnicon	2	1	6	100-140	Medium
Newvicon	5	1	4	100-150	Medium

*After Rowlands, J.A. "Television Camera Design and Specification" in *Specification, Acceptance Testing and Quality Control of Diagnostic X-ray Equipment,* J.A. Seibert, G.T. Barnes, and R.G. Gould (Eds.), AAPM monograph No. 20, AIP Publications: Woodbury, NY 1994.

Video camera characteristics that affect fluoroscopic imaging include lag, noise characteristics and sensitivity, dynamic range, accuracy of the grayscale, spatial resolution, and spatial distortion and uniformity. The selection of a camera depends on its clinical application. Low lag tubes are used in most angiographic settings although some dedicated neuroangiographic rooms use tubes with moderate lag.

Although no such intensifier is available, IIs having an integrated video camera have been proposed. In this design, optical coupling to the camera would be eliminated and the output screen of the II would be the target surface of the video camera. This design would reduce or eliminate veiling glare and reduce the length of the II-video camera combination but lack the aperture for controlling light levels to the camera. However, a CCD camera might function well in this arrangement.

Video Raster

Since the video chains used in fluoroscopy are closed circuit systems, they take advantage of vast technological improvements that have occurred since the development of commercial television. Specifically, they are not constrained to a particular line or frame rate. For many years, fluoroscopic video systems have used high line rates, now commonly 1023 horizontal lines, and static images during angiographic runs have been obtained at 1024^2 resolution. Another difference from standard video is the use of progressive rather than interlaced readout by the pickup tube and often for display.

Non-interlaced readout has the advantage of eliminating field-to-field variations that occur when bright horizontal objects are imaged or when the radiation to the intensifier is pulsed (Figure 6). The later occurs not only during angiographic runs but also during pulsed fluoroscopy which is now available on most new angiographic rooms.

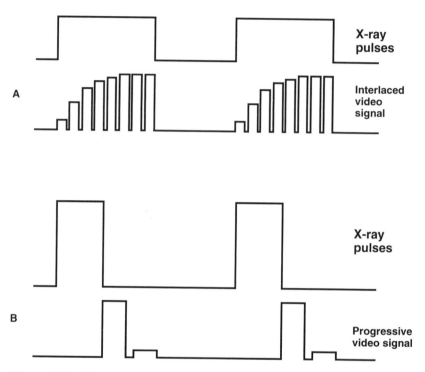

Figure 6. The effect of progressive versus interlaced video target readout on the output signal. The progressive readout would normally take twice as long as the time to readout a single field during interlaced readout (1/30 second). However, high line-rate readout systems may take more time. A "scrub" frame is also shown for the progressive readout system.

The disadvantage of specialized video systems is that they increase equipment costs. For example, should it be desired to record a fluoroscopic sequence, a standard VCR cannot be used unless the system has been purchased with a relatively expensive RS-170 standard video port (which would provide much poorer spatial resolution as well). Indeed, video recorders generally are not available for high line rate systems.

Digital Video Processors (DVPs)

Digital technology has altered the way angiography is done, allowing procedures of greater complexity and shortening procedure times compared to cut-film methods. To make use of this technology, the video signal is digitized, stored, processed, and output as an analog video signal, all at essentially video rates. Digitization in current equipment is 10 to 12 bits and can be at a 512^2 or 1024^2 matrix size although at least one commercial unit is capable of 2048 resolution (the unit is sold with a video camera).

Once in digital form, a number of processing algorithms can be applied rapidly by the DVP to the images, the principal one is subtraction of a mask image. If the mask image is acquired prior to iodinated contrast entering the FOV, subtraction will remove all structures but the iodine-filled vessels from images taken when contrast medium is present. To linearize the subtraction, the video images must first be logarithmically amplified either digitally or prior to digitization.

The above assumes that the only change that has occurred between the acquisition of the mask image and that of the opacified image is the inflow of the iodinated medium into the FOV. However, any slight amount of patient motion that occurs will result in the appearance of motion artifacts which can be very visible, particularly if a high contrast object, such as bone, has moved. Thus, a second important task of the DVP is to shift the mask and the contrast image relative to one another. Perhaps surprisingly given the possible complexity of patient motion, pixel shifting can be very effective even when done in only the x and y directions. More elaborate pixel shifting schemes have been implemented including rotation and image stretching but generally are no more effective than simple bi-directional shifting. However, the pixel shifting must be on a sub-pixel basis. Because these images are large, typically 1024^2 by 10+ bits, sub-pixel shifting is computationally intensive and, in order to perform this task quickly, most DVPs use custom processing boards for image processing rather than standard computer systems. The DVP is also used for image smoothing, sharpening, and image contrast enhancement, the latter being by means of a look-up table that maps pixel values to gray shades. DVPs contain standard digital storage devices such as hard disks or MODs for short-term image storage. Fairly recently, Digital Imaging in Communications in Medicine (DICOM) compliant image ports are available for sending images to PACS.

DVPs are sometimes used during fluoroscopy for the purpose of noise reduction, described below, and for "road-mapping" where a mask image containing iodinated contrast is continuously subtracted from the live fluoroscopic image. The "road-map" image then shows the moving catheter superimposed on the image of the vessels.

Image Acquisition Using Image Intensifiers

Fluoroscopy

As described, fluoroscopy is done at low x-ray exposure rates for the purpose of viewing dynamic events. Even at low exposure rates, the fluoroscopic dose to the patient can be substantial and methods to reduce patient and operator exposure are desirable.

If dose reduction is achieved by lowering the instantaneous exposure rate, image quality suffers. However, some improvement in image quality can be achieved by noise reduction using the digital processor. Specifically, weighted frame averaging methods can be effective where the most current image is weighted most heavily and the weighting of prior frames falls exponentially.

The problem with frame averaging is the same as with camera lag, i.e., motion becomes blurred. To avoid this problem, some DVPs compare, on a pixel-by-pixel basis, the pixel values in the current image to those in the incoming image. If the difference exceeds some set threshold, the difference is assumed to be caused by a change in the object and the new pixel value is substituted for the current value and output for the viewed image. If the difference is below the threshold, the difference is assumed to be noise and the new value is averaged with the current value. Significant dose reduction can also be achieved by using last image hold (LIH). This feature works well with frame averaging techniques and permits the fluoroscopist to stop fluoroing yet remain oriented to the image of the patient. The last image acquired is presented continuously on the monitor until fluoro is once again activated.

Pulsed fluoroscopy has been shown to reduce patient exposure by 30% to 50%. Rather than operate the x-ray tube continuously at a low current, the tube is pulsed at less than 30 frames per second, usually 15 but sometimes lower. The video camera must operate in a progressive scan mode with readout occurring between pulses. The video signal is sent to the DVP and output at the standard video rate of 30 images per second to avoid flicker. Thus, for a pulse rate of 15 per second, each image would be shown twice in display. This example would appear to halve the dose rate. However, because the eye integrates images with a time period of 0.2 seconds, only 3 pulses of radiation would form the discerned image, and noise in the image could be a problem. To overcome this noise, the exposure per pulse can be increased (by increasing the mA), reducing the dose savings but improving the image quality. As long as the mAs remain below the continuous mAs, patient (and operator) dose are reduced. Pulsed fluoro systems, are more expensive than non-pulsed systems in part because equipment is needed for switching the x-ray beam on and off. Grid-controlled x-ray tubes produce the sharpest pulses but are expensive.

Angiography

Angiography involves the imaging of blood vessels subsequent to the injection of iodinated contrast into those vessels using a catheter. Angiography has become highly specialized both in terms of the equipment and who performs the procedure. While all angiography involves some fluoroscopy, mainly to help in the guidance of catheters into the desired location, the images recorded are static ones, acquired with short exposures at radiographic dose levels (high x-ray tube currents). Many angiographic procedures involve multiple iodinated contrast injections (runs) with 10 to 20 images acquired per run in body or neuro angiography and over a hundred in cardiac procedures.

Cardiac angiography uses equipment with relatively small diameter intensifiers, often only 25 cm in diameter and low lag video cameras. Image acquisition rates of 30 images per second are needed and image subtraction is not normally used. Most cardiac facilities are single plane. Cardiac digital systems can acquire 1024^2 images (usually 8 bit) at 30 frames per second, which generates an enormous amount of data. Handling, manipulating and storing this digital data is difficult. The current trend is to create a CD ROM for each case. Images are viewed using PCs with CD players, replacing 35 mm projectors.

One advantage of digital images for cardiac imaging is that quantitative measurements are easily made, for example, ventricular volumes, ejection fractions, and degree of vessel constriction (% stenosis). Processing systems sold for cardiac imaging have a large package of image analysis software and measurement results can be stored with the digital images. Most cardiac angiographic systems are not on networks, certainly not hospital-wide networks, and are not DICOM compliant (although for sales purposes they may have a DICOM port). However, the tremendous volume of digital data complicates strict compliance. For example, lossy compression using wavelet technology (and therefore not DICOM consistent) for image storage would be of great benefit. The fact that cardiac systems are operated by cardiologists adds a political complication to incorporating these systems into system-wide PACS.

Neuroangiographic imaging is done with larger intensifiers (30-35 cm), fine focal spot x-ray tubes, and bi-plane systems. Image acquisition rates seldom exceed 4 to 5 images per second and are usually no more than 4 per second. High quality subtraction images are paramount. Body angiographic imaging is done with large IIs (35-40 cm) and only a single plane is needed. Acquisition rates are the same as for neuro imaging and both subtracted and non-subtracted images are obtained.

Typically, the digital systems for neuro and body angiographic systems are similar. Maximum image acquisition capabilities for 1024^2 images are usually no more than 7.5 per second and may be 15 or less 512^2 images. Within an angiographic run, the frame rate is usually varied, beginning fast and slowing to only 1 or 2 images per second at the end of the run. If image subtraction is to be done, it is important that the angiographic system maintain a consistent output and response throughout the run even with changes in the frame rate. Video cameras may have difficulty remaining consistent when the frame rate changes. Less frequently than in cardiac imaging, quantitative measurements are also made from neuro and body angiographic images. For example, aneurysm sizing can be an important measurement in neuro imaging.

A recent development in body and neuro angiography is the use of rotation of the gantry during a run. As iodinated contrast is injected into the FOV, the gantry supporting the x-ray tube and image intensifier is rotated as fast as 30° per second while imaging at a fixed and rapid rate, usually at least 7.5 images per second. The images are played back at 30 images per second (as a movie) with the result that the observer has a strong sense of the 3D aspects of the vasculature. If subtraction images are desired, a full rotational mask run is obtained prior to the injection run. The angiographic system will acquire images in the injection run at the same angular positions as in the mask run. This subtraction procedure is analogous to leg "run-offs" where the patient table is stepped and/or the gantry moved along the legs during image acquisition. Subtraction images are obtained by obtaining a separate mask run. In both cases, the patient dose is doubled by the mask run whereas, for a stationary sequence, mask images are obtained from only one or two exposures out of the sequence of more than ten images.

The volume of digital data in neuro and body imaging, while less than in cardiac procedures, is still large. For example, a neuro procedure consisting of 12 runs with 16 images of a 1024^2 matrix would produce 300 Mbytes of data.

PACS Issues

While most angiographic systems have a DICOM image port, very few have been incorporated into a PACS. The reasons for this are many, starting with the large volume of data angiographic procedures generate. As is the case when angiographic runs are filmed, one way to reduce the data volume would be to store only key images. That is, from the original image data, only a summary series of key and critical images would be transferred to the PACS. Some equipment manufacturers allow operators to create summary series, sometimes by transferring the data to a workstation where images are viewed and sorted to create the desired series. Images are then sent to the PACS from the workstation. Indeed, a workstation is often the DICOM port for angiographic systems: images are not obtained directly from the imaging equipment but pass through the workstation (which, of course, costs extra) into the PACS. Part of the reason the workstation route is often used is that most angiographic digital processors are highly specialized, serial processors and not standard computer systems. Thus, running standard software programs on these units is sometimes not possible. It should also be noted that it might not be possible to create summary series on all runs. For example, a rotational angiographic run needs to be viewed with all its images.

It should be possible to compress angiographic images, particularly subtraction images where much of the background is uniform, to a large degree without loss of diagnostic information. If, for example, a compression ratio of 20:1 can be achieved, a level shown to work for more complex CR images without compromising diagnostic content, the data volume becomes much more feasible; DICOM compliance would be lost however.

A second issue for PACS is how to handle subtraction images. Generally, PACS displays cannot do subtraction or can do so without the needed features of pixel shifting and rapid mask selection. A problem is created when unsubtracted images are stored locally on the angiographic systems and these "raw data" images, which are the acquired images, are those sent to PACS. Clearly, this problem goes away if the angiographic system can queue up and send the subtracted, pixel-shifted, processed images.

The PACS must also capture any quantitative data produced by the specialty software of an angiographic system. This problem is common to independent workstations that send images to a PACS and is usually handled by adding images to the procedure image file. In this case, the quantitative data could be burned into the images rather than exist as an overlay.

Finally, a Radiology Information System (RIS) interface to the imaging equipment, providing a worklist of scheduled patients and their demographic data, is desirable. Entry errors at the operator control and, in some cases, inadequate information entry, specifically the inability to enter an exam accession number, can cause problems in transferring images to PACS. However, since angiographic rooms are not high throughput rooms, lack of this RIS interface is less problematic than for other types of imaging equipment.

Conclusion

Angiographic equipment is evolving. It is becoming more specialized on both the hardware and software sides. In most institutions, digital angiography is used to the exclusion of cut-film in body and neuro imaging and most new angiographic equipment does not support film changers. Cardiac angiography is increasingly digital although the high cost of these digital systems is a deterrent. Cardiac systems, in part because they are operated by cardiologists and in part because of their huge digital data volume, are not now connected to PACS. On the other hand, neuro and body systems are being connected to PACS resulting in many challenges.

A promising future development for angiography is flat-panel detectors. Their small size compared to image intensifiers makes them attractive for interventional procedures. Their potential ability to operate near and in MR facilities may also open up a new area for imaging. But the image intensifier will be hard to displace. Its high image quality, its dynamic range as reflected in its ability to do both fluoro and static imaging, its relatively high detection efficiency, and its low cost in comparison to the current outlook for flat-panel systems assure the intensifiers place in radiology for years to come.

References

Rowlands, J.A. "Television Camera Design and Specification." In: *Specification, Acceptance Testing and Quality Control of Diagnostic X-ray Imaging Equipment.* Seibert, J.A., Barnes, G.T., Gould, R.G. (Eds.) AAPM Monograph No. 20, AIP, Woodbury, NY. 461-481; 1994.

Bibliography

Bushberg, J.T., Seibert, J.A., Leidholdt, E.M., Boone, J.M. *Fluoroscopy. The Essential Physics of Medical Imaging,* Baltimore, MD: Williams & Wilkins; 169-192; 1994.

de Groot, P.M. "Image Intensifier Design and Specifications." In: *Specification, Acceptance Testing and Quality Control of Diagnostic X-ray Imaging Equipment.* Seibert, J.A., Barnes, G.T., Gould, R.G. (Eds.) AAPM monograph No. 20, AIP, Woodbury, NY. 429-460; 1994.

Krestel, E. (Ed.) "X-ray Diagnostics." *Imaging Systems for Medical Diagnostics.* Munich: Siemens Aktiengesellschaft; 318-387; 1990.

Shepard, S.J. "Road Mapping, Last-Image Hold and Pulsed Fluoroscopy." In: *A Categorical Course in Physics: Technology Update and Quality Improvement of Diagnostic X-ray Imaging Equipment.* Gould, R.G., Boone, J.M. (Eds.) Oak Brook, IL: RSNA Publications. 111-118; 1996.

Suleiman, O.H., Spelic, D.C. "Technology Overview of Fluoroscopic Systems." In: *A Categorical Course in Physics: Technology Update and Quality Improvement of Diagnostic X-ray Imaging Equipment.* Gould, R.G., Boone, J.M. (Eds.) Oak Brook, IL: RSNA Publications

Film Digitizers and Laser Printers

J. Anthony Seibert, Ph.D.
Department of Radiology
University of California Davis Medical Center
Sacramento, California 95817

Introduction

In the migration to all-digital imaging and PACS in the radiology department, a bridge from analog screen-film systems is necessary. The film digitizer and the laser printer provide the transition from analog film to digital images, and digital images to analog film, respectively. Even in an all-digital department with "filmless" operation, the ability to get analog images from outside sources, and likewise, the ability to provide analog film images to outside entities without digital capabilities is essential. This overview covers the important operational characteristics and requirements of film digitizers and laser film printers in a digital imaging/PACS environment. Interface issues are reviewed. Finally, periodic quality control procedures, needs analysis, and Digital Imaging and Communications in Medicine (DICOM) version 3.0 standard conformance/compliance issues are discussed.

Film Digitizers

Film digitizers convert the continuous optical density (OD) variations on analog film into a digital image, based upon the discrete sampling and quantization of transmitted light from a scan of the film. There are several types of film digitizers. Drum scanner digitizers provided the first high resolution, high-quality digital images that could be used on digital computers. These digitizers required a significant amount of time and effort to acquire the digital data. Although still in use, they are not practical for clinical use. Camera-based digitizers, "camera-on-a-stick" models, were introduced in the early to mid 1980's to provide an easy and quick digital image of a film mounted on a lightbox. Manual focusing and aperture adjustments are required to ensure the proper signal levels to the analog vidicon or charge coupled device (CCD) cameras. Camera resolution (e.g., ~1000 or ~500 lines or pixels per side) relative to the scanned field of view is a limitation of these systems (particularly for large format films). Light scatter and glare significantly reduce the useful dynamic range of the camera, which is extremely limited compared to the range of light intensities commonly encountered in a radiographic film from 0.15 - 3.6 OD. This represents a transmitted light intensity variation of over 1000 to 1, which is often beyond the linear operating range of the typical camera photosensor and/or electronics. Because of these inadequacies and the small number of these systems in current clinical use, they are not covered in this review, and frankly should not be used. Details can be found elsewhere (Trueblood, 1993). What follows is a review of laser and CCD linear array film digitizers comprising the majority of systems now in clinical use. Operational characteristics, measures of image quality, and acceptance/quality control tests are discussed. Considerations of DICOM printer issues are included.

Laser Film Digitizers

The laser film digitizer comprises a laser source, mirror deflection components, focusing lenses, a transmission light collection chamber, photomultiplier tube, analog logarithmic amplifier, analog to digital converter (ADC), and film translation mechanics. These components are controlled with a computer and peripherals to capture the output digital image one line at a time. Timing of the laser beam deflection and translation speed of the film determines the specific spatial position of the laser spot on the film, encoded into the digital image matrix in the horizontal (laser scan) and vertical (film translation) directions. Figure 1 diagrams the basic components of a laser film digitizer.

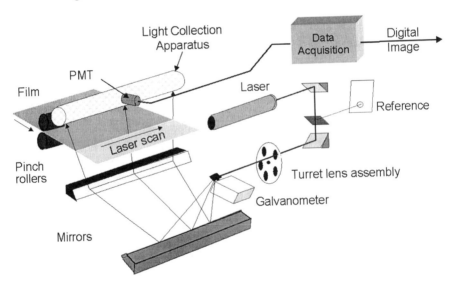

Figure 1. Diagram of a typical laser film digitizer. This is one representation of several laser film digitizer designs, all of which function in a similar way.

Laser sources include the HeNe gas laser of 633 nm wavelength or a solid-state diode laser of 670 to 690 nm. The path of the laser beam (which is focused by lenses not shown in the diagram) is directed by mirror optics and partially deflected to a reference detector, which compensates for intensity variations over time. In some sophisticated laser scanners that offer multiple spatial resolutions, a turret lens assembly further refines the focus of the laser beam according to the selected output resolution. Rapid sweeping of the laser beam is accomplished with either a galvanometer (oscillating planar mirror) or polygonal (multifaceted) mirror. The resultant moving beam is then deflected off stationary mirrors and projected perpendicular to the film. A light collection device captures the transmitted light through the film, the intensity of which is sensed by a photomultiplier tube (PMT) (or solid-state photodiodes) and converted to a proportional electronic signal. Non-linear amplification (typically a logarithmic conversion) is applied, followed by digitization (sampling and quantization) with an ADC. Finally, the digital values are stored in computer memory. In this geometry, a *diffuse* optical density measurement is made, similar to the measurements made with a densitometer.

CCD-based Film Digitizers

The CCD film digitizer comprises a collimated, diffuse light source, a lens to focus the transmitted light onto a linear CCD detector, signal collection electronics, ADC, and computer subsystem. Illumination of the film and the transmitted light intensity occurs continuously during the translation of the film through the optical coupling stage. Light incident on the CCD array produces a proportional number of electrons in discrete detector elements on the CCD, which are read out during the translation of the film. Signals are acquired, processed with a linear response, and converted to a digital image. The maximum optical density range that is achieved is limited by the noise of the CCD camera, as well as the few digital numbers allocated at high OD. Diffuse optical density is measured for this geometry, similar to the laser system mentioned previously. A typical schematic and inner workings of a CCD-based digitizer is shown in Figure 2.

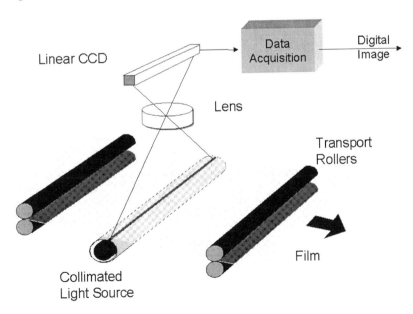

Figure 2. Schematic diagram of a CCD-film digitizer and major components are illustrated (Trueblood 1993).

Laser versus CCD Signal Processing

In the previous section, it was pointed out that laser and CCD digitizers have different attributes for signal acquisition and conversion to a digital image. Most laser systems use *analog* logarithmic amplification of the electronic signal voltage prior to digitization. CCD digitizers capture the transmitted light signal linearly, and digitize the linear signal. The signal responses to the optical density variations are illustrated in Figure 3.

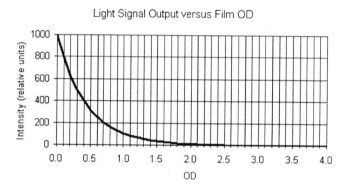

Figure 3. The response of a film digitizer (laser or CCD) in relative output intensity to optical density (OD) variations on film is shown.

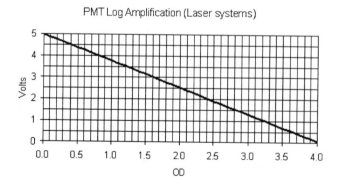

Figure 4. The response of a laser-based digitizer output after analog logarithmic amplification of the transmitted signal through the film.

Since OD = $\log_{10}$ (1/T), where T is the transmittance, then T=10^{-OD} and the logarithmic amplification linearizes the recorded optical density variations on the film as shown in Figure 4. Digital values are directly proportional to optical density across the full dynamic range of the system. In this situation, for a 12-bit digitization, each digital number is adjusted to provide 0.001 OD units, which gives an OD range of 0 to ~ 4.0. However, at high OD values the light intensity is weak, and the signal competes with the noise characteristics of the electronics, which limits the upper range to a typically useful value of ~3.6 OD. Film digitizers typically operate with a reversed look-up-table (LUT) (Figure 5) to mimic the response of film, with the noise greatest in the highest OD regions.

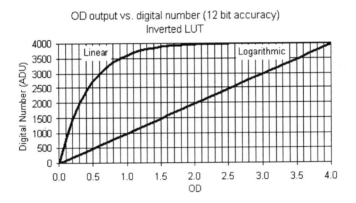

Figure 5. Optical density to digital number relationship for a linearly and a logarithmically digitized signal for a 12-bit ADC.

For the linearly acquired signal, the digitization produces a nonlinear distribution of digital numbers relative to optical density. While *digital* logarithmic amplification is possible, the number of digital numbers assigned to the high optical density range is very small. This results in very few values representing the variations in OD, particularly with a limited number of ADC bits to encode the signal. Table I lists the allocation of analog to digital units (ADU) for a 12-bit and 14-bit ADC. At high optical densities, a severely limited number of digital values are available to encode the variations. However, with extremely low noise linear CCD arrays and large bit depths (e.g., 16 bits, which encodes ~65,000 levels), higher maximum OD can be obtained. There are now several manufacturers producing CCD digitizers that claim a maximum of ~ 3.6 OD.

Table I. Distribution of digital numbers in the linearly acquired optical density range.

OD Range	Signal Range	# ADU, 12 bits	# ADU, 14 bits
0 to 1	100% - 10%	3700	15000
1 to 2	10% - 1%	370	1500
2 to 3	1% - 0.1%	37	150
3 to 4	0.1% - 0.01%	~4	~15

Measures of Film-digitizer Image Quality

Contrast Response

Contrast response refers to the ability of the digitizer to accurately render the optical density variations. This is the most likely aspect of film digitizers to vary over time. The accuracy is dependent on the calibration of the system and the optical density range of the film—as mentioned earlier, the response for some laser systems is linear with respect to optical density. In this situation, the calibration of 0.001 OD unit per digital number should provide a detection sensitivity of 0.02 OD at the mid-range density. A slope of 1.0 ± 5% should be obtained over the specified OD range for a calibrated film step wedge. Causes for failure include misadjustment of the laser or light source, PMT, photodiodes, or ADC from the electronic components. Dust on the mirrors, lenses, or light collection devices is a common problem, particularly with older vintage laser systems. Film scratches, artifacts, excessive glare, or light leaks also contribute to poor response.

Spatial Response

Spatial resolution of film digitizers depends upon the effective sampling pitch (space between samples) and the sampling aperture (the effective laser spot or the CCD pixel dimensions) in the horizontal and vertical directions on the film. The bandwidth of the electronics (sampling rate) also can affect the spatial resolution. Film transport speed is set to provide equal effective sampling pitch in the horizontal and vertical directions. Most systems have variable resolution—each setting should be evaluated quantitatively, with sinusoidal or square-wave resolution test patterns. Measuring the modulation as a function of the sinusoid frequency or determining the standard deviation within a region of interest (ROI) over the square-wave test pattern (Droege, 1983) can provide a reasonable estimate of the modulation transfer function (MTF) as a function of spatial frequency. The digitizer should provide resolution up to the Nyquist frequency, equal to $1/(2 \times$ sampling aperture) in both directions. For instance, a nominal 100 μm *effective* aperture will provide $1/(2 \times 0.1$ mm) = 5 lp/mm resolution.

Central and peripheral resolution should be similar. Evaluation on a digital monitor requires an understanding of the limitations imposed by the video display card and the cathode ray tube relative to the matrix size of the image being displayed.

Geometric Accuracy

Geometric accuracy is dependent on two components of the digitized image. The horizontal distance (x) is dependent on the beam sweep and optical accuracy, while the vertical (y) distance is dependent on line timing and film transport speed. Diagonally, the accuracy is a combination of the vertical and horizontal distances. Spatial linearity, stability, aspect ratio, and pixel calibration effect absolute distance accuracy in the digitized image. Absolute accuracy should be within ±5% and typically within (2% throughout the image. Geometric accuracy in the periphery of the image is often less than in the central area, particularly for laser digitizers.

Density Variability and Noise Uniformity

Variation in the density response of the digitizer occurs mainly in the horizontal direction. Some systems have a reproducible intensity fall-off from the center to the periphery due to the signal collection apparatus. Corrections are implemented by acquiring calibration scans in air and using the data in a "flat-field" procedure, which applies a correction map to make the response uniform and independent of horizontal position. Other sources of density non-uniformity include signal aliasing (high frequency signals beyond the Nyquist frequency that are folded into the low frequency spectrum, e.g., moiré patterns caused by grid lines), electrical interference/instability, and source-illumination variations during the scan. Transient responses such as these are not easy to correct. Noise signatures are also unique for given digitizer types. Stationary noise patterns can result from inadequate calibration and dust/debris on mirrors. Noise should be greatest at highest OD, and should be uniform for a specific OD level independent of x - y position.

Veiling Glare and Persistence

Veiling glare is a low frequency degradation affecting the dark areas in the digitized image. Stray light (lens flare) and/or dusty mirrors (light diffusion) cause glare. Both x and y directions in the output image are affected where light diffuses from the bright areas into the dark areas. *Persistence* is caused by inadequate recovery of the sensor or the electronics from overload conditions, and is presented as a trailing high signal region along the x direction. Both glare and persistence reduce the detector contrast and have greatest impact near large density transitions. These degradations are more apparent with image contrast and brightness adjustments of the digital image. Severe persistence and lag can mask underlying contrast variations in the image.

Specifications, Film Digitizer Systems

Digitizer System Performance and Siting

There are over 20 current manufacturers of film digitizers. Specific information on any particular digitizer, both laser-based and CCD-based, is often available on the Internet (see www.neoforma-ra.com for example and search for film digitizers). Film digitizers have various capabilities, costs, and siting requirements. Specifications should include spatial resolution, contrast dynamic range, and film-scanning rate, among others. Resolution can be categorized as fine (≤100 µm), medium (100 to 200 µm), and coarse (>200 µm) pixel pitch, with a corresponding effective sampling aperture. In general, laser-based film digitizers have a greater optical density range (~0.1 to 3.6 OD), better optical density accuracy, and higher signal-to-noise ratio compared to CCD-based film digitizers (~0.1 to 3.2 OD). This is in part due to logarithmic amplification of the analog signal before digitization, and the wider dynamic range of the electronic components in the signal acquisition chain of laser digitizers. However, recent technological enhancements have extended the dynamic range to up to 3.6 OD in CCD-based systems, making them competitive in this area. Some CCD digitizers can attain extremely fine resolution (down to ~20 microns in some digitizers) with excellent geometric accuracy. In addition, the CCD digitizers, in general, are less complex, require less maintenance, have less temperature sensitivity, and are less expensive to purchase and operate. All newer laser imagers, whether laser or CCD based, have enhanced stability and reduced preventive maintenance needs. Modular components make system repair less complicated for both CCD and laser digitizers.

Film scan speed is an important consideration for specific applications. Large format 35×43 cm (14" × 17") films can require from ~20 to ~70 seconds, depending on the type of digitizer and spatial resolution selected. An integrated film feeder that can automatically bulk-load several size films is optional on many digitizers. For remote outpatient or low-volume teleradiology needs, a single-feed, low scan-speed system is probably sufficient. For high throughput needs (e.g., in a film library) however, a higher throughput system with a bulk-load feeder device is preferable.

Size and space requirements for the digitizer and the associated computer workstation must be considered. Some systems are extremely heavy, and cannot easily be placed on a desktop. In addition, film digitizer environmental requirements and ambient lighting should not be ignored. For some digitizers, high illumination in the room area can increase signals and reduce quality of the digitized image.

Computer Interface and Software

The film digitizer is typically interfaced to a personal computer system for the acquisition, storage, and transfer of the digitized images. Software functionality should include control of the film digitizer parameters, selection of image resolution, film size, and look-up-table transformations. Typical software features include the ability to select sub-image areas and to process the images with spatial filtering and window/level controls. In addition, a TWAIN interface and selectable image formats for output such as TIFF, JPEG, BMP, etc., are features to be strongly considered.

A DICOM conformant computer workstation is part of the film digitizer system that allows image transmission to the PACS via an attached local area network or teleradiology application. Raw image data is acquired from the digitizer system via proprietary or standard image formats. The software specifies the interface parameters of the film digitizer, acquires the digital images, and appends patient demographic and examination data to generate *secondary capture* information object in DICOM 3.0 format. Information Object Descriptor (IOD) for the secondary capture DICOM object includes patient demographics, modality specific information, image look-up-tables, image size, image compression, and other details on DICOM specific attributes as described in these proceedings (Kennedy et al., 1999). Software should support input of patient demographic data, provide for whole or partial selection of the digitized image, allow selection of lossless or lossy image compression, and have image manipulation and processing capabilities for a full 12-bit image. At the minimum, the digitizer computer system must have *Service Class User* (SCU) functionality for image storage that can interoperate with the existing imaging PACS network hardware and software. Enhanced DICOM functionality should include *Service Class Provider (SCP) and Query/Retrieve* abstract classes to enable the workstation to function as a standalone image review system and PACS information terminal.

Acceptance Testing

Acceptance tests verify performance characteristics of the film digitizer, and set benchmark levels for periodic quality control. If possible, request any available quality control (QC) test films and software, and get a written report indicating the specifications of the unit, the tests performed, and the results. Implement a standard set of QC films to benchmark optimal performance for contrast response, spatial resolution, contrast uniformity and noise, and x-y distance accuracy/aspect ratio. The test films should include a calibrated density step wedge, a density/noise uniformity area, a high-resolution test chart for horizontal and vertical directions, and a method to assess distance accuracy. A film densitometer and a quantitative computer analysis package are essential items. Commercial or "home-grown" analysis films are acceptable, as long as they can stress the system sensitivity with subtle tests. In general, homegrown laser-generated films are typically produced with 8-bit grayscale, and have possibly variable uniformity accuracy. Commercial films are, for the most part, precision made and calibrated—much better than can be achieved with homegrown test patterns produced on an 8-bit laser camera. In addition, associated software for quantitative analysis is also available (of course at additional cost, but in many cases well worth it). Other acceptance tests include validation of the film feeder device, barcode reader, digital interfaces, vendor software specifications, DICOM conformance and compatibility for the Secondary Capture IOD, and interoperability with the PACS archive. Image workstation monitors and system configurations also fall under the acceptance testing and periodic QC guidelines for the film digitizer unit. Keep in mind that the monitor quality and calibration is a critical component, and must be included in the overall QC program.

Periodic Quality Control

Quality control frequency is based on the historical operational characteristics, the use of the system, and the variability in the response of the tests. In general, tests should be initially accomplished frequently, and after a break-in period, less frequently performed according to the results. There are several articles in the literature that review pertinent tests for film digitizers (Lim 1996, Esser et al. 1991, Meeder et al. 1995, Yin et al. 1992). Recommended quality control tests and their initial frequency are outlined below.

Daily
1. Digitize a calibrated density step wedge that spans an OD range of at least 0.1 to 3.0, and plot the accuracy and reproducibility in the form of a characteristic curve (signal response function). The system should be able to reproduce densities within 5% from day to day. Films can be commercially provided or homegrown. Manufacturers should be able to supply these films at a nominal cost. The Society of Motion Picture and Television Engineers (SMPTE) (Gray et al. 1985) or Halpern (Halpern 1995) patterns are examples of films that can be used to evaluate the density values and simple resolution.

2. Track the values graphically, and indicate the limits (±5%) to determine acceptable performance for the day.

3. Verify data acquisition and image transmission to PACS/Teleradiology systems (as part of the network). This includes assessment of the attributes of the secondary capture object in DICOM to ensure proper transmission of data to the archive, and to verify image recall from the archive with the image information intact and correct. QC of DICOM issues aspects is covered in these proceedings (Oskin, et al., 1999).

Weekly
1. Density uniformity and noise analysis is performed with a uniformly exposed film. The digital number average is obtained within a ~100×100 pixel region of interest in the center and peripheral quadrants of the digital image. This test determines the possibility of drifts of the digital response. Noise signatures can be evaluated as a function of optical density by evaluating the standard deviation within an ROI and plotting versus step number. Here, the noise should increase with optical

density. Anomalous noise patterns or trends indicate problems with the digitizer, requiring adjustment or repair.

2. System MTF is measured with evaluation of square wave test patterns (e.g., in the SMPTE or Halpern test films) and analyzing the modulation response as a function of spatial frequency. An alternative is to estimate the modulation as a function of spatial frequency by measuring the standard deviation within a ROI (Droege, 1983), which can be used as an indicator of modulation amplitude.

3. White to black and black to white transition accuracy can be obtained by plotting the image profile response in the rapidly changing areas on the film. Look for trailing signals that indicate improper electronic adjustments, particularly for white to black transitions, and inadequate response from a sharp black to white transition.

4. Characteristic curve analysis and gamma response function can be plotted from the evaluation of the density. The gamma function is calculated as the derivative of the characteristic curve, and can improve the sensitivity of discovering system drifts, component malfunction, and calibration settings.

Monthly/Quarterly
1. Horizontal and vertical distance accuracy and aspect ratio accuracy can be determined from the SMPTE or Halpern test films. Absolute distance should be within ±3%, and the aspect ratio within ±5%.

2. Adjustments of the digitizer should be accomplished according to manufacturer recommendations. This includes such tasks as PMT/Laser adjustments, and more importantly for older laser digitizer systems, mirror, and lens cleaning.

General Comments regarding QC

Many of the QC tests recommended above can be automated with commercial software available from several vendors with database reporting tools to track performance over time and to verify digitizer performance. Certainly, the frequency of any of these tests should be matched to the likelihood of finding anomalous results. Therefore, a logical approach is an initial high-test frequency to establish reproducibility. Then the testing frequency is adjusted to a rate that provides the desired sensitivity in picking up anomalous performance levels. When automated routines can be used to evaluate, log, and document digitizer performance, testing can and should be frequent.

Preventive Maintenance and Operational Issues

Routine maintenance for digitizer systems includes simple cleaning of the covers, and where accessible, cleaning of the film transport pinch-rollers. Often, labels from the films are stuck on the transport rollers or in the film path, causing subsequent film jams or other difficulties. For laser systems, mirror cleaning and equipment dusting are important to minimize artifacts and glare. Improved digitizer designs are less prone to dust by strategically placing mirrors in a configuration that minimizes settling. Periodic (e.g., quarterly) cleaning and electronic adjustments should be left to service personnel or advanced users who are more adept at understanding and maintaining the system and performance levels.

All digitizers degrade with time, including laser output and light bulb intensity (CCD systems). Automatic compensation circuits can maintain optimal performance with the use of feedback circuits, automatic gain control, and self-calibrating electronics throughout the lifetime of the component.

Operational issues of the digitizer include the following:

1. Obtain the latest operational software from the manufacturer; improvements can dramatically enhance system performance.

2. Install and operate the digitizer in a "clean" environment.

3. Maintain low ambient light and stable room temperature.

4. Allow 30 minutes of warm-up time to allow electronics, CCD detectors, laser amplifiers, etc., to become thermally stable prior to first use.

5. Preventive maintenance and periodic quality control tests are essential to ensure proper operation of the film digitizer.

Film Digitizer Summary

Film digitizers are available in different designs, and have varying levels of performance, siting requirements, and costs. Laser-based and CCD-based systems have relative advantages and disadvantages. The appropriate choice is highly dependent on the intended use of the equipment. One might consider a high throughput, quantitatively accurate, fast scan rate system for a film library transition to a digital archive, or a cost-effective, low maintenance, yet adequate digitizer for a remote teleradiology application. Interaction in a PACS environment requires an additional understanding of DICOM conformance and compatibility matters, which are covered by others within these proceedings.

Laser Film Printers

Over the past two decades, a significant growth of digital imaging modalities has occurred, spurred by the introduction of computed tomography and magnetic resonance imaging and the rapid growth of computed radiography imaging systems and ultrasound. This has led to a corresponding need to provide hard-copy images for viewing, diagnosis, and archiving of such images. Early on, this capability was provided by analog video-based multiformat cameras, which have subsequently been supplanted for the most part by laser camera imagers. This section covers the functional and operating characteristics of laser printers, including wet (external chemical) processing and dry (internal, self) processing systems.

Historically, the first laser printer was introduced in 1983 as part of the Fuji Computed Radiography system model 101 (Sonoda et al. 1983). A stand-alone laser imaging system was first introduced in 1984 by 3M, St. Paul, MN (now Imation, part of Eastman Kodak Corporation) (Anderson 1987). Since then, several models by various manufacturers of a wide range of capabilities have been introduced. Throughput, resolution, contrast range, printing speed, film formats, modality interfaces, DICOM conformance, and costs are among several aspects of the laser camera that must be considered for purchase, installation, use, periodic maintenance, and quality control. Technological advances continue, particularly in the area of dry process systems, based upon silver halide, carbon, ink, and tinted wax deposition methods. Extension of the DICOM standard to provide print service class implementations in 1997 has enhanced the flexibility of laser printers to provide hard-copy images over a PACS network. Until soft-copy readout becomes the norm, radiologists and referring physicians will continue to rely heavily on these printer technologies as an integral part of the radiological imaging chain and an indispensable part of a PACS. With current filmless operations, approximately 10-15% of images are still printed on film for various reasons (Young 1999). These include sending images to referring physicians without softcopy display, to the operating room, to orthopedics for image measurements, etc., as well as a variety of other reasons. It is anticipated that film or paper will continue to be necessary well into the future. Thus, considerations for network printing are extremely important.

Laser cameras comprise both hardware and software features that enable the reproducible and reliable printing of film. Characteristics of laser film (wet and dry processed), acceptance tests, quality control, and PACS interoperability requirements are reviewed.

Laser Imager Equipment Design

A laser imager "generic" design is illustrated in Figure 6. Most imagers resemble units designed for xerography and laser printers. Major components include the laser source, beam shaping optics, a laser modulator, a deflecting mirror assembly, shaping lenses, a cylindrical reflection mirror, a film bin of unexposed film, transport mechanics for the film, and an exposed film receptor. Film is mechanically transported through the optical stage, where the laser beam is deflected rapidly in the horizontal scan direction by reflection from a polygonal mirror. The laser power is instantaneously modulated by the digital image values in order to produce a corresponding optical density at the specific x-y position on the film. At the end of the sweep, the laser beam deflection is repeated from the next surface of the multi-faceted mirror assembly to write the next line on the film. Continuous transport of the film through the optical stage results in a raster scan writing pattern. Certain requirements for the beam size and the transport speed are necessary to ensure uniform response and spatial resolution, as explained later. After the film has passed through the system, it continues to the processor with either wet or dry methods to render the final image.

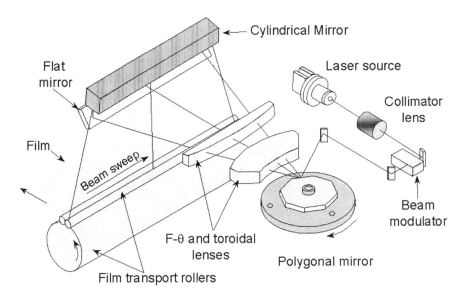

Figure 6. Basic components of a laser film digitizer are illustrated.

As environmental concerns and costs mount to maintain wet chemical processing, an increase in "dry" systems is likely to occur, particularly in light of the anticipated decrease in film usage as PACS and soft-copy reading becomes more prevalent. Dry processing is explained in further detail later in this review. For non-docked processor systems, film is stored in a light-tight cassette and subsequently taken to a darkroom for rapid processing.

Laser sources for film imagers include helium-neon (633 nm), solid state diode (~670 nm), and infrared (780 - 820 nm) wavelengths. The laser beam is shaped with specialized optics to maintain a specific beam profile, most typically Gaussian in shape with a diameter specified by the manufacturer. This is typically 75 to 85 µm but can range from 50 to 100 µm, depending on the application and characteristics of the laser system. Mirrors in the beam path reflect the beam through various lenses, and modulate the laser beam power according to the input digital number and corresponding optical density. Sweep of the beam across the film typically occurs with a polygonal reflecting mirror assembly with several facets (usually 8), where each facet prints a successive line on the film. Beam reflection is passed through an f-theta and toroidal lens assembly to ensure a consistent shape, intensity, and speed across the width. Cylindrical mirrors in the laser path also help to maintain a consistent beam diameter. Without these lenses, resolution would be inferior at the edges of the film.

Laser beam intensity modulation controls the optical density on the film. Accurate rendition of the optical density proportional to digital number is extremely important in the final image. Coarse modulation can result in grayscale contouring (uniform banding), which significantly decreases image quality. Gas lasers usually require an external modulator, whereas diode lasers can be directly modulated. External acousto-optical modulators use a mechanical vibration of an optical grating to vary the intensity of a constant-power laser beam. The laser power and modulation units can be balanced separately in this design. Direct modulation with solid-state diode lasers can be implemented by controlling either the laser output intensity or the exposure duration. Applied current to the diode laser controls the intensity output. Pulse width modulation or pulse count modulation is used to control the duration of exposure time for each pixel on the film. Pulse width methods vary the pixel printing time, while pulse count methods vary the number of pulses occurring for a fixed exposure time per pixel.

Laser beam power is configured to deliver the desired maximum optical density on film according to the type of film, processing conditions, beam filters, and mirrors/lenses in the beam path. In the externally acousto-optical modulated system, a reference detector/feedback loop system maintains a constant beam power, independent of temporal fluctuations. A different maximum density can be selected for a specific type of film dependent on the reference diode sensitivity setting. For the directly modulated system, the rotation of a polarized beam splitter determines the maximum laser-light intensity to the film. Feedback circuitry provides an excellent reproducibility in either case.

Resolution of Laser Imagers

Resolution and quality of the output image are determined by the pixel pitch, laser spot size, laser spot shape, and beam modulation characteristics. Pixel pitch is the center-to-center spacing of the pixel areas on the film. This determines the maximum theoretical resolution that can be attained (the cutoff frequency) in a discretely sampled system, equal to 1/(pixel pitch). The spatial frequencies that are *accurately* transmitted depend on the effective pixel aperture as determined by the effective laser-spot size and shape. In a system with the pixel pitch equal to the pixel aperture, the Nyquist frequency (maximum frequency that can be accurately rendered in the output image) is equal to $1/(2 \times$ effective pixel aperture). The pixel pitch is slightly different in the fast (laser sweep) and slow (film transport) directions.

Pixel pitch defines the number of images that can be recorded on the film. Pixel replication and interpolation produces magnified images, and sub-sampling or down sampling of the digital image data produces minified images. Laser spot size is controlled by the scanning optics and laser modulation methods, and is influenced by the pixel pitch. Because the final printed image is accomplished with raster scan methods, the raster visibility must be balanced with the output resolution. While a small laser-spot size will provide better resolution, it will also result in undesirable raster-line visibility. On the other hand, blurring out the raster lines reduces the spatial resolution capabilities of the camera. Incorrect balance of the size and shape of the spot can also result in image banding. Additionally, the moving laser beam in the fast scan direction blurs and makes the effective spot size somewhat larger than the actual spot size, which does not occur in the slow scan direction. Laser cameras that use pulse-width modulation have spot sizes that depend on the digital number (longer exposure is required for digital numbers that code for higher optical density).

Miscellaneous Equipment Considerations

Other considerations for laser imager hardware include the number and type of input channels, the amount of on-board random-access memory, and the size of the hard disk (if any). For a laser imager that requires connections to several imaging modalities, manufacturers offer computer systems (e.g., digital multi-formatters) that interface to the modalities through dedicated point-to-point channels. These external interfaces convert the image data from the modality into the formats that the specific laser printer requires. Each vendor implements a printer protocol that is often proprietary. DICOM conformant network print servers that interface directly to a laser printer port and have network printing capability are becoming available in greater numbers, and are obviously desirable in a PACS environment. Although the throughput is somewhat reduced compared to a point-to-point hardwired connection because of network bandwidth limitations, the flexibility and redundancy of the network printing capability are a reasonable tradeoff. As the number of printed films are reduced with the growth and experience of soft copy, this will become less of an issue.

Laser Imager Software

Software drives the hardware and provides features that control image quality and calibration settings. The number one setup issue for a laser camera is to ensure that the printed image matches the image(s) on the display workstation. Adjustment of the digital numbers representing the input image must occur, since display monitors have varying characteristic curves and contrast responses. Before the image is stored for printing, a LUT transformation curve must be applied to correct for these variations. In the case of a DICOM network printer, each of the workstations connected to the printer must have proper DICOM header information that will allow the printer to properly apply a given LUT to the data. The number of bits of grayscale information must also be considered. Most printers have an 8-bit range of grayscale values that encode the optical density. For images with 10, 12, 14 or 16 bits, a conversion to 8 bits must occur in addition to the adjustment for brightness/contrast variations. In general, the quality of the printed film using the network printing capability is less than the corresponding point-to-point connection to the printer. This is chiefly due to the lack of experience and tuning of the DICOM print management services standards implemented for these tasks. Advanced DICOM standards for (laser film) printing are being introduced over the next several years.

All laser cameras have internal calibration components that compensate for variations in the laser film sensitivity and processor conditions. Calibration films are printed by the laser beam subsystem at known power levels encoded by the minimum to the maximum digital numbers. The film OD values are linearized with a LUT procedure. An example is illustrated in Figure 7. On newer systems, a built-in densitometer accomplishes this automatically. Calibration establishes and maintains the desired optical density range. The amount of compensation to ensure the proper operating range should be tracked during periodic quality control. Catastrophic failures can occur when the laser adjustment can no longer compensate for other, more serious problems, such as processor chemistry contamination, temperature problems, and/or low chemistry activity. Whenever the laser camera or film processor is serviced, it is important to recalibrate the laser camera. Fortunately for newer systems, this is a straightforward and simple procedure.

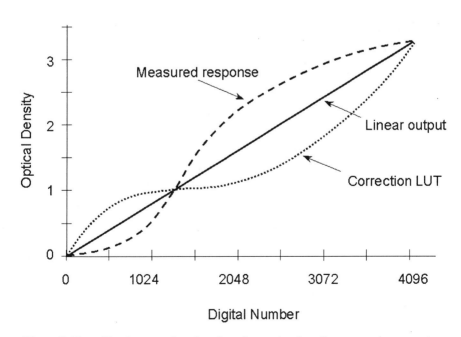

Figure 7. The calibration procedure for a laser imager involves the measured response to a known input laser power determined by the input digital number (long-dashed line), determination of an inverse correction (short-dashed line) and the output linear response (solid line). Adapted from Bogucki (Bogucki, 1996).

Laser Films

Conventional (Wet Processing) Laser Films

In conventional laser imagers, the film image is recorded when the laser beam deposits energy on the silver halide emulsion coating. This releases electrons, which reduce silver ions in the crystalline matrix into silver atoms and form latent image centers. Subsequent development of the film amplifies the remaining silver atoms at each latent image center, resulting in the deposition of metallic silver. Fixing stops film development and removes the excess undeveloped silver halide emulsion. The result is a pattern of optical density variations on the film substrate that correspond to the digital image. Film designed for laser cameras have a single-emulsion coating and have sensitivities matched to the wavelength (energy) of the laser beam obtained by adding organic dyes to the emulsion. The unexposed film is sensitive to either red or infrared wavelengths, and cannot be used in darkrooms designed for diagnostic film. Additionally, laser imagers require a specific type of laser film; for instance, infrared diode lasers will not properly expose films designed for red-wavelength HeNe gas lasers.

Dry (Self-processing) Laser Films

"Dry" imagers use film media that do not require external processing. Several methods exist to produce a "dry" processed image, including thermal transfer, sublimation transfer, and direct thermal recording. For medical imaging applications in which a transparent film is produced from the digital data and grayscale encoded, thermal processing is used most. There are several different mechanisms for thermal processing, including the use of silver-based emulsions that are heat sensitive, the use of heat permeable dye microcapsules, and carbon based "adherographic" printing technologies.

Silver Emulsion Thermal Processing

The photo-thermographic process is based on thermally activated silver-halide based compounds, which enables the amplification and processing of a latent image with the local deposition of heat. This "dry" silver halide technology was first introduced to the medical imaging field by 3M-Imation in 1995, based upon a silver behenate developer (Morgan, 1991). When exposed to heat (either by laser energy deposition or heat transfer from a thermal head), silver behenate diffuses *only at latent image centers* in the silver halide layer, and releases silver to form visible silver grains. Where there are no latent image centers created during the film exposure, the compound remains unchanged and does not release silver. In this instance, light transparency is maintained. Characteristics of the processed film are sensitometrically similar to wet-processed films, and have an optical density range from about 0.2 to 3.2 OD.

Since all of the chemicals remain in the "developed" film, a potential for unprocessed chemicals continuing the development process is a concern. A term called "print-up" has been coined that describes the continued darkening of films subjected to high heat conditions. In this situation, the higher optical densities fade and the lower optical densities increase. Technological improvements in the chemistry of the materials have solved the majority of these early problems, and image stability even in high heat conditions is not of as much concern. However, storage conditions of unexposed films are more severe in terms of tolerable humidity and temperature. Shelf life is also much shorter than conventional wet-processed silver-halide films.

Microcapsule Dye Technology

Another method of producing a grayscale image is based on heat permeable microcapsules that allow surrounding developer agents to enter and react with the dye to produce a color center (Hosoi, 1998). A thermal head composed of a linear array of discretely controlled thermal elements is used to modulate and deliver the heat to the film over very small areas (~85 μm or ~300 dots per inch). When the film passes over the heat elements, the microcapsules containing up to six different color precursor dyes become permeable to the developer, and form a black color with an opacity characteristic of silver grains. As cooling occurs, the capsules become impermeable, and the reaction is stopped. Smooth gradation performance that mimics the characteristic curve of silver-halide films is enhanced by the presence of microcapsules with two different color-forming temperatures, so that fine-tuning can occur with temperature control. Similar to the silver-based dry film processing, high storage temperatures of the processed films can increase image density changes with time.

Adherographic Processing

An alternative dry processing method is based upon the selective adhesion of carbon particles in an intricate binary writing process onto a transparent or reflective plastic base with a subsequent protective sealer added. This dry laser technology was introduced by Polaroid Medical Imaging Systems (now Sterling Diagnostic Imaging) in 1993 (Cargill 1994). The film comprises an imaging layer containing carbon in a polymeric matrix and a laser-sensitive layer sandwiched between the film base and polyester base. A gallium-arsenide laser is focused at the interface of the two layers, which causes adhesion at the interface. The two layers are separated, producing an image and its negative from the selective transfer of the carbon particles. Lamination of the polyester base with a cover sheet protects the final film image.

Image creation is a binary process—the carbon is transferred to the image base through the application of laser energy that just exceeds a threshold to cause adhesion. In order to achieve continuous tone-scale images, each pixel is subdivided into many "pels," typically with a dimension of 5 μm on a side. Pixel optical density is determined by the number and pattern of pels that are activated within the pixel, which can range from 0.01 to 3.2 OD. (Cargill 1994). Dithering patterns are used to achieve a gradation tonescale that mimics the characteristic curve response of film. In addition, with nonoverlapping pels and pixels, the intrinsic resolution is extremely high and MTF curves closely mimic a sinc function (e.g., nearly ideal response). Artifacts such as banding can occur when pels are mispositioned or the image is shifted during the layer separation process (Bogucki 1996).

Summary—Dry Laser Film Technology

Printing technologies are continuously changing—innovative methods (hardware and software) to produce diagnostic quality films in an inexpensive and environmentally responsible way are being constantly offered. One thing is certain—the wet processing methods will give way to dry processing, particularly as the throughput of dry lasers and the stability of the output images matches that of conventional laser imager systems.

Acceptance Testing and Quality Control for the Laser Imager

Acceptance testing verifies adherence to the purchase agreement, delivery of all equipment, proper installation, and determination of baseline performance levels for the laser imager. Baseline values include measurements of contrast response, spatial resolution, low-contrast sensitivity, and line structure. Published specifications and specifications agreed upon in the purchase contract should be verified, such as film throughput rate and density adjustment capabilities. Film processor and modality to printer interfaces should also be tested. The latter verifies the implementation of proper LUT curves to match the "properly calibrated" CRT image display as close as possible to the printed film on a lightbox. This is the most critical aspect of the laser printer—modality interface. It is also extremely important to have the laser imaging system correctly calibrated for the laser source, laser film, and film processor. Subsequent calibrations and system performance indices use the initial calibration step tablet for baseline values. (See the section on software issues and Figure 7.)

Quality control is performed to ensure that the laser (film) imager is operating at peak performance levels. The imager should be checked once daily, with an internally generated sensitometry strip and densitometric evaluation of the results. Reproducibility of the steps should be within (5% of previous values. Densitometric results should be used to recalibrate the imager when close to or out of tolerance. For laser systems with wet processing, the most temperature sensitive films should be used to measure the reproducibility and stability of the laser system. The speed point (the film's most temperature sensitive point) best analyzes processor performance, and an upper density point (~3.0 OD) best measures the stability of the laser subsystem (Bogucki 1996). Correct monitor adjustment for brightness and contrast settings is also very important, so that digital window/level adjustments are correctly portrayed and printed on the output film. Laser printers typically have an 8- or 10-bit digital-to-analog converter. Proper printing is extremely dependent on the correct implementation of LUT conversions. This *must be* adjusted correctly at acceptance, and verified with continuous quality control checks.

More complete testing is recommended by the International Electrotechnical Commission (IEC) for laser imagers, which includes grayscale pattern analysis, image geometry, spatial resolution, contrast sensitivity, and line structure (International Electrotechnical Commission 1994). The SMPTE test pattern (Figure 8) meets the criteria specified by the IEC, and has been previously recommended for the acceptance and quality control tests for video multiformat cameras (Gray et al. 1985, 1993).

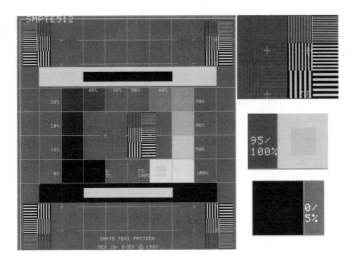

Figure 8. The Society of Motion Picture and Television Engineers (SMPTE) test pattern. On the left is the test pattern, and on the right are magnified sub-images of the high-contrast resolution chart and the low-contrast patches at 95-100% and 0-5% of the digital driving levels.

Densitometric analysis of the individual steps corresponding to digital driving levels from 0 to 100% in steps of 10% allows gray-level reproducibility analysis. Limiting spatial resolution at 100% and lower contrast levels (bar patterns found at the corners of the test image) are qualitatively verified by visual inspection. The matrix size of the SMPTE pattern should be equal to the largest matrix size that is clinically printed. Geometrical and aspect ratio accuracy can be measured directly on the printed film from the lines delineating the contrast steps. Contrast sensitivity at the lowest (0-5%) and highest (95-100%) digital driving levels can be densitometrically measured for reproducibility. Optical density measurements at the transition from white to black and black to white edges can show lag effects, which reduce and increase the optical density levels from ideal values.

Also extremely important for laser imagers is the evaluation and verification of correct line spacing as well as uniformity in the output image, which can be accomplished by printing a uniform image of OD $\cong 1$. Uniformity of the image response and the lack of visible raster lines demonstrate proper performance. Variations in the film transport speed, mechanical vibrations of the camera, focusing problems with the laser optics, laser power fluctuations, and problems with the laser deflection mirror can lead to banding and/or uniformity problems. These subtle degradations are often masked by clinical or test patterns, and can degrade printed film quality significantly.

DICOM Conformance for Laser Printers

DICOM Print Management Service Class (PMS) has rapidly evolved over the past several years to encompass the needs of a PACS to provide print services. In 1997, basic print services were implemented as part of the DICOM 3 standard for print management. In this standard, diagnostic quality printing to hardcopy printers on film or paper via the network is supported for grayscale (black and white) and color images, among other attributes. Sample DICOM conformance statements are available on the Internet (Agfa 1999). Network print servers from various manufacturers have been designed to achieve this capability.

Historically, laser printers have been operable in a point-to-point direct connection with the modalities, sharing ports, and modality-specific print formats. In these situations, the modality must be able to implement the proprietary vendor printing protocol to print. In this situation, siting flexibility is minimal and alternatives for laser printer downtime are nonexistent. With DICOM network printing, flexibility of siting laser printers, easy sharing by many imaging modalities, redundancy, and off-site printing are all possible in a properly configured PACS environment. Printing is invoked by a Service Class User (SCU) Application Entity (AE), which means that the imaging modality has chosen to print a study to a specific printer with a given AE title as a target. The SCU (imaging modality) makes use of the Service-Object Pair (SOP) classes defined for print management for the Service Class Provider (SCP), which is the printer server connected to the printer. In other words, the modality defines a film session that sends instructions to format the printer and print the film. Returned from this interaction is the status of the printer (e.g., printed, out of film, jam, etc.) Of course, the requisite modality to printer configuration (SOP Class) is necessary, which requires DICOM compatibility between the user and the provider. DICOM conformance statements specify the compliance of the Print Management Service Class with the DICOM standard, but do not necessarily guarantee interoperability, particularly when integrating medical equipment from one manufacturer with other equipment supporting the DICOM protocol. **Additional validation tests are essential to ensure accurate data exchange between the service class user (the modality), and the service class provider (the printer server and printer).** More details regarding the DICOM standard and implementation are covered in another presentation (Kennedy et al. 1999, Oskin et al. 1999). A simplified block diagram in Figure 9 illustrates the relationship between the SCU and SCP for print management. A typical PACS configuration for DICOM print services is illustrated in Figure 10. Several options exist for printing as shown in the figure. Direct, converter box, and third party solutions exist from the modality to DICOM to the printer.

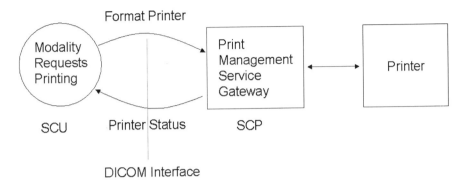

Figure 9. A block diagram of modality-printer Service-Object Pair DICOM print session is shown. The modality (SCU) requests print services from the PMS Gateway (SCP), which determines the requested formatting, and interfaces to the printer via proprietary formats. Returning from the SCP to the modality is the printer status.

So, what *is* needed for network printing via DICOM? A laser printer must have an interface to a print manager workstation for image formatting, and must have the minimal capability of providing 8-bit (256 grayscale) image rendition. The Print Management Service Class workstation should be DICOM conformant *and* compatible for the SOP class Unique IDentifiers (UIDs) that explicitly define the association between the modality and the printer. DICOM compatible software on the modality (SCU) for print services must also be available. In addition, AE titles for the specific printers to be targeted by the modality are necessary. There is a lot of information "under the hood" in the conformance statement for Print Management Services, as well as other DICOM issues. It is highly recommended that the physicist seek assistance from Information Services individuals and the PACS manager for assistance in dealing with and understanding these issues. Details of printer configuration, modality, resolution, film size, image size, polarity, rotation, input/output look-up-tables, minimum density, maximum density, and many other descriptors are beyond the scope of this work. For the medical physicist involved in quality assurance of PACS and printing capabilities, these underlying details are usually not necessary to explicitly know. Further information on the DICOM standard is posted on the web at www.nema.org/nema/medical/dicom/html/intro.html.

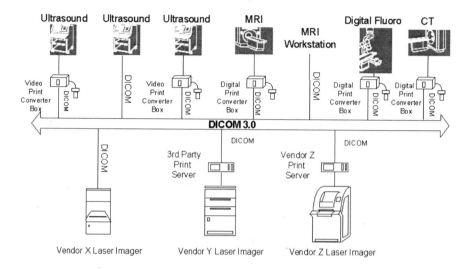

Figure 10. A typical PACS and network printing architecture. Shown are various modality–DICOM interfaces, and DICOM-laser imager interfaces. Adapted from presentations at the Society of Photooptical Instrumentation Engineers '99 PACS Workshop, San Diego. (Simon, 1999).

New DICOM Directions for Print Management

DICOM Print Store, added to the standard in 1998, allows the printer SCP to archive the profile and reprinting of film copies. This capability includes new DICOM objects "Stored Print Storage" (the print profile), "Hardcopy Grayscale or Color Image Storage," and "Preformatted Secondary Capture Image." Additionally, query/retrieve services are implemented to interface to the archive for the use of these objects. In late 1999, the "Presentation Look-Up-Table (LUT)" and "Print Configuration and Basic Overlay" objects should be added. The former object specifies a LUT that maps the image pixel values into a specified range of luminance values according to DICOM supplement 28: Grayscale Standard Display Function (DICOM 1998). This optimizes the "Just Noticeable Differences" based upon the human visual model, and enhances the visual consistency between various laser imagers. Implementation occurs in conjunction with the Basic Print object. The latter capability uses printer characteristics obtained from the network (e.g., grayscale, color, film-format size, portrait or landscape configuration, and display information) to optimize the output image. Simple overlays are also added to the Basic Print functionality, extremely useful for foreign character sets, which are otherwise very difficult and unwieldy to implement.

Summary

Film digitizers and laser printers are increasing in importance and presence in the diagnostic radiology department as the progression to an all-digital, soft-copy based PACS environment occurs. Consequently, the medical physicist must be at the forefront of basic knowledge of film digitizers and laser imagers, their functional attributes, and their integration into a PACS. The underlying details of DICOM are beyond the "practical" knowledge base of the medical physicist and certainly require input from PACS-savvy individuals from the institution as well as from the vendors. So, it is very important for the medical physicist to take an active role in understanding *basic* PACS concepts and terminology. This will enable the melding of the basic physics expertise with the clinical requirements and practical aspects of ensuring optimal equipment performance and patient care in the "New World" of PACS.

References

Agfa Medical Imaging, DICOM Conformance Statement, Print Management Service Class, available from the internet at http://medical.agfa.com/dicom/cs.html, 1999.

Anderson, W.F. "A laser multiformat imager for medical applications." *Proc SPIE* 767:516-523, 1987.

Bogucki, T.M. "Laser Cameras," In *Syllabus: A Categorical Course in Physics—Technology Update and Quality Improvement of Diagnostic X-ray Imaging Equipment,* Gould, R.G., and Boone, J.M., (Eds) RSNA publications, Oak Brook, IL, pp.195-201, 1996.

Cargill, E.B., Habbal, F. "Characteristics of the new Helios imaging platform." Polariod Medical Imaging Systems, Newton, MA, 1994.

DICOM Supplement 28: Grayscale Standard Display Function. Rosslyn, VA. The National Electrical Manufacturers Association, 1998. This document is available from ftp://ftp.nema.org/medical/dicom/Final, filename: sup28_ft.pdf.

DICOM Standards Committee current documentation can be accessed via the World Wide Web at "www.nema.org/nema/medical/dicom", all documents current as of 1999.

Droege, R.T. "Method to monitor resolution in digital images." *Medical Physics* 10: 337-343, 1983.

Esser, P.D., Halpern, E.J., Amis, E.S. Jr. "Quality assurance of picture archiving communications systems with laser film digitizers." *J Digital Imaging* 4: 241-247, 1991.

Hosoi, N., Yoneda, J. Fuji Computed Radiography, Technical Review No. 7. Development of Fuji Medical Dry Film DI-AT. Fuji Photo Film Co. Ltd, Tokyo, Japan, 1998.

Gray, J.E, Anderson, W.F., Shaw, C.C., Shepard, S.J., Zeremba, L.A., Lin, P.J.P. "Multiformat video and laser cameras: history, design considerations, acceptance testing, and quality control." Report of AAPM Diagnostic X-Ray Imaging Committee Task Group Number 1. Med Phys 20, 427-438, 1993.

Gray, J.E., Lisk, K.G., Haddick, D.H., Harshbarger, J.H., Oosterhof, A., Schwenker, R. "Test pattern for video displays and hard-copy cameras." *Radiology* 154: 519-527, 1985.

Halpern, E.J. "A test pattern for quality control of laser scanner and charge-coupled device film digitizers." *J Digital Imaging* 8: 3-9, 1995.

International Electrotechnical Commission. "Evaluation and routine testing in medical imaging departments: constancy tests-hard copy cameras." International Standard, Geneva Switzerland: Bureau Central de la Commission Electrotechnique International, 1994.

Kennedy, R.L., Oskin, M.H., Seibert, J.A., Hecht, S.T. "Introduction to DICOM." In *Practical Digital Imaging and PACS,* 1999 AAPM Summer School Proceedings (this monograph), Seibert, J.A., Filipow, L., Andriole, K.P., 1999.

Lim, A.J. "Image Quality in Film Digitizers: Testing and Quality Assurance," In *Syllabus: A Categorical Course in Physics—Technology Update and Quality Improvement of Diagnostic X-ray Imaging Equipment,* RSNA, Gould, R.G. and Boone, J.M. (Eds.) publications, Oak Brook, IL, 1996. pp.183-193.

Meeder, R.J.J., Jaffray, D.A., Munro, P. "Tests for evaluating laser film digitizers." *Med Phys* 22:635-642, 1995.

Morgan, D.A. "Dry silver photographic materials." In: *Handbook of Imaging Materials.* Diamond, A.S., (Eds.) New York, N.Y., Marcel Dekker, 1991.

Oskin, M.H., Seibert, J.A., Kennedy, R.L. "Diagnostics and Acceptance Testing for DICOM Networks: Experience at the University of California Davis Medical Center." In *Practical Digital Imaging and PACS,* Seibert, J.A., Filipow, L., Andriole, K.P., 1999. AAPM Summer School Proceedings (this monograph), 1999.

Sonoda, M., Takano, M., Miyahara, J., Kato, H. "Computed radiography utilizing scanning laser stimulated luminescence." *Radiology* 148: 833-838, 1983.

Simon, D.A. "DICOM Print Management." Presentation at the Society of Instrumentation Engineers (SPIE) '99 DICOM Workshop, San Diego, CA. February 23, 1999.

Trueblood, J. "Radiographic Film Digitization" In *Digital Imaging*, Hendee, W., Trueblood, J., (Eds.) AAPM Summer School, AAPM Monograph #22, pp. 99-122., 1993.

Yin, F.F., Giger, M.L., Doi, K., Yoshimura, H., Xu, X.W., Nishikawa, R.M. "Evaluation of imaging properties of a laser film digitizer." *Phys Med Biol* 37: 273-280, 1992.

Young, J. Presentation at the Medical University of South Carolina PACS conference, Charleston, SC, March, 1999.

Computed Radiography Overview

Katherine P. Andriole, Ph.D.
Assistant Professor, Department of Radiology
University of California at San Francisco
and Department of Bioengineering
University of California at Berkeley
530 Parnassus Avenue CL158 Box 0628
San Francisco, CA 94143-0628
Kathy.Andriole@Radiology.ucsf.edu
(415) 476-3924 FAX (415) 502-3217

Introduction

Computed Radiography (CR) refers to projection X-ray imaging using photostimulable or storage phosphors. In this modality, X-rays incident upon a photostimulable phosphor-based image sensor or imaging plate produce a latent image that is stored in the imaging plate until stimulated to luminesce by laser light. This released light energy can be captured and converted to a digital electronic signal for transmission of images to display and archival devices. Unlike conventional screen-film radiography in which the film functions as the imaging sensor, or recording medium, as well as the display and storage media, CR eliminates film from the image recording step, resulting in a separation of image capture from image display and image storage. This separation of functions potentiates optimization of each of these steps individually. In addition, CR can capitalize on features common to all digital images; namely, electronic transmission, manipulation, display, and storage of radiographs. Other terms synonymous with storage phosphor-based CR include photostimulable phosphor radiography, digital luminescence radiography, storage phosphor radiography, and radioluminography (Bogucki 1995).

Recent technological advances in CR have begun to make this modality more prevalent in the clinical arena, at large and small institutions, community hospitals, private practices, etc. Hardware and software improvements in the photostimulable phosphor plate, in image reading-scanning devices, in image processing algorithms, and in the cost and utility of image display devices have contributed to the increased acceptance of CR as the digital counterpart to conventional screen-film projection radiography. The purpose of this chapter is to provide an overview of the state-of-the-art in CR systems. A basic description of the data acquisition process will be given, followed by a review of system specifications, image quality, and performance including signal-to-noise, contrast, and spatial resolution characteristics. Advantages and disadvantages inherent in CR, and a comparison with conventional screen-film radiography will be discussed.

The types of CR equipment presently available will be listed. An explanation of the image processing algorithms that convert the raw CR image data into useful clinical images will be provided. The image processing algorithms to be discussed include image segmentation or exposure data recognition and background removal, contrast enhancement, spatial frequency processing including edge enhancement and noise smoothing, dynamic range control (DRC), multiscale image contrast amplification (MUSICA), and dual energy subtraction. This will be followed by a discussion of the uses of CR in Picture Archiving and Communication Systems (PACS), key features for successful clinical implementation, and the medical physicist's role in the process. Examples of several types of artifacts potentially encountered with CR are given along with their causes and methods for correction or minimization of these effects. A summary will address future trends and briefly mention other digital projection radiography devices.

Review of the Fundamentals

Process Description

A CR system consists of a screen or plate of a stimulable phosphor material that is usually contained in a cassette and is exposed in a manner similar to traditional screen-film cassettes. The photostimulable phosphor in the imaging plate (IP) absorbs X-rays that have passed through the patient, thus "recording" the X-ray image. Like the conventional intensifying screen, CR plates produce light in response to X-ray, at the time of exposure. However, storage phosphor plates have the additional property of being capable of storing some of the absorbed X-ray energy as a latent image; approximately half of the incident X-ray intensity is lost as luminescence (Kodak 1992). Plates are typically made of an europium-doped barium-fluoro-halide-halide crystallized matrix. Electrons from the dopant ion become trapped just below the conduction band when exposed to X-rays. Irradiating the imaging plate at some time after the X-ray exposure with red or near-infrared laser light liberates the electrons into the conduction band stimulating the phosphor to release some of its stored energy in the form of green, blue or ultraviolet light—the phenomenon of photostimulable luminescence. The intensity of light emitted is proportional to the amount of X-ray absorbed by the storage phosphor (Bogucki 1995), which is to say that the CR imaging plate is a linear detector.

The readout process uses a precision laser spot scanning mechanism in which the laser beam traverses the IP surface in a raster pattern. The stimulated light emitted from the IP is collected and converted into an electrical signal, with optics coupled to a photomultiplier tube (PMT). A special optical filter must be used in front of the PMT to block the stimulating light which typically is a factor of 10^8 higher intensity than the light emitted from the IP (Kodak 1992). The PMT converts the collected light from the IP into an electrical signal, which is then amplified, sampled to produce discrete pixels of the digital image, and sent through an analog-to-digital converter (ADC) to quantize the value of each pixel (i.e., a value between 0 and 1023 for a 10-bit ADC or between 0 and 4095 for a 12-bit ADC).

Not all of the stored energy in the IP is released during the readout process. Thus, to prepare the imaging plate for reuse and another exposure, the IP is briefly flooded with high intensity (typically fluorescent) light. This erasure step ensures removal of any residual latent image.

A diagram of the process steps involved in a CR system is shown in Figure 1. In principle, CR inserts a digital computer between the imaging plate receptor (photo-stimulable phosphor screen) and the output film. This digital processor can perform a number of image processing tasks including compensating for exposure errors, applying appropriate contrast characteristics, enhancing image detail, and storing and distributing image information in digital form.

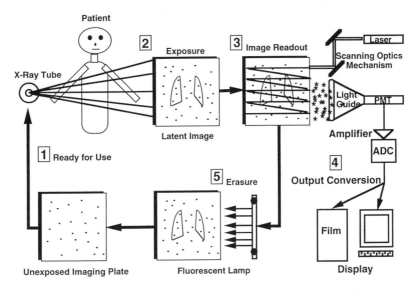

Figure 1. The image production steps involved in CR. The imaging plate is exposed to X-ray, read out by a laser scanning mechanism and erased for reuse. A light guide collects the photostimulated luminescence and feeds it to a photomultiplier tube (PMT) that converts the light signal to an electrical signal. Amplification, logarithmic conversion, and analog-to-digital conversion produce the final digital signal that can be displayed on a cathode ray tube monitor or sent to a laser printer for image reproduction on film.

System Characteristics

One of the most important differences between CR and screen-film systems is in exposure latitude. The exposure response of a digital imaging system relates the incident X-ray exposure to the resulting pixel value output. System sensitivity is the lowest exposure that will produce a useful pixel value and the dynamic range is the ratio of the exposures of the highest and lowest useful pixel values (Barnes 1993). Storage phosphor systems have extremely wide exposure latitude, approximately 10^4 times wider than the latitude of the widest dynamic range conventional X-ray system (Kodak 1992). The latitude of screen-film systems is limited by the saturation ("shoulder") and threshold ("toe") portions of its sigmoidal characteristic Hurter & Driffield (H&D) curve. Since film serves as both the acquisition and the display medium, there is also a design tradeoff that must often be made between exposure latitude and visual contrast in screen-film systems. The wide latitude of storage phosphor systems, and effectively linear detector characteristic curve, allows them to capture a wider range of exposure information in a single image than is possible with any screen-film system. In addition, the wide dynamic range of CR allows it to be used under a broad range of exposure conditions without the need for changing the basic detector. This also makes CR an ideal choice for applications in which exposures are highly variable or difficult to control as in portable radiography. The digital image processing in CR systems can usually create a diagnostic image out of under- or over-exposures via appropriate look-up table correction, that would have necessitated retakes with a screen-film system.

Dose requirements of a medical imaging system depend on the system's ability to detect and convert the incoming signal into a usable output signal (i.e., to absorb and convert incident X-rays into film optical density or electrical light upon a PMT). It is important to stress that CR systems are *not* inherently lower dose systems than screen-film. In fact, some dual-screen, screen-film systems have higher X-ray absorption leading to better dose utilization than CR, and several studies have demonstrated a higher required exposure for CR to achieve equivalent optical density on screen-film (Wilson 1993, Andriole 1994). However, the wider latitude of storage phosphor systems makes them much more forgiving of under- or over-exposure. As in any digital radiography system, when dose is decreased, the noise due to quantum mottle increases (Kodak 1992). Reader tolerance of this noise tends to be the limiting factor on the lowest acceptable dose.

Image Quality

DQE

Objective descriptors of digital image quality include the detective quantum efficiency (DQE) and spatial resolution response of the image capture process, as well as the exposure response and the dynamic range. DQE is a measure of the fidelity with which a resultant digital image represents the transmitted X-ray fluence pattern (i.e., how efficiently a system converts the X-ray input signal into a useful output image), and includes a measure of the noise added (Barnes 1993). Also taken into account are the input/output characteristics of the system and the resolution response of unsharpness or blur added during the image capture process. The linear, wide-latitude input/output characteristic of CR systems relative to screen-film, leads to a wider DQE latitude for CR, which implies that CR has the ability to convert incoming X-ray quanta into "useful" output over a much wider range of exposure than can be accommodated with screen-film systems (Kodak 1992).

Spatial Resolution

The spatial resolution response or sharpness of an image capture process can be expressed in terms of its modulation transfer function (MTF) which, in practice, is determined by taking the Fourier Transform of the line spread function (LSF), and relates *input* subject contrast to *imaged* subject contrast as a function of spatial frequency (Barnes 1993). The ideal image receptor adds no blur or broadening to the input LSF, resulting in an MTF response of one at all spatial frequencies, faithfully reproducing the input throughout the image. A real image receptor adds blur, typically resulting in a loss of MTF at higher spatial frequencies.

The main factors limiting the spatial resolution in CR, similar to screen-film systems, is X-ray scattering within the phosphor layer. However, it is the scattering of the stimulating beam in CR, rather than the emitted light as in screen-film, that determines system sharpness (Matsuda 1993, Kodak 1992). Broadening of the laser light spot within the IP phosphor layer spreads with the depth of the plate. Thus, the spatial resolution response of CR is largely dependent on the initial laser beam diameter and on the thickness of the IP detector. Other factors that improve CR system response characteristics also tend to have adverse effects on the overall signal. For example, the intensity of the stimulating laser, which affects the amount of stored signal extracted from the plate, is inversely proportional to image sharpness (i.e., higher laser power, which increases the amount of signal extracted, yields lower sharpness) (Kodak 1992). The reproducible spatial frequency of CR is also limited by the sampling utilized in the digital readout process. The spatial resolution of CR is less than that of screen-film, with CR ranging from 2.5 to 5 line pairs per millimeter (lp/mm) versus the 10 lp/mm or higher spatial resolution of screen-film.

Contrast Resolution

The contrast or grayscale resolution for CR is much greater than that for screen-film. Since overall image quality resolution is a combination of spatial and grayscale resolution, the superior contrast resolution of CR can often compensate for its lack of inherent spatial resolution. By manipulating the image contrast and brightness, or window and level values respectively, small features often become more readily apparent in the image. More work needs to be done to determine the most appropriate window and level settings with which to initially display a CR image. Lacking the optimum default settings, it is often useful to "dynamically" view CR softcopy images with a variety of window and level settings.

Noise

The types of noise affecting CR images include X-ray dose-dependent noise and fixed noise (independent of X-ray dose). The dose-dependent noise components can be classified into X-ray quantum noise, or mottle, and light photon noise (Matsuda 1993). The quantum mottle inherent in the input X-ray beam is the limiting noise factor, and it arises in the process of absorption by the imaging plate, with noise being inversely proportional to the detector X-ray dose absorption. Light photon noise arises in the process of photoelectric transmission of the photostimulable luminescence light at the surface of the PMT, and is inversely proportional to the number of photoelectrons, with the noise power being inversely proportional to the incident X-ray dose, the X-ray absorptivity of the imaging plate, the light condensing efficiency of the light guide which collects the photostimulable luminescence (PSL) light, with photoelectric conversion efficiency of the PMT, etc. (Matsuda 1993).

Fixed noise sources in CR systems include IP structural noise (the predominant factor), noise in the electronics chain, laser power fluctuations, quantization noise in the analog-to-digital conversion process (Matsuda 1993, Kodak 1992). IP structural noise arises from the nonuniformity of phosphor particle distribution, with finer particles providing noise improvement. Note that for CR systems, it is the *noise* sources that limit the DQE system latitude, whereas in conventional X-ray systems, the DQE latitude is limited by the narrower e*xposure response* of screen-film.

Comparison with Screen-Film

Table 1 summarizes the comparison of CR systems with conventional screen-film and Table 2 lists the advantages of CR, including all the benefits of digital images which can be electronically processed, manipulated, distributed, displayed, and archived. The extremely large latitude of CR systems makes CR more forgiving in difficult imaging situations such as portable examinations, and enables decreased retake rates for improper exposure technique. The superior contrast resolution of CR can compensate in many cases for its lesser spatial resolution. Cost savings and improved Radiology Departmental workflow can be realized with CR and the elimination of film.

Table 1. Summary Comparison of CR with Conventional Screen-Film.

	Conventional X-Ray	CR
Receptor	screen-film	photostimulable phosphor
Characteristic Curve	sigmoidal H&D curve	linear; wide dynamic range (10^4)
High kV	decreased contrast	contrast does not vary
Low kV	increased contrast	contrast does not vary
High mAs	increased density	uniform density
Low mAs	decreased density	uniform density, coarse grain
Spatial Resolution	superior, 10-15 lp/mm	3-5 lp/mm
Contrast Resolution	inferior, fixed	superior, manipulable
Display	film	film & monitor
Archival	film	film & digital storage device

Table 2. Summary of Advantages of CR.

• Digital images capable of being electronically processed, manipulated, distributed, displayed, and archived.

• Large latitude system allowing excellent visualization of both soft tissue and bone in the same exposure image.

• Superior contrast resolution can compensate for lack of spatial resolution.

• Decreased retake rate.

• Cost savings if film is eliminated.

• Improved radiology department workflow with elimination of film handling routines.

Available CR Systems

Historical Perspective

Photostimulable luminescence, the phenomenon in which a phosphor releases trapped energy as light when re-excited by infrared or visible light of a wavelength longer than the stimulus, has been known for centuries, but did not capture the interest of scientific researchers until 1603 with the discovery of the Bolognese stone in Italy (Kato 1991). The notion of optical de-excitation was not described until 1867 by Becquerel (Krongauz 1974). In 1926, Hirsch proposed a means of retaining the fluorescent image for prolonged periods, using storage phosphors to record the image, heat to re-stimulate the image for viewing in a dark room or for exposing film, and a red light to erase the image so that the phosphor screen could be reused (Hirsch 1926).

Most of the progress in storage phosphor imaging has been made post World War II (Berg 1947). In 1975, Eastman Kodak Company (Rochester, NY) patented an apparatus using infrared-stimulable phosphors or thermoluminescent materials to store an image (Luckey 1975). In 1980, Fuji Photo Film (Tokyo, Japan) patented a process in which photostimulable phosphors were used to record and reproduce an image by absorbing radiation, and then releasing the stored energy as light when stimulated by a helium-neon laser (Kotera 1980). The emitted phosphor luminescence was detected by a PMT and the electronic signal produced, which reconstructed the image.

Fuji was the first to commercialize a storage phosphor-based CR system in 1983 (as the FCR 101) and published the first technical paper (in *Radiology*) describing CR for acquiring clinical digital X-ray images (Sonoda 1983). The central processing type second-generation scanners (FCR 201) were marketed in 1985 (Matsuda 1993). Third-generation Fuji systems marketed in 1989 included distributed processing (FCR 7000) and stand-alone (AC-1) types (Matsuda 1993). Fuji systems in the FCR 9000 series are improved, higher speed, higher performance third-generation scanners. Current Fuji systems in the 5000 series include an upright chest unit (5501) and a multi-plate autoloader.

In 1992, Kodak installed its first commercial storage phosphor reader (Model 3110) (Bogucki 1995). Their current model, the KESPR (Kodak Ektascan Storage Phosphor Reader) Model 400 or CR 400 Plus includes an autoloader device. In 1994, Agfa-Gevaert N.V. (Belgium) debuted its own CR system design (the ADC 70) (Agfa 1994). In 1997, Agfa showed its ADC Compact with greatly reduced footprint. This product will be sold exclusively after the beginning of 1999. In 1998, Lumisys presented its low-cost, desktop CR unit (the ACR 2000) with manual-feed, single plate reading. Agfa also introduced a low-cost, entry-level single plate reader (the ADC Solo) in 1998, appropriate for distributed CR environments such as clinics, trauma centers, intensive care units (ICUs), etc.

Several other companies have been involved in CR research and development including: N.A. Philips Corp., Konica Corp., E.I. DuPont de Nemours & Co., 3M Co., Hitachi, Ltd., Seimens AG, Toshiba Corp., General Electric Corp., Kasei Optonix, Ltd., Mitsubishi Chemical Industries, Ltd., Nichia Corp., GTE Products Co., and DigiRad Corp. (Kodak 1992). However, the four distinct state-of-the-art commercially available CR systems include Agfa's, Fuji's, Kodak's, and Lumisys'.

Recent Technological Advances

Major improvements in the overall CR system design and performance characteristics include a reduction in the physical size of the reading units, increased plate reading capacity per unit time, and better image quality. These advances have been achieved through a combination of changes in the IPs themselves, in the image reader or scanning devices, and in the application of image processing algorithms to effect image output. These technological modifications will be detailed in this and the following sections.

Photostimulable Phosphor Plate

The newer (Fuji) type-V imaging plates developed for the latest CR systems, as well as for use in previous models, have higher image quality (increased sharpness) and improved fading and residual image characteristics. In order to permit use of a visible light semiconductor laser in the latest Fuji IP readers (discussed below), in place of the helium-neon laser of older models, the photostimulable phosphor plate had to be modified to accommodate a reading light wavelength of 680 nanometers (nm), as opposed to 633 nm for earlier generation readers. This was achieved by changing the plate material from a europium-doped barium-fluoro-bromide (BaFBr:Eu)-phosphor to a europium-doped barium-fluoro-bromo-iodide (BaF(Br,I):Eu)-phosphor (Matsuda 1993).

Higher image quality has resulted from several modifications in the imaging plate phosphor and layer thickness. Smaller phosphor grain size in the type-V IP (down to approximately 4 microns (μm)) diminishes fixed noise of the imaging plate, while increased packing density of phosphor particles counteracted a concomitant decrease in photostimulable luminescence (Matsuda 1993). A thinner protective layer is utilized in the type-V plates tending to reduce X-ray quantum noise, and in and of itself, would improve the spatial resolution response characteristics of the plates as a result of diminished beam scattering. However, in the newest IPs, the quantity of phosphor coated onto the plate is increased for durability purposes, resulting in the same response characteristic of previous imaging plates (Ogawa 1995).

Image Scanning Devices

An historical review of CR scanning units chronicles improved compactness and increased processing speed. The first Fuji unit (FCR 101) from 1983 required roughly

6 square meters of floor space to house the reader and could only process about 45 plates per hour, while today's Fuji models (i.e., FCR 9000s) occupy less than one square meter and can process approximately 110 plates per hour (Matsuda 1993). This is a decrease in apparatus size by a factor of approximately one sixth and an increase in processing capacity of roughly 2.5 times.

The use of a high-output visible light semiconductor laser (versus the older model helium-neon gas laser) and polygon mirror scanning apparatus permits the attainment of higher speeds in the current scanners by avoiding a reduction in PSL intensity of the imaging plates. The laser spot has a Gaussian profile and is 100 µm in diameter at the plate plane (Bogucki 1995). A scanning lens appropriate for polygonal mirror scanning was developed to create an ultra-wide beam deflection angle (of 90 degrees), minimizing optical deviation to secure uniform beam diameter, and improving laser power utilization efficiency (Matsuda 1993). Shortened reading time per pixel via improved PMT and analog circuit system response and analog-to-digital conversion speed also contributed to high-speed processing.

An additional reading device design requirement is the need for a highly efficient light condensing system and a light detector of high photoelectric conversion efficiency and low noise. In Fuji CR systems, a single sheet of acrylic resin (approximately 8 mm in thickness) is heated and bent to yield 100% reflectivity of incident light from the acrylic edge surface within the plate, thereby achieving the highest light collecting efficiency for guiding the light into a PMT (Matsuda 1993). In the latest Kodak CR reader (Model 400) five PMTs sitting directly above the plate are utilized versus one PMT in the earlier model (Bogucki 1995).

Achievement of high processing speed necessitated an improved IP handling mechanism. This was accomplished by parallel execution of the following steps: IP feeding and loading, image reading, image erasure, and image processing (Matsuda 1993). A redesign of the erasure unit, which restores the imaging plate to a reusable state after image reading, to a two-stage method, has been adopted in the current model Fuji CRs. The combination of high-brightness fluorescent tubes, with an ultraviolet cutoff filter for a two-stage irradiation process facilitates high-speed erasure with a low power consumption, compact device (Matsuda 1993).

Image Output Formats

CR imaging plate sizes, pixel resolutions, and their associated digital file sizes are roughly the same across manufacturers for the various cassette sizes offered. For example, the 14" by 17" (or 35 cm by 43 cm metric equivalent) plates are read with a sampling rate of 5-5.81 pixels per mm, at a digital image matrix size of roughly 2K by 2K pixels (1760 by 2140 pixels for Fuji (Matsuda 1993) and 2048 by 2508 pixels for Agfa and Kodak (Bogucki 1995). Fuji images are quantized to 10 bits (for 1024 gray levels), and Agfa and Kodak images have a 12-bit logarithmic quantization (for

4096 gray levels). Thus, total image file sizes range from roughly 8 megabytes (MB) to 11.5 MB. The smaller plates are scanned at the same laser spot size (100 microns) and the digitization rate does not change, therefore, the pixel size is smaller (Bogucki 1995). The 10" by 12" (24 cm by 30 cm) plates are typically read at a sampling rate of 6.7-9 pixels per millimeter (mm) and the 8" by 10" (18 cm by 24 cm) plates are read at 10 pixels per mm (Matsuda 1993, Bogucki 1995).

All sizes of Fuji images are typically printed on one size (10" by 14") film. If they are printed in the one-on-one image display format, the images from 14" by 17" and the 14" by 14" plates are reduced by two-thirds, unless the new HQ acquisition 4K by 5K image capture is utilized and the resulting 32 MB image printed on 14" by 17" film. This high resolution image capture improves the spatial resolution and overall image quality at a cost of greatly increased digital file size, complicating data handling, transmission, storage, and softcopy display. Agfa and Kodak print the larger (35 cm by 43 cm) 2K by 2.5K images on 14" by 17" film and the smaller files on 10" by 14" film. CR images can also be printed in a two-on-one format for a side-by-side display of the default processed image and an edge enhanced image, for example. If this display format is used, 8" by 10" images are reduced by six-sevenths, 10" by 12" images are reduced by two-thirds, and 14" by 17" images are reduced by one half.

Image Processing Algorithms

CR images are acquired over four decades of exposure (0 to 10^4) so some image processing must be performed to optimize the radiograph for output display. Each manufacturer has its own set of proprietary algorithms which can be applied to the image for printing on laser film or display on their own proprietary workstations. Prior to the Digital Imaging and Communications in Medicine (DICOM) standard, only the raw data could be directly acquired digitally. Therefore, to attain the same image appearance on other display stations, the appropriate image processing algorithms (if known) had to be implemented somewhere along the chain from acquisition to display. Now image processing parameters can be passed in the DICOM header, and algorithms applied to CR images displayed on generic workstations. In general, the digital image processing applied to CR consists of a recognition or analysis phase, followed by contrast enhancement and/or frequency processing.

Image Segmentation

In the image recognition stage, called exposure data recognizer (EDR) by Fuji (Matsuda 1993) and segmentation by Kodak (Kodak 1994), the region of exposure is detected (i.e., the collimation edges are detected), a histogram analysis of the pixel gray values in the image is performed to assess the actual exposure to the plate, and the appropriate look-up table specific to the region of anatomy imaged and chosen by the X-ray technologist at the time of patient demographic information input is selected.

Proper recognition of the exposed region of interest is extremely important as it affects future processing applied to the image data. For example, if the bright white areas of the image caused by collimation at the time of exposure is not detected properly, its very high gray values will be taken into account during histogram analysis, increasing the "window" of values to be accommodated by a given display device (softcopy or hardcopy), thus decreasing contrast in the image. Fuji has greatly improved their recognition technique (EDR—exposure data recognition) through the use of neural network pattern matching; such that even off-angle collimation (problematic in the past) is properly recognized (Takeo 1994). Agfa's and Kodak's segmentation algorithms, in addition to detection of collimation edges in the image, enable users to blacken the region outside these edges, in the final image if so desired (Bogucki 1995, Kodak 1994). This tends to improve image appearance by removing this bright white background in images of small body parts or pediatric patients. The photo in Figure 2 demonstrates this feature of "blackened surround," which also allows multiple exposures on a single IP.

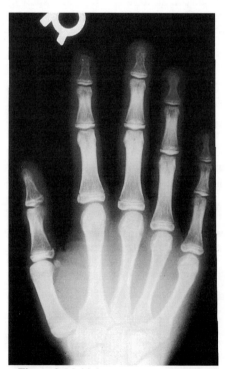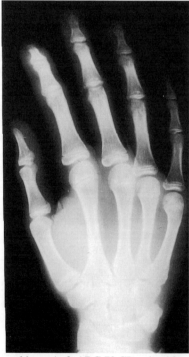

Figure 2. Multiple exposures on a single IP processed in an Agfa ADC 70 CR unit with "blackened surround" applied.

Contrast Enhancement

Conventional contrast enhancement, called gradation processing by Fuji (Matsuda 1993), tone scaling by Kodak (Bogucki 1995, Kodak 1994), latitude reduction by Agfa (Agfa 1994), is performed next. This processing amounts to choosing the best characteristic curve (usually a nonlinear transformation of X-ray exposure to image density) to apply to the image data. These algorithms are quite flexible and can be tuned to satisfy a particular user's preferences for a given "look" of the image (Gingold 1994). Look-up tables are specific to the region of anatomy images. Figure 3 shows an example of the default adult chest look-up table (3A) applied to an image (Kodak Model 400) and the same image with high contrast processing (3B). A reverse contrast scale or "black bone" technique in which what was originally black in the image becomes white, and what was originally white in the image becomes black, is sometimes felt to be beneficial for identifying and locating tubes and lines.

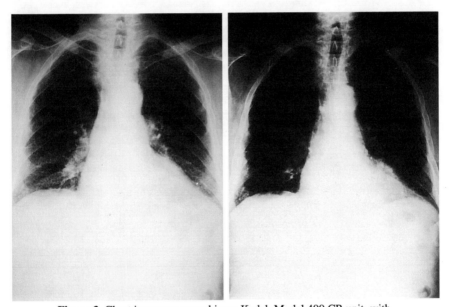

Figure 3. Chest image processed in an Kodak Model 400 CR unit, with
A. default mode and **B**. high contrast algorithm applied.

Spatial Frequency Processing

The next type of image processing usually performed is spatial frequency processing, sometimes called edge enhancement. These algorithms adjust the frequency response characteristics of the CR systems, essentially implementing a high or band pass filter operation to enhance the high spatial frequency content contained in edge information. Unfortunately, noise also contains high spatial frequency information and can be exacerbated by edge enhancement techniques. To lessen this problem, a nonlinear unsharp masking technique is typically implemented serving to suppress noise via a smoothing process. (Unsharp masking is an averaging technique that, via summation, tends to blur the image. When this is subtracted from the original image data, the effect is one of noise suppression.) Specific spatial frequencies can be preferentially selected and emphasized by changing the mask size and weighting parameters. For example, low frequency information in the image can be augmented by using a relatively large mask, while high frequency or edge information can be enhanced by using a small mask size (Matsuda 1993). The photos in Figure 4 depict frequency processing for edge enhancement (in 4B) versus the Agfa default chest algorithm (in 4A) (Model ADC 70).

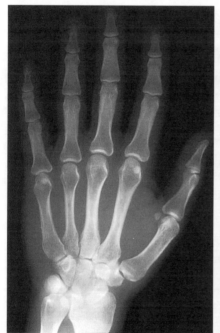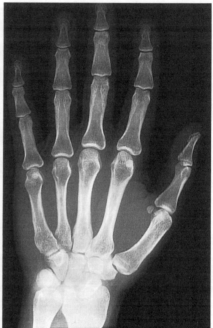

Figure 4. Hand image processed in an Agfa ADC 70 CR unit, with **A**. default mode, **B**. edge enhancement algorithm applied.

DRC

An advanced algorithm by Fuji, for selective compression or emphasis of low-density regions in an image, independent of contrast and spatial frequency is known as dynamic range control (DRC) processing (Ishida 1993). The algorithm consists of performing an unsharp mask for suppression of high spatial frequency information, then application of a specific look-up table mapping to selected regions (i.e., low density areas). This mask is then added back to the original data with the overall result being improved contrast in poorly penetrated regions, without loss of high frequency and contrast emphasis. In a clinical evaluation of the algorithm for processing of adult portable chest exams, DRC was found to be preferred by five thoracic radiologists in a side-by-side comparison, providing improved visibility of mediastinal details and enhanced subdiaphragmatic regions (Storto 1995).

MUSICA

Multiscale image contrast amplification (MUSICA) is a very flexible advanced image processing algorithm developed by Agfa (Agfa 1994, Vuylsteke 1997). MUSICA is a local contrast enhancement technique based on the principle of detail amplitude or detail strength, and the notion that image features can be striking or subtle, large in size or small. MUSICA processing is independent of the size or diameter of the object with the feature to be enhanced. The method is carried out by decomposing the original image into a set of detail images, where each detail image represents an image feature of a specific scale. This set of detail images, or basis functions, completely describes the original image. Each detail image representation and the image background are contrast equalized separately; some details can be enhanced and others attenuated as desired. All the separate detail images are recombined into a single image, and the result is diminished differences in contrast between features regardless of size, such that all image features become more visible. Figure 5 shows CR images processed with the Agfa default processing (5A) and the same image MUSICA enhanced (5B).

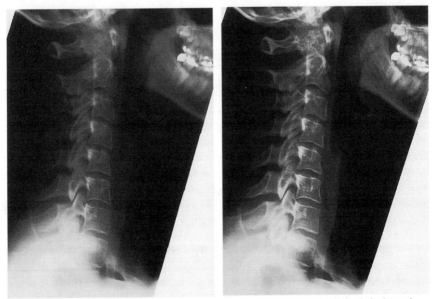

Figure 5. C-Spine image processed in an Agfa ADC 70 CR unit with **A**. default mode, **B**. MUSICA algorithm applied.

Dual Energy Subtraction

Another processing algorithm offered by Fuji, which requires both hardware and soft-ware modifications to the FCR 9000 units, is the single exposure, dual-energy subtraction technique (Ishida 1993, Bacarini 1994). In this method, X-ray energies are separated by the insertion of a copper filter between two IPs such that a low-energy image is recorded on the front IP and a high-energy image is recorded on the back IP (Ishida 1993). Manipulation of these different energy images can be done to achieve a soft tissue (bone subtracted) image and a bone (soft tissue subtracted) image. It is felt that this dual-energy subtraction technique may provide improved lung nodule detection, among other applications.

CR in PACS

Uses

CR can be utilized for the digital image acquisition of projection radiography exam-inations into a PACS. As a result of its wide exposure latitude and relative forgiveness of exposure technique, CR can improve the quality of images in difficult imaging situations, such as in portable or bedside examinations of critically ill or hospitalized patients. As such, CR systems have been successfully utilized in the ICU setting, in the emergency room (ER) or trauma center, as well as in the operating room (OR). CR can also be cost effective for a high volume clinic setting, or in a low volume site as input to a teleradiology service.

Key Features for Clinical Implementation

CR, as for any digital image acquisition device, is the first point of entry into a PACS. Errors may propagate from here, with the quality of the PACS output being directly dependent on the quality of the signal in. In addition to image quality, essential features for successful clinical implementation of CR systems for a PACS include the follow-ing: DICOM conformance of the modality is essential and includes compliance with the image data and header format, as well as the DICOM communication protocol. Equally critical is interfacing to the radiology information system (RIS)/hospital infor-mation system (HIS). Integration of the CR system with the RIS/HIS can reduce human errors on patient demographic information input and improve efficiency.

Ease of integration of the device into the daily workflow routine and simplicity and robustness of the user interface are very important. Reliability, fault tolerance, and capabilities for error tracking are also major issues to consider as are CR system speed and performance.

Medical Physicist's Role

Among the many roles of the medical physicist in incorporating the CR imaging modality into the diagnostic imaging department are acceptance testing of the device and quality assurance (QA) / quality control (QC). The medical physicist should be involved in the citing and planning of the CR system, as well as the installation, testing and tuning, and training. Substantial efforts have been underway to standardize CR QA/QC, such as the American Association of Physicists in Medicine (AAPM) Task Group #10 draft document "Computed Radiography Acceptance Testing and Quality Control." See also (Seibert 1994) and (Willis 1995). In spite of the fact that CR is more forgiving of a broad range of exposures, the use of this modality is not an excuse to employ poor radiographic technique. CR exposures should be routinely monitored as well as the image quality on a per exam type basis.

Image Artifacts

The appearance and causes of image artifacts that can occur in current CR systems should be recognized and logged by the medical physicist. Artifacts can arise from a variety of sources including those related to the imaging plates themselves, to image readers, and to image processing. Several types of artifacts potentially encountered with CR have been minimized with the latest technology improvements, but may still be seen in older systems.

Lead backing added to the aluminum-framed, carbon-fiber cassettes has eliminated the so-called light-bulb effect, darkened outer portions of a film due to backscattered radiation (Solomon 1991). High sensitivity of the CR plates renders them extremely susceptible to scattered radiation or inadvertent exposure, thus routine erasure of all CR plates on the day of use is recommended as is the storing of imaging plates on end, rather than the stacking of cassettes one on top of the other (Volpe 1996). The occurrence of persistent latent images after high exposures or after prolonged intervals between plate erasure and reuse (Solomon 1991, Oestman 1991) has been lessened by the improved efficiency of the two-stage erasure procedure utilized in the latest CR systems (Volpe 1996). Improved recognition of the collimation pattern employed for a given image through the incorporation of neural network processing (in the Fuji FCR 9000), allows varied (including off-angle) collimation fields and, in turn, improves histogram analysis and subsequent processing of the imaged region (Volpe 1996), although these algorithms can fail in some instances.

The new standard version V (ST-V) and high resolution V (HR-V) type imaging plates achieve higher spatial resolution than earlier versions, due in part to their thinner phosphor and surface-protection layers. They are, however, more susceptible to damage, such as plate cracking, from wear-and-tear and can create troublesome artifacts as depicted in (Volpe 1996).

Inadvertent double exposures can occur with the present CR systems, potentially masking low-density findings such as regions of parenchymal consolidation, or leading to errors in interpreting line positions. Examples are included in (Volpe 1996). Such artifacts are more difficult to detect than with screen-film systems because of CR's linear frequency processing response, optimizing image intensity over a wide range of exposures (i.e., due to its wide dynamic range).

Laser scanning artifacts can still occur with current CR readers and are seen as a linear artifact across the image, caused by dust on the light source (Volpe 1996). Proper and frequent cleaning of the laser and light guide apparatus as well as the imaging plates themselves can prevent such artifacts.

The ability of CR to produce clinically diagnostic images over a wide range of exposures is dependent on the effectiveness of the image analysis algorithms applied to each data set. The specific processing parameters used are based on standards tuned to the anatomic region under examination. Incorrect selection of diagnostic specifier or inapropriate anatomic region can result in an image of unacceptable quality. Understanding the causes of some of these CR imaging artifacts as well as maintaining formal, routine quality assurance procedures can help to recognize, correct, and avoid future difficulties.

Summary

Technological advances in CR hardware and software have contributed to the increased acceptance of CR as the current counterpart to conventional screen-film projection radiography, making the use of this modality for clinical purposes more widespread. CR is compatible with existing X-ray equipment, yet separates out the functions of image acquisition or capture, image display, and image archival versus traditional screen-film, in which film serves as the image detector, display, and storage medium. This separation in image capture, display, and storage functions by CR enables optimization of each of these steps individually. Potential expected benefits are improved diagnostic capability (via the wide dynamic range of CR and the ability to manipulate the exam through image processing) and enhanced Radiology Department productivity (via networking capabilities for transmission of images to remotely located digital softcopy displays and for storage and retrieval of t digital data).

Other digital projection radiography imaging sensors, also called flat panel detectors, include the various types of indirect conversion methods in which light is first generated using a scintillator or phosphor and then detected by charge-coupled devices (CCDs) or thin-film-transistor (TFT) arrays in conjunction with photodiodes; and direct digital radiography (DDR) devices such as Sterling's DR (originally E.I. DuPont de Nemours & Co., Medical Products Department, Wilmington, DE), which consists of a thin-film pixel array, selenium X-ray photoconductor, dielectric layer, and top electrode (Lee 1995). DDR devices offer direct energy conversion of X-ray for immediate readout. These detectors have high efficiency, low noise and good spatial resolution, wide latitude, and all the benefits of digital or filmless imaging.

These sensors are not yet widely used clinically because of their high cost of production and their one-room-at-a-time technology as well as portability issues and other impracticalities. The ease of use, straight forward integration, and relative reliability of CR systems versus DDR systems adds to their attractiveness as a replacement for screen-film systems in general radiography, in a PACS digital imaging network. It is likely that CR and DDR devices will coexist for some time.

Several technical limitations still remain such as CR's decreased spatial resolution compared to conventional screen-film methods, preventing its use in certain clinical applications, such as mammography. Meeting the cost competitiveness of screen-film systems is difficult unless film printing is eliminated from the cost equation. Future improvements in image processing algorithms, with a better understanding of optimum display settings for soft copy viewing have the potential to greatly facilitate and standardize softcopy reading. High performance diagnostic digital workstations for display of CR are still expensive and cumbersome to operate but becoming better. Improved display station graphical user interface (GUI) design, increased familiarity with and greater confidence in soft copy reading should drive CR systems to filmless operation. At the present time, CR appears to be the primary candidate for replacing screen-film systems for general projection radiography in a filmless radiology department.

References

Agfa. "The Highest Productivity in Computed Radiography." *Agfa-Gevaert N.V. Report*, Belgium, 1994.

Andriole, K.P., Gooding, C.A., Gould, R.G., and Huang, H.K. "Analysis of a High-Resolution Computed Radiography Imaging Plate Versus Conventional Screen-Film Radiography for neonatal Intensive Care Unit Applications." *SPIE Physics of Medical Imaging* 1994; 2163:80-97.

Bacarini, L., Granieri. G.F., La Torre, E., Giacomich, R., and Saccavini, C. "Dual Energy Subtraction with Single Exposure By CR." *SCAR '94 Computer Applications to Assist Radiology*, J.M. Boehme, A.H. Rowberg, and N.T. Wolfman, (Eds.) June 12-15, 1994, pp. 737-738.

Barnes, G.T. "Digital X-Ray Image Capture with Image Intensifier and Storage Phosphor Plates: Imaging Principles, Performance and Limitations." *Proceedings of the AAPM 1993 Summer School: Digital Imaging.* University of Virginia, Charlottesville, VA, AAPM Monograph 22 (Madison: Medical Physics Publishing, 1993), 23-48.

Berg, G.E. and Kaiser, H.F. "The x-ray storage properties of the infra-red storage phosphor and application to radiography." *Journal of Applied Physics* 1947; 18:343-347.

Bogucki, T.M., Trauernicht, D.P., and Kocher, T.E. "Characteristics of a Storage Phosphor System for Medical Imaging." *Kodak Health Sciences Technical and Scientific Monograph*, No. 6, New York, Eastman Kodak Co., July 1995.

Gingold, E.L, Tucker, D.M., and Barnes, G.T. "Computed radiography: user-programmable features and capabilities." *Journal of Digital Imaging* 1994; 7(3):113-122.

Hirsch, I.S., "A new type of fluorescent screen." *Radiology* 1926; 7:422-425.

Ishida, M. *Fuji Computed Radiography Technical Review,* No. 1, Tokyo, Fuji Photo Film Co., Ltd., 1993.

Kato, H. "Photostimulable Phosphor Radiography Design Considerations." *Proceedings of the AAPM 1991 Summer School: Specification, Acceptance Testing and Quality Control of Diagnostic X-Ray Imaging Equipment.* UC Santa Cruz, Santa Cruz, CA. July 15-19, 1991; Vol. II, pp. 860-898.

Kodak. "Digital Radiography Using Storage Phosphors." *Kodak Health Sciences Technical and Scientific Monograph*, New York, Eastman Kodak Co., April 1992.

Kodak. "Optimizing CR Images with Image Processing: Segmentation, Tone Scaling, Edge Enhancement." *Kodak Health Sciences Technical and Scientific Manuscript*, New York, Eastman Kodak, March 1994.

Kotera, N., Eguchi, S., Miyahara, J., Matsumoto, S., and Kato, H. Method and Apparatus for Recording and Reproducing a Radiation Image. U.S. Patent 4,236,078. 1980.

Krongauz, V.G., and Parfianovich, I.A. "Photostimulated Luminescence of Phosphors." *Journal of Luminescence* 1974; 9:61-70.

Lee, D.L, Cheung, L.K., and Jeromin, L.S., "A New Digital Detector for Projection Radiography." *Proceedings of SPIE Physics of Medical Imaging*, San Diego, CA, Feb. 26-27, 1995, 2432:237-249.

Luckey, G. Apparatus and Methods for Producing Images Corresponding to Patterns of High Energy Radiation. U.S. Patent 3,859,527. June 7, 1975. Revised No. 31847. March 12, 1985.

Matsuda, T., Arakawa, S., Kohda, K., Torii, S., and Nakajima, N. *Fuji Computed Radiography Technical Review*, No. 2, Tokyo, Fuji Photo Film Co., Ltd., 1993.

Oestman, J.W., Prokop, M., Schaefer, C.M., and Galanski, M. "Hardware and software artifacts in storage phosphor radiography." *RadioGraphics* 1991; 11:795-805.

Ogawa, E., Arakawa, S., Ishida, M., and Kato, H. "Quantitative analysis of imaging performance for computed radiography systems." *SPIE Physics of Medical Imaging 1995*; 2432:421-431.

Seibert, J.A. "Photostimulable Phosphor System Acceptance Testing." In: Seibert, JA, Barnes, GT, and Gould, RG, (eds.) *Specification, Acceptance Testing and Quality Control of Diagnostic X-ray Imaging Equipment. Medical Physics Monograph No. 20*. Woodbury, NY: AAPM. 771-800; 1994.

Solomon, S.L., Jost, R.G., Glazer, H.S., Sagel, S.S., Anderson, D.J., and Molina, P.L., "Artifacts in computed radiography." *AJR* 1991; 157:181-185.

Sonoda, M., Takano, M., Miyahara, J., and Kato, H. "Computed radiography utilizing scanning laser stimulated luminescence." *Radiology* 1983; 148:833-838.

Storto, M.L., Andriole, K.P., Kee, S.T., Webb, W.R., and Gamsu, G. "Portable Chest Imaging: Clinical Evaluation of a New Processing Algorithm in Digital Radiography." *81st Scientific Assembly and Annual Meeting of the Radiological Society of North America*, Chicago, November 26 - December 1, 1995.

Takeo, H., Nakajima, N., Ishida, M., and Kato, H. "Improved automatic adjustment of density and contrast in FCR system using neural network." *SPIE Physics of Medical Imaging 1994;* 2163:98-109.

Volpe, J.P., Storto. M.L., Andriole, K.P., and Gamsu, G. "Artifacts in chest radiography with a third-generation computed radiography system. *AJR* 1996; 166:653-657.

Vuylsteke, P., Dewaele, P., and Schoeters, E. "Optimizing Radiography Imaging Performance." *Proceedings of the 1997 AAPM Summer School,* pp 107-151.

Willis, C.E., Leckie, R.G., Carter, J., Williamson, M.P., Scotti, S.D., and Norton, G. "Objective Measures of Quality Assurance in a Computed Radiography-Based Radiology Department." In *Proceedings of SPIE*. 2432:588-599; 1995.

Wilson, A.J. and West, O.C. "Single-exposure conventional and computed radiography: The hybrid cassette revisited." *Investigative Radiology* 1993; 28(5):409-412.

Computed Radiography: QA/QC

Charles E. Willis, Ph.D., DABR
Department of Radiology
Baylor College of Medicine

Introduction

Computed Radiography (CR), also known as storage-phosphor radiography, photo-stimulable-phosphor radiography, is a relatively new imaging method for projection radiography (Kato 1994). More hospitals are introducing CR into routine service, fielding multiple CR units, and extending its practice beyond bedside examinations. As CR is introduced into general radiology, quality assurance (QA) programs must evolve to accommodate the characteristics of this new technology. Although CR affords a greater degree of control over the appearance of the plain x-ray image, it presents a challenge to the technologist, who must substantially change his practice, and to the radiologist, who must adapt to images with a substantially different appearance. CR also presents a challenge to the physicist, who must provide guidance on adjustment of practice to preclude and correct nondiagnostic examinations. Because 70% of the department's workload is ordinary radiography, mastery of CR technology is a prerequisite for establishing a totally digital radiology department.

Quality Assurance Principles

QA, which is more recently known as quality improvement (QI) or performance improvement (PI), includes all those activities that seek to answer the question "Are we operating our medical devices properly?" As such, QA includes all quality control (QC) activities to ensure the devices are operating properly, and a large portion of clinical engineering activities to ensure that the devices are properly supported. QA provides a systematic approach to ensure consistent, maximum performance from the physician and the imaging facilities (NCRP 1988). Unless devices are reliably maintained and performance is reliably controlled, QA indicators will provide ambiguous data.

Comprehensive QA is labor-intensive and expensive, even when we rely on automation to gather data. QA programs must be tailored to the characteristics of the imaging technology, to the specific local implementation of the technology, and to the local resources available.

QA monitors are usually focused on sensitive indicators of performance decrement. These indicators have been developed from long-term institutional experience and shared experiences of many institutions. The experience base needed to correctly identify sensitive indicators, to establish action limits, and to take appropriate corrective action does not yet exist for CR (Willis et al. 1994).

It is important to appreciate that CR technology was developed and is most widely used in Japan, where socialized health care is very different from the environment in most American hospitals. The radiologist's role in interpretation of images is secondary to the clinician's in Japan—about half the radiologists have strictly administrative duties. The training and expertise of technologists is more extensive and includes independent research and QA responsibilities assumed by medical physicists in the United States. In fact, there is an absence of diagnostic radiological physicists in Japanese hospitals. CR products are developed by a staff of imaging engineers, typically educated at the masters level, who rely on feedback from clinical sites rather than from firsthand clinical experience. It is reasonable to expect that wider practice of CR in the United States. coupled with competition from three additional manufacturers will lead to substantial improvements in CR products and practice.

A reasonable approach to dealing with new imaging technology like CR would be to conduct thorough acceptance testing (AT) to establish a performance baseline, conduct a periodic subset of AT to determine deviations from baseline, and to adapt QA methods from conventional technology to CR (Seibert 1994). A limitation to this approach is that CR technology is constantly changing, and the performance baseline must be frequently reestablished (Dobbins et al. 1995). Performance characteristics of CR also vary between different equipment vendors.

CR is not just a detector. CR affects every step of the imaging chain from acquisition of the radiographic projection to interpretation of the image (Willis et al. 1996). Comprehensive QA needs to address how changes at each step affect the efficient production and utilization of diagnostic information.

Changes Introduced by CR

Capture of the Radiographic Projection

The challenges brought on by the introduction of CR are superimposed on the usual QA problems experienced in a conventional radiology setting: patient motion, inappropriate technique selection, improper positioning, improper alignment of the x-ray beam and grid, inadequate or incorrect patient identification can still adversely affect the ultimate quality of the CR image. However, the impact of these errors can be more or less significant than with screen/film (SF) radiography.

Although the projection of the radiographic image onto the imaging plate is still an analog process, the fact that the image will later be digitized imposes special considerations on the radiographic examination. Unlike SF, smaller format CR cassettes provide better spatial resolution than large format CR cassettes because of reduced pixel dimensions at the same matrix size. Although one would expect to encounter worse noise characteristics and less contrast detectability with smaller pixels, smaller cassettes are used to overcome historical criticism of CR for its limited spatial frequency resolution. The autoranging and contrast rescaling features of CR help offset detectability losses from noise.

Obtaining multiple images on one plate, a good conventional practice, is counterproductive with CR because it requires a larger format cassette, and the single digital image file cannot be independently manipulated by view. Use of multiple collimation fields on a plate may confuse image processing software that is important in developing the digital image. Different views sometimes require individualized processing. Unlike conventional radiography, technologists must take care to distinguish which view each CR cassette contains for multiple view examinations.

Unless the display device is sophisticated, images captured on different-sized cassettes are displayed at different default magnifications. This complicates comparisons between views within an exam or with historical exams acquired on different-sized cassettes (Willis et al. 1998).

The position of the radiation field on the cassette affects the CR image, therefore, collimation and light-field convergence are more critical to image quality than in SF imaging. The position and orientation of the patient, as well as the extent of the anatomy that is included within the collimation field, affects the appearance of the processed image (Nakajima et al. 1993). Interference with the collimation boundary, such as misplacement of a letter marker, intersection of the boundary by a metallic implant, collimation nonparallel to the cassette edges, off-center collimation, or even nonperpendicular collimation can cause errors.

Association of patient demographics with the image can be a source of error. Manual data entry is prone to error. Isolated electronic systems for demographics require duplicate data entry. Newer CR systems include interfaces to the radiology information system (RIS) to retrieve patient demographics. These systems can be augmented with bar code scanners to further reduce errors. The latest systems include Digital Imaging and Communications in Medicine (DICOM) Modality Worklist functions. Demographics for exams that are scheduled in the RIS are automatically available to the resource where the exam will be performed. The Modality Worklist is of limited value for unscheduled exams, and may be too specific when resources are reallocated. When incorrect identification occurs, it is important to aggressively correct the data or purge the digital image to preclude proliferation of incorrectly identified electronic copies.

Development of the Image

A new class of errors arises from incorrect image acquisition processing, post-acquisition processing, and management of processing parameters (Oestmann et al. 1991). Selection of the wrong exam type or view can have dramatic effects on the image. When this mistake involves post-acquisition processing, the effects are reversible. When the mistake involves acquisition processing, such as pattern recognition and histogram analysis, the effects are often unrecoverable. Successive generations of Fuji (Fuji Photo Film Co. Ltd., Tokyo, Japan) hardware and software have reduced the system's susceptibility to artifacts. For example, in Fuji scanners prior to the model AC1, the results of acquisition processing of a preliminary low-intensity scan of the imaging plate determined the gain settings for the main scan of the plate. AC-series and FCR 9000-series devices acquire the image under a fixed gain and then use the results of acquisition processing to remap the acquired data to a smaller number of bits per pixel. When this remapping is erroneous, data can be lost. In order to render acquisition processing errors recoverable, the newest FCR 5000 device retains all of the acquired data. Agfa (Ridgefield Park, NJ) maintains the capability to reprocess its CR image at a QC processing station, however, once the image is released as a DICOM image, recovery by reprocessing is limited. Eastman Kodak (Rochester, NY) CR also depends on pattern recognition for determining the meaningful part of the image, so these devices are also subject to processing errors, some of which may be irreversible.

There are 5040 total post-acquisition processing parameter entries for 3 renditions each of 240 exam types in the standard Fuji CR software. An additional 3 parameters are needed for each rendition and exam type if "dynamic range control" (DRC) is implemented. These basic exam types are typically augmented with a multitude of customized exam types (89 in one hospital). Subtle differences in numerical values of parameters, such as the difference between -0.50 and -0.05, are difficult for a human observer to discern, but can have pronounced effects on the resulting image. The parameter values can be different from one individual machine to another. These parameters can be modified by unsupervised personnel unless precautions are taken to prevent changes without service intervention. The parameters can also change when new software is introduced into the scanner. The magnitude of the complexity and variability demands a method of automated management of parameter values. Fuji service engineers can download and upload parameters via a laptop computer.

Agfa has a similar magnitude of complexity with regard to processing parameters. On the surface, each examination and view is specified by 4 processing parameter values, a default look-up-table (LUT), and 2 window offsets. Beyond this, the exam and view has a default speed class, erasure time, and default pattern recognition for collimation. Agfa service and applications personnel customize and manage the configuration of each machine with a laptop computer, however, software for inspecting this large number of parameters is lacking.

There is no general agreement on which processing algorithms are optimal. A recent survey of Japanese hospitals shows a wide variation in processing values in clinical use (JSRT 1995). A lack of deviation from the manufacturer's standard set does not always indicate satisfaction: variation in practice means that some exams are seldom or never used in certain hospitals. Processing parameters are sometimes changed capriciously when the actual source of image quality problems is inappropriate technique, improper equipment calibration, or technologist error. New exam types that are created by the user should be based on exams for similar anatomy, otherwise acquisition processing errors are likely. The important point in terms of QA is that the modification of default processing should be approached in a deliberate manner, should ultimately be a radiologist's decision; and it should be well-documented and reexamined later to ensure that the change resulted in a net improvement.

CR images passed from the acquisition system may not even include the post-acquisition processing, depending on the interface between the CR and the Picture Archiving and Communication System (PACS). CR systems were initially designed to produce hard-copy images. Many early interfaces depended on the Digital Acquisition System Manager (DASM) from Analogic Corporation (Peabody, MA). The DASM converts the proprietary Fuji DMS communications into industry standard SCSII (Small Computer Standard for Information Interchange). Unfortunately, the image data passed by the DASM is "raw, ranged data," which includes the effects of acquisition processing, but not post-acquisition processing. By either reverse engineering (Templeton et al. 1992) or by licensing agreements, interface manufacturers have been able to apply post-acquisition processing according to instructions passed in the file header. As a result, soft-copy diagnosis at some PACS installations does not benefit from the image enhancement. Even when the standard CR image file is processed, the presence of processing depends on proper configuration of the interface.

Correction of Suboptimal Images

Technologists expect for the first image to be acceptable. Corrections tend to be by "trial-and-error." Modifications that make good sense with SF imaging do not work the same way with CR. Increasing mAs improves only noise, not density or contrast. Changing kilovolt peak value affects contrast, penetration, scatter, and plate efficiency, all of which interact to affect the processing that determines the ultimate image. Even with full-functionality postprocessing workstations, quality-control technologists are likely to depend only on speed shift and contrast shifts when trying to recover suboptimal images.

While there are clear reasons why the technologist needs the ability to reorient and annotate the image at a quality control workstation, there are other reasons why routine modification of the image by the technologist may be counterproductive. Even if care is taken to provide identical viewing conditions for the technologist and radiologist, the technologist is only trained to recognize anatomy, rather than pathology. Because inappropriate image processing can mask important clinical features, and some image processing can be irreversible after the image is released, powerful reprocessing functions should be reserved to the radiologist. A technologist should use image processing as a last resort in order to recover a nondiagnostic image in order to avoid a repeated examination.

In a setting where primary diagnosis is made from the laser-printed CR image, wasted film is a key quality-assurance indicator. The sources of wasted film can be repeated examinations, or reprinted examinations that require no additional radiation exposure to the patient to correct a nondiagnostic image. Exams that are often reprinted are candidates for modification of processing parameters. Collimation errors are a new source of positioning repeats.

New artifacts are observed with CR, some of which have correspondence with SF artifacts (Oestmann et al. 1991; Solomon et al. 1991; Volpe et al. 1996; Willis 1999). These include dust particles on the imaging plates, scratches or cracks in the plate, and dust on light collection optics. Some CR scanners track the unique identity of each imaging plate, and in this case it is straightforward to select and examine the suspected plate for debris or permanent damage. In scanners where the identity of the plate is not followed, some hospitals have marked each plate in a peripheral location with a unique identifier. In systems where the imaging plate is not habitually associated with an individual cassette, isolating problems with the cassette is more difficult.

Aliasing and *moiré* patterns due to interactions of fixed grid lines and the sampling matrix have been reported. This effect can also be accentuated by inopportune selection of magnification factor during display of the digital image. The sampling matrix differs among manufacturers, models, and cassette sizes. Some pixel dimensions are non-square, so effects can be apparent in one cassette orientation and absent in another. These artifacts can be eliminated by matching the cassette size with a grid line rate that is either high enough not to be resolved by the sampling matrix or low enough to be well-resolved. The former solution is expensive and may require more radiation exposure to the patient. The latter puts grid lines on the image, which radiologists are accustomed to since the introduction of scatter reduction grids, but may be accentuated by image processing.

A combination of the increased sensitivity of CR to scattered radiation and the lack of lead backing on early CR cassettes produced the "tombstone" artifact, which was the image of a clip on the back of the imaging cassette (Tucker et al. 1993). This clip is also clear evidence of another error, namely, reverse cassette orientation during exposure. On cassettes that do not have the clip, other features of the reverse of the cassette may be a sign of reverse orientation. Otherwise, there is an unusually low signal acquired from the reverse exposure of the "single emulsion" imaging plate, especially if the primary beam has to traverse lead backing. The "lightbulb" effect, artifactual darkening of the periphery in obese patients, has also been attributed to the increased sensitivity of CR to scatter (Solomon et al. 1991). Increased sensitivity to scatter increases the consequences of poor practice such as storing cassettes inside fluoroscopic examination rooms, and it encourages the use of grids on all patients regardless of size.

Double exposures can arise from the traditional source, but they can also be caused by erasure failure secondary to lamp failure or overexposure. Double exposures can also be associated with interrupted power and data communications errors.

Other artifacts include accentuation of the edges of photodetectors caused by unsharp masking, clipping of data in the hilar regions of the lung caused by inappropriate gradation processing, and clipping of data in the clavicular region associated with overexposure.

Control of Exposure Factor Selection

In conventional radiography, the primary indicator of incorrect technique is a film that is too dark or too light. This indicator is not useful with CR, because of the density equalization that CR provides (Freedman et al. 1993). Routine QA must monitor a digital indicator of exposure to the imaging plate (see Figure 1) (Willis et al. 1995). There are many factors that affect the absolute accuracy of this exposure indicator. Thus, the numerical indication of improper exposure is a derived quantity subject to interpretation. It is clear that the distribution of the exposure index is much narrower with phototimed examinations than those using manual technique; this finding suggests that the indicator is a valid index of radiation exposure.

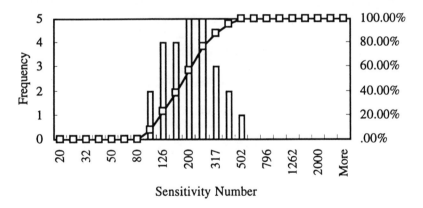

Figure 1. The frequency distribution of the exposure index, "Sensitivity." The data was collected from 1206 clinical CR images including 43 different exam types acquired using manual technique without guidance as to exposure index. The x-axis shows the maximum Sensitivity (S number) of the histogram interval. The "Frequency" axis shows the number of images within each interval. The right-hand axis is the key for the cumulative distribution (curved line). The linear version reveals little about the distribution. The log-linear version (shown) resembles a symmetric normal distribution. The log-normal model facilitates the use of descriptive statistics. The mean for this distribution is 245. The distribution is mesokurtic and slightly skewed to the right. Subpopulations of the data set can be compared to the parent distribution to assess the statistical significance of differences as an indicator of systematic overexposure or underexposure. When the exposure index is reported as part of the image file header, this data can be collected and analyzed automatically.

The wide exposure latitude of CR has been credited with substantial reductions in repeats, especially in portable exams which lack automatic exposure control (Sagel et al. 1990). This feature also means that CR is more tolerant of overexposure than SF imaging; this increased tolerance is another possible explanation for the reduced repeat rate (Schaefer et al. 1989). Other factors that can cause a decreased repeat rate include systematic under-reporting and reluctance to repeat an examination without confidence that the repeated exam will yield substantially improved quality.

Although the notion of overexposure in CR was raised in the context of management of patient radiation exposures, it is not obvious that overexposure can have a negative impact on image quality. Although the autoranging function of CR allows compensation over a wide range of exposures, there is a limit of adjustment. At the point where the range of subject contrast in the image can no longer be accommodated by the remaining dynamic range of the system, data is clipped at the extremes. Thus, over-exposure can result in loss of light areas and dark regions.

In practice, underexposure is less of a problem, because radiologists begin to complain about the "quantum mottle" in the image at one-half to one-fourth of the usual exposure. This effect may be modulated by the quantity and kernel size of edge enhancement applied to the image. Lower exposures, which contain more noise, can generally tolerate less enhancement than high exposures.

The literature is equivocal about the radiographic speed of CR relative to SF imaging (Dobbins et al. 1992). A recent report correlated observers' evaluation of noise with the exposure indicator to establish a speed for CR exams (Huda et al. 1996). Direct comparisons of CR and SF in the literature are of limited value because they neglect to address how the scanners were calibrated. These reports lack details to show that the SF was operating at the proper speed, and they compare the two systems using the SF technique chart. The absorption of energy by the imaging plate is very different from most conventional screens (Boguki et al. 1995); therefore the technique chart may be quite different from that used in conventional radiology. For example, the appropriate kVp for a SF receptor with a k-edge of 50 keV might need to be reduced by 10 kVp to accommodate CR with a k-edge of 37 keV. The disparity between SF and CR technique is most apparent when a hospital reverts to SF temporarily because of CR equipment downtime.

CR imaging plates come in different varieties and generations of manufacture. There are two general speed classes: thick plates (standard type, general purpose) and thin plates (high resolution, high definition) that require two to three times more radiation exposure to produce the same signal as the thick plates. Recent high resolution options introduced by Fuji and Agfa provide higher definition images by modified sampling of standard type plates. As with SF, it is possible for the technologist to confuse the speed classes and their associated techniques, but with CR the autoranging compensates for this mistake. Within the speed classes there have been six commercial generations of

Fuji plates, three Agfa types, and at least two Kodak types. Because the sensitivity to radiation and light output varies among generations, mixed generations of plates introduces undesired variability. It is important to calibrate the CR scanner for the particular imaging plates to be used. In early generations of imaging plates, the output varied widely among individual plates, to such an extent that each plate needed to be tested. Our experience with later generations is that manufacturing quality control has improved to the degree that such comprehensive testing may no longer be necessary.

Adjustment of phototimers is also problematic, because there is no widely accepted method for setting phototimers for use with CR. Phototimers are usually adjusted by using a standard technique and phantom to obtain a particular density on SF images. In normal operating modes, CR autoranging delivers a uniform density regardless of phototimer setting. Phototimers could be set up by the conventional method (with SF) and then used for CR. This does not take into account the different composition and backscatter characteristics of the CR cassette and plate, much less any differences in speed. Typically, institutions that use SF phototimer setup also use +2 density steps to acquire satisfactory exams. Phototimers could be adjusted in normal CR operating modes by disregarding density and targeting either a value of the exposure index or a specific entrance exposure. The validity of the exposure index in normal operating modes depends to a large extent on how faithfully the phantom approximates human anatomic structures in terms of subject contrast. Phototimers can be adjusted in CR test modes to achieve desired density or pixel value, exposure index, or entrance exposure. In this case, an anthropomorphic phantom is not necessary: an American National Standards Institute (ANSI) or Center for Devices and Radiological Health (CDRH) phantom can be used (Conway et al. 1984). The problem is in extrapolating CR performance in test modes to normal operating conditions.

Interpretation of the Image

Reduced display formats of the 26 cm × 36 cm hardcopy output and "two-up" format complicate measurements and comparisons to historical SF images and other views. As mentioned above, different magnification of CR exams and views can also cause confusion. Conventional alternators need masking to accommodate the smaller format films. Manufacturers are moving to 14 × 17 inch (35 × 43 cm) hard-copy output, but different magnification remains a complication for soft-copy display of CR.

Radiologists are often uncertain about whether a difference in appearance on CR is a true clinical feature or the result of image processing. Radiologists report the subjective impression that they are overcalling interstitial lung disease because of the accentuation of lung markings in CR. No single rendering seems appropriate for low contrast and high frequency features, which was the original motivation for the "two-up" format. There is a tendency to regard the image presentation problem as transitory, because when fully-functional digital workstations are available, the observer will be able to modify the image at will. However, even with soft-copy diagnosis, the initial presentation of the image is likely to be important in expediting review of normal studies and in raising the radiologist's level of suspicion to a point where he will employ additional tools to enhance the presentation of subtle clinical features. Any system that routinely depends on the QC technologist or the radiologist to adjust the appearance of the image does not make efficient use of imaging resources.

The technical literature reflects concern about the detectability of cortical bone lesions (Prokop et al. 1990), pleural effusions, obstructive disease, pneumothorax, interstitial disease, parenchymal masses with CR (Blume and Jost 1992; Chotas and Ravin 1992). Basically, most radiologists have not yet established a "comfort level" with CR. A major goal of any QA plan must be to provide the radiologist with assurance that the images being viewed contain all the relevant clinical features.

Elements of a Comprehensive QA Program

Acceptance Testing

Gray and Stears (1994) describe AT as a part of the process of acquisition of medical imaging equipment. They recommend that AT for imaging devices should measure image quality of the system rather than simple conformance to engineering specifications. The clinical significance of performance variations in CR is largely undocumented, unlike SF radiography. Standardization of tests and criteria for abnormal performance are sorely needed. To this end, the American Association of Physicists in Medicine (AAPM) chartered Task Group Number 10, whose recommendations are available in draft form. The Task Group's recommendations are based on pioneering work by Seibert (1994), results from 16 individual scanners fielded by the U.S. Military (Willis et al. 1994), the experiences of task group members (Huda et al. 1995), other academicians (Jafroudi et al. 1995), and information provided by CR manufacturers (Boguki 1997).

In addition to ensuring that the device and accessories match the contract and constituting a baseline for QC measurements, thorough AT provides an opportunity to become familiar with device functions and controls. It is especially worthwhile to test manufacturer's claims of performance that are critical to your particular institution. For example, throughput may have been an important consideration in the selection or configuration of the CR hardware, and in this case, AT should reflect this.

Because of automatic image processing, test objects that worked well with SF may not adequately simulate the human anatomy with CR, leading to erroneous interpretations (Chotas and Ravin 1992). Definitive physical measurements of imaging performance are too complex for routine clinical use (Metz et al. 1995). While new test objects have been developed specifically for CR, their practical value remains to be established in routine clinical practice (Cowen et al. 1993; Workman and Cowen 1993). Agfa provides three specialized test objects, with software for automatic interpretation of two. Fuji recently introduced their first CR test object.

Physicists should oversee installation and configuration of the CR hardware. They should ensure that the alphanumeric data recording features are configured to uniquely identify the scanner and to report the exposure index. They should make sure the hard-copy recording or soft-copy display devices are properly adjusted. They should ensure that the light-collection systems are calibrated according to manufacturer's specifications.

Before acceptance testing, medical physicists should ensure that the test equipment is within calibration and that there is access to an x-ray generator that has accurate and reproducible output. Physicists should review the manufacturer's documentation and develop a plan. They should coordinate his plan with the vendor's service personnel and with the radiology department so that the room and scanner can be monopolized for the duration of testing.

The first phase of AT is to conduct a component inventory and inspection. Each imaging plate should be inspected and the serial number, size, and type should be recorded. A bar code scanner can expedite this process. Each plate should be cleaned and erased before introduction into clinical use. The condition and external markings of each cassette should be inspected, and the cassette serial number and type should be recorded. The scanner's error log should be viewed and contents recorded. The settings of user-programmable parameters should be verified and recorded. The software version and serial numbers of all hardware end-items should be recorded.

AT of image output devices should precede any checks of the scanner. This testing can be accomplished by checking the laser printer and processor by means of internal test patterns or sensitometry. The soft-copy display can be calibrated by means of a digital Society of Motion Picture and Television Engineers (SMPTE) test pattern (Gray 1994). The display can be matched to the laser printer output using the SMPTE test pattern or the CR image of a step wedge.

Image checks should be conducted to verify CR calibration, autoranging, and uniformity. Variations in the mechanical motions of the scanner can be checked from the radiographic projection of two metal straightedges oriented along each scanning axis. The dynamic range of the scanner can be determined from multiple exposures of a step wedge at different mAs on the same imaging plate. The limit of spatial resolution is determined from the image of two lead bar patterns oriented along the two scanning axes. Contrast detectability is measured from the image of a contrast detail test object, such as the University of Alabama–Birmingham (UAB) phantom (Wagner and Barnes 1991) or Leeds TO.16 (Cowen et al. 1993; Workman and Cowen 1993), using standard beam conditions. Image checks of anthropomorphic chest, skull, and extremity phantoms (abdomen, if available) are made using clinical technique, positioning, phototiming, and image processing. Image checks can also be performed using special test objects provided by the manufacturer.

System checks include measurement of throughput under steady-state conditions. They also include functional checks of exam and patient data interfaces, image data output interfaces, image processing functions, and operator controls. It is also important to check the function of all cassette formats, which can be accomplished during the image checks.

Maintenance

Operator maintenance tasks that have considerable impact on CR image quality include cleaning of the laser printer, processor, and imaging plates. It is important to use the cleaning solvent recommended by the manufacturer, because screen cleaners or aqueous alcohol solutions may damage the protective layer of the imaging plate. Unlike SF radiology, cleanliness needs to be maintained outside the darkroom in the vicinity of the CR scanner and cassette storage areas. Cassettes, themselves, must be kept clean to avoid introducing dust, tape, letter markers, contrast agents, and blood into the scanner via the cassettes. Older CR cassettes have not proven as sturdy as SF cassettes, however new cassette designs may prove to be more durable. Scanner jams are more complex than jams in either automatic film processors and daylight loaders, and they require service intervention.

Organizational maintenance tasks that affect CR image quality include convergence of light and x-ray fields, scanner sensitivity calibration, periodic scanner maintenance, and software upgrades. It is important to perform tests to verify CR performance following any major service event, including relocation of the scanner, any software upgrade, any change in the type of imaging plate, and any service of the laser or light collection system. It is essential to maintain a comprehensive log of downtime for each scanner, and to record routine operator maintenance, preventive maintenance, and software configuration changes. The capital investment in each scanner is such that, unlike film processors, redundancy is not always possible; so the impact of downtime is critical to the department's function. For this reason, it is wise to consider arranging for factory training of in-house clinical engineering personnel for first-call purposes.

Quality Control

QC has several aspects: concurrent assessments by the technologist as images are produced, periodic tests at regular intervals, retrospective assessments in which data collected from many images are analyzed for trends, and incidental tests conducted to troubleshoot problems or follow up corrective actions.

Technologists inspect the image when it is produced to determine whether the patient can be released or whether the view must be repeated. Although the premier consideration is the appearance of the image and the clinical question to be addressed, numeric guidance based on exposure index is helpful to the technologist in reaching a decision (Table 1). The intent of the inspection is to prevent nondiagnostic images from being forwarded to the radiologist for interpretation. It is important that the viewing conditions be similar for both the technologist and the radiologist. Where image modification is possible, the technologist should attempt to recover nondiagnostic images before repeating the exposure. There is little to be gained by repeating a view without a significant change in kVp value, collimation, patient positioning, or examination type. In a filmless environment, nondiagnostic images can conveniently disappear without a trace. Repeats should be recorded according to examination type, reason for repeat, exposure index, and technologist. These records form the basis for retrospective assessments (Table 2). Unexplained nondiagnostic images should be retained for use in consultations with vendor applications personnel.

Table 1. Reasons for repeated examinations. Percentages of the total of 1043 repeated examinations. These data were collected from analysis of repeated examinations from a one-month period in a hospital using CR.

REASON	NUMBER	PERCENTAGE (%)
Positioning	489	46.9
Overexposed	122	11.7
Underexposed	105	10.1
Reprinted	89	8.5
Motion	57	5.5
Wrong exam code	54	5.1
Over-collimated	40	3.8
Artifact	23	2.2
No exposure	21	2.0
Double exposed	17	1.6
No marker	10	1.0
Marker over part	8	0.8
Other	8	0.8
TOTAL	1043	

Table 2. QC evaluation based on exposure index.

SENSITIVITY (S NUMBER)	AGFA (lgM)	KODAK (Exposure Index)	INDICATION
>1000	<1.45	<1250	Underexposed -repeat view
601-1000	1.45-1.74	1250-1549	Underexposed -QC exception required
301-600	1.75-2.04	1550-1849	Underexposed -QC approval required
150-300	2.05-2.35	1850-2150	Acceptable range
75-149	2.36-2.65	2151-2450	Overexposed -QC approval required
50-74	2.66-2.95	2451-2750	Overexposed -QC exception required
<50	>2.95	>2750	Overexposed -repeat view

Periodic tests should include a subset of image checks that are also used in AT. The uniformity check is useful in demonstrating proper calibration and the condition of the light collection optics. The contrast detectability check should be the most sensitive method for detecting noise problems in the system, but it is limited by the subjectivity and variability of scoring by human observers. Images of appropriate anthropomorphic phantoms help show problems in image processing that might otherwise go undetected.

Periodic tests include operator checks and adjustment of laser printer output devices. Although laser output devices incorporate self-adjustment mechanisms, these are not without problems, even when used judiciously (Huda et al. 1993). Because laser printers do not indicate how much they have self-adjusted, they may mask a chemistry problem until the problem becomes catastrophic. Another problem arises when there is a discrepancy between the internal density measurement and an external densitometer.

Technologist Training

CR technology is not included in the curriculum of the usual training program for radiologic technologists. When CR devices are installed, the vendor usually provides some initial applications training. Thereafter, applications assistance is available from the vendor or from other sources at additional cost. Even if novice users are sophisticated enough to internalize the initial training, retention of knowledge gained in initial training is transient, and personnel turnovers are frequent. Institutions using CR must develop their own internal training programs.

The training program needs to address initial orientation of new technologists and continuing education for existing technologists. New technologists need to have a general overview of CR technology, information on the specific practice of CR at the local institution, and hands-on training with the CR hardware that is supervised by an experienced technologist for at least one week. At the end of this period, the supervisor should be able to certify the technologist's clinical competency to perform CR examinations independently.

In addition to the usual recurring technologist topics, in-service training should review CR technology, the effect of CR autoranging on As-Low-As-Reasonably-Achievable (ALARA) principles, operator maintenance functions, acquisition processing and collimation rules, post-acquisition image processing, CR artifacts, problem examinations including measurement and positioning, and bedside examinations including alignment of grid and x-ray beam. Every effort should be made to encourage participation and feedback from the technologist audience. Training that incorporates a practicum is especially effective. Video training films should be considered, especially when the content of a topic is relatively constant. These videos can be used for individual remedial training when necessary. Reference materials including applications manuals, reference books, and selected journal articles need to be readily available to technologists.

Radiologist Oversight and Feedback

Active participation by the radiologist is often overlooked as a key element to the success of any QA program. All too often the radiologist's valuable incidental guidance corrects only immediate problems in image quality without addressing habitual deficiencies. The radiologist's film critique is a mechanism for documenting the causes and frequency of substandard imaging. A list of codes is provided to each radiologist to dictate into the report. The codes include comments on both image availability and quality. When transcribed into the RIS, automated reports can be generated to establish individual responsibility for service and monitor improvement.

Conclusions

The inherent complexity of CR demands additional initial training and continuing education for technologists, radiologists, clinical engineers, and physicists. Existing QA resources must be redirected and additional QA resources are required. Detailed backup planning is required for system downtime. Redundancy should be considered in the form of duplicate hardware or networking. Realization of the anticipated economic benefit of CR may be adversely affected.

CR is the only credible technology available that supports large-scale PACS or high-volume teleradiology. CR obviates image contention between radiologists and clinicians by enabling electronic distribution of images and providing unlimited reprint capability. CR provides more consistent quality of portable examinations. CR allows post-acquisition image manipulation. CR affords lost image recovery by reprinting and allows daylight processing of plain radiographs. Only through conscientious, comprehensive QA efforts can we realize the full benefits of CR technology.

References

Blume, H. and Jost, G. "Chest imaging within the radiology department by means of photostimulable phosphor computed radiography: a review." *J Dig Imag.* 5:67-78; 1992.

Boguki, T.M., Trauernicht, D.P., and Kocher, T.E. Characteristics of a Storage Phosphor System for Medical Imaging. Technical and Scientific Monograph No. 6. Rochester, NY: Eastman Kodak. 5; 1995.

Boguki, T.M. Acceptance Testing and Quality Control of Computed Radiography Systems. Technical and Scientific Bulletin. Cat No. 879 2038. Rochester, NY: Eastman Kodak 1997.

Conway, B.J., Butler, P.F., Duff, J.E., Fewell, T.R., Gross, R.E., Jennings, R.J., Koustenis, G.H., McCrohan, J.L., Rueter, F.G., and Showalter, C.K. "Beam quality independent attenuation phantom for estimating patient exposure from x-ray automatic exposure controlled chest examinations." *Med Phys* 11(6): 827-832; 1984.

Chotas, H.G. and Ravin, C.E. "Digital chest radiography with storage phosphor systems: potential masking of bilateral pleural effusions." *J Dig Imag.* 5: 14-19; 1992.

Cowen, A.R., Workman, A., and Price, J.S. "Physical aspects of photostimulable phosphor computed radiography." *Brit J of Radiol.* 66: 322-345; 1993.

Dobbins, J.T. III, Rice, J.J., Beam, C.A., and Ravin, C.E. "Threshold perception performance with computed and screen-film radiography: implications for chest radiography." *Radiology* 183: 179-187; 1992.

Dobbins, J.T. III, Ergun, D.L., Rutz, L., Hinshaw, D.A., Blume, H., and Clark, D.C. "DQE(f) of four generations of computed radiography acquisition devices." *Med Phys.* 22(10): 1581-1593; 1995.

Freedman, M., Pe, E., Mun, S.K., Lo, S.C.B., and Nelson, M. "The potential for unnecessary patient exposure from the use of storage phosphor imaging systems." *Proc SPIE.* 1897: 472-479; 1993.

Gray, J.E. and Stears, J.G. "Acceptance testing of diagnostic x-ray imaging equipment: considerations and rationale." In: *Specification, Acceptance Testing and Quality Control of Diagnostic X-ray Imaging Equipment.* Seibert, J.A., Barnes, G.T., and Gould, R.G., (Eds.) Medical Physics Monograph No. 20. Woodbury, NY: American Association of Physicists in Medicine. 1-9; 1994.

Gray, J.E. "Multiformat video and laser camera acceptance testing (and quality control)." In: *Specification, Acceptance Testing and Quality Control of Diagnostic X-ray Imaging Equipment.* Seibert, J.A., Barnes, G.T., and Gould, R.G., (Eds.) Medical Physics Monograph No. 20. Woodbury, NY: American Association of Physicists in Medicine. 955-964; 1994.

Huda, W., Jing, Z., and Hoyle, B.A. "Film density calibration for computed radiography systems: is the standard three-point procedure accurate?" *Radiology* 188: 875-877; 1993.

Huda, W., Arreola, M., and Jing, Z. "Computed radiography acceptance testing." *Proc SPIE.* 2432: 512-521; 1995.

Huda, W., Slone, R.M., Belden, C.J., Williams, J.L., Cumming, W.A., and Palmer, C.K. "Mottle on computed radiographs of the chest in pediatric patients." *Radiology* 199:249-252; 1996.

Jafroudi, H., Steller, D., Freedman, M., and Mun, S.K. "Quality control on storage phosphor digital radiography systems." *Proc. SPIE.* 2432: 563-577; 1995.

Kato, H. "Photostimulable phosphor radiography design considerations." In: *Specification, Acceptance Testing and Quality Control of Diagnostic X-ray Imaging Equipment.* Seibert, J.A., Barnes, G.T., and Gould, R.G., (Eds.) Medical Physics Monograph No. 20. Woodbury, NY: American Association of Physicists in Medicine. 731-770; 1994.

Metz, C.E., Wagner, R.F., Doi, K., Brown, D.G., Nishikawa, R.M., and Myers, K.J. "Toward consensus on quantitative assessment of medical imaging systems." *Med Phys.* 22(7): 1057-1061; 1995.

Nakajima, N., Takeo, H., Ishida, M., and Nagata, T. "Automatic setting functions for image density and range in the FCR system." Fuji Computed Radiography Technical Review No. 3. Tokyo, Japan: Fuji Photo Film Co., Ltd. 23; 1993.

National Council on Radiation Protection and Measurements. "Quality assurance for diagnostic imaging." NCRP Report No 99. Bethesda, MD. 1; 1988.

Seibert, J.A. "Photostimulable phosphor system acceptance testing." In: *Specification, Acceptance Testing and Quality Control of Diagnostic X-ray Imaging Equipment.* Seibert, J.A., Barnes, G.T., and Gould, R.G., (Eds.) Medical Physics Monograph No. 20. Woodbury, NY: American Association of Physicists in Medicine. 771-800; 1994.

Oestmann, J.W., Prokop, M., Schaefer, C.M., and Galanski, M. "Hardware and software artifacts in storage phosphor radiography." *RadioGraphics* 11: 795-805; 1991.

Prokop, M., Galanski, M., Oestmann, J.W., von Falkenhausen, U., Rosenthal, H., Reimer, P., Nischelsky, J., and Reichelt, S. "Storage phosphor versus screen-film radiography: effect of varying exposure parameters and unsharp mask filtering on the detectability of cortical bone defects." *Radiology* 177: 109-113; 1990.

Sagel, S.S., Jost, R.G., Glazer, H.S., Molina, P.L., Anderson, D.J., Solomon, S.L., and Schwarber, J. "Digital mobile radiography." *J Thorac Imag.* 5(1): 36-48; 1990.

Schaefer, C.M., Greene, R.E. Oestmann, J.W., Kamalsky, J., Hall, D.A., Llevellyn, H.J., Robertson, C., Rhea, J., Rosenthal, H., Ruebens, J.R., Shepard, J., and Templeton, P.A. "Improved control of image optical density with low-dose digital and conventional radiography in bedside imaging." *Radiology* 173: 713-714; 1989.

Society of Radiological Technology. Processing of CR in current practice. *Computed Radiography.* Chapter 11. 6: 106-136; 1995. (Japanese).

Solomon, S.L., Jost, R.G., Glazer, H.S., Sagel, S.S., Anderson, D.J., and Molina, P.L. "Artifacts in computed radiography." *AJR.* 157(1): 181-185; 1991.

Templeton, A.W., Wetzel, L.H., Cook, L.T., Harrison, L.A., Eckard, D.A., Anderson, W.H., and Hensley, K.S. "Enhancement of storage phosphor plate images: a C-language program." *J Dig Imag.* 5(1): 59-63; 1992.

Tucker, D.M., Souto, M., and Barnes, G.T. "Scatter in computed radiography." *Radiology* 188: 271-274; 1993.

Volpe, J.P., Storto, M.L., Andriole, K.P., and Famsu, G. "Artifacts in chest radiography with a third generation computed radiography system." *AJR.* 166: 653-657; 1996.

Wagner, A.J. and Barnes, G.T. "Assessing fluoroscopic contrast resolution: a practical and quantitative test tool." *Med Phys.* 18: 894-899; 1991.

Willis, C.E., Weiser, J.C., Leckie, R.G., Romlein, J., and Norton, G. "Optimization and quality control of computed radiography." *Proc. SPIE.* 2164: 178-185; 1994.

Willis, C.E., Leckie, R.G., Carter, J., Williamson, M.P., Scotti, S.D., and Norton, G. "Objective measures of quality assurance in a computed radiography-based radiology department." *Proc. SPIE.* 2432: 588-599; 1995.

Willis, C.E., Mercier, J., and Patel, M. "Modification of conventional quality assurance procedures to accommodate computed radiography." 13th Conference on Computer Applications in Radiology. Denver, Colorado. pp. 275-281; 1996.

Willis, C.E., Parker, B.R., Orand, M., and Wagner, M.L. "Challenges for pediatric radiology using computed radiography." *J Dig Imag.* 11 (3) Suppl 1 (August):156-158; 1998.

Willis, C.E. "Chapter 7. Computed radiography imaging and artifacts." *Filmless Radiology.* Siegel and Kolodner eds. New York: Springer-Verlag. 137-154; 1999.

Workman, A. and Cowen, A.R. "Signal, noise, and SNR transfer properties of computed radiography." *Phys Med Biol.* 38: 1789-1808; 1993.

Digital Mammography

Martin J. Yaffe, Ph. D.
Imaging/Bioengineering Research
Sunnybrook and Women's College Health Sciences Centre
and Departments of Medical Imaging and Medical Biophysics,
University of Toronto,
Toronto, Canada

Introduction

Breast cancer is a major killer of women. Approximately 179,000 women were diagnosed with breast cancer in the United States in 1998 and 43,500 women died of this disease (Landis et al. 1998).

Mortality from breast cancer can be reduced if the cancer is detected *in situ* (within the ductal system) or when it is minimally invasive and before metastasis has occurred to the point that treatment is ineffective (Smart et al. 1995, Tabar et al. 1995). This is most likely to be the case when the cancer is small and the most effective means currently available for detecting small cancers is x-ray mammography.

Mammography is used both for investigating symptomatic patients (diagnostic mammography) and for screening of asymptomatic women in selected age groups. It is also used for pre-surgical localization of suspicious areas and in the guidance of needle biopsies.

Challenges in Imaging the Breast

To provide visualization of the key signs of disease, the imaging system must precisely measure the transmitted x-ray intensity through all regions of the breast and must amplify the small level of attenuation contrast to produce visible signals. Important information is contained in the fine detail associated with microcalcifications and thin fibers radiating from the tumor mass, and, therefore, the spatial resolution of the imaging system must be very high. Because of these requirements, mammography is one of the most technically demanding radiological imaging techniques.

Screen-film Mammography

Screen-film mammography is, and will continue to be a valuable tool for detection and diagnosis of breast cancer and is the only tool that, up to now, has been demonstrated to have a role in reducing mortality from this disease through early detection as part of a routine screening program. Screen-film mammography has several distinct advantages including:

(a) The technology is relatively inexpensive and robust.

(b) The receptor provides very high spatial resolution—in excess of 20 line-pairs/mm limiting resolution.

(c) Images are conveniently displayed using viewbox technology. Multiple images can be displayed simultaneously.

(d) Film provides an inherent logarithmic compression of dynamic range onto the available optical densities of the film. This often provides an acceptable rendition of information acquired in the mammogram in a single presentation, without the need to adjust display parameters.

Limitations of *Screen-film Mammography*

In screen-film mammography the film must act as an image acquisition detector as well as a storage and display device. It performs very well in providing excellent spatial resolution of high contrast structures and is an efficient medium for long-term storage of image data. As in any situation, however, where many jobs must be done simultaneously, certain compromises result and these are discussed below.

Contrast/latitude

Breast tumors and microcalcifications are visualized in the mammogram due to differential x-ray attenuation between these structures and normal breast tissue. The overall displayed contrast of structures on the mammogram results from this "attenuation contrast" combined with the photographic (optical density) gradient of the mammographic film.

Figure 1 shows measured x-ray attenuation coefficients of fibroglandular breast tissue, fat and breast carcinoma versus x-ray energy (Johns et al. 1987). The very small differences between these curves illustrate why mammography is such a challenging imaging task, particularly when the tumor is surrounded by fibroglandular tissue. As shown in Figure 2, attenuation contrast decreases rapidly with increasing x-ray energy. In order to maximize attenuation contrast, mammography is conventionally carried out with low energy x-ray spectra, typically using a molybdenum anode x-ray tube operated at a potential of approximately 26 kVp with additional molybdenum beam filtration. The breast attenuates x-rays very strongly at these energies, and, therefore, to obtain adequate signal from the image receptor, a relatively high dose compared to general radiography (>1 mGy mean glandular dose per image) is received by the breast.

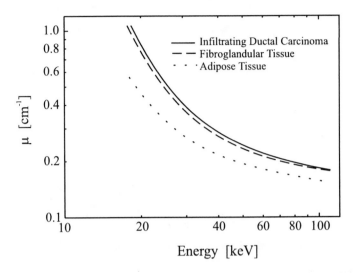

Figure 1. Linear attenuation coefficients of breast tissue types versus x-ray energy.

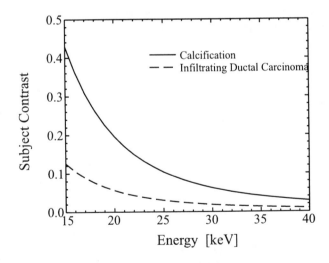

Figure 2. Attenuation contrast for tumor and microcalcification versus x-ray energy.
From (Johns and Yaffe 1987).

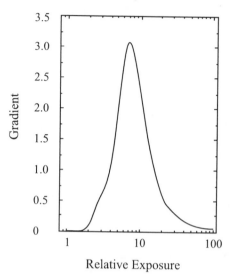

Figure 3. Gradient of mammography film.

The display contrast properties of the radiographic film are described by the gradient of its characteristic curve. Because of its sigmoidal shape, the range of x-ray exposures over which the film display gradient (Figure 3) is significant, i.e., the image latitude, is limited to a factor of about 25. This may be a problem—depending on the composition of the breast, the maximum range of transmitted exposures can be 100:1 or more. If a tumor is located in a very lucent or opaque region of the breast, then, even though the x-ray attenuation contrast is significant, the final contrast displayed to the radiologist may be considerably reduced because of the limited gradient of the film. This is particularly a concern in patients whose breasts contain large amounts of fibroglandular tissue, the so-called DY type breast as defined by Wolfe (Wolfe 1976).

Noise

All radiological images contain random fluctuation or noise due to the statistics of x-ray quantum absorption. This noise can limit the reliability of detection of small or subtle structures. In addition, other sources of noise, due to the structure of the fluorescent screen and the granularity of the film emulsion used to record the image, compound this problem. An ideal imaging system is "quantum-limited," meaning that x-ray quantum noise is the dominant source of random fluctuation. Generally, existing mammographic screen-film systems are not quantum-limited, because at high spatial frequencies, noise in the imaging system is dominated by film granularity and screen structure, not by the number of x-ray quanta recorded.

An imaging system can be made quantum-limited by reducing intrinsic noise sources and by using more x-rays to form the image. For a fixed system speed, the latter is best accomplished by increasing the x-ray interaction efficiency of the screen. When a system is x-ray quantum-limited, further reduction in noise requires an increase in the number of x-rays incident on the imaging system, i.e., an increase in patient dose.

Compromise between resolution and efficiency

Another key limitation of screen-film mammography is the tradeoff between spatial resolution and detector x-ray interaction (detection) efficiency. In a fluorescent screen used with film, spatial resolution is determined mainly by the amount of blur due to diffusion of light travelling from the point of x-ray interaction in the screen to the film. Screen blur increases as the thickness of the screen is increased. To maintain high spatial resolution, mammographic screens must be kept relatively thin. For this reason, the detection efficiency of mammographic systems is compromised, necessitating an increase in radiation dose.

Inefficiency of scatter rejection

Even at the low x-ray energies used in mammography, Compton x-ray scattering is an important process of interaction between the x-ray beam and the breast. The magnitude of scattered x-ray quanta incident on the imaging system is comparable to the intensity of directly transmitted primary radiation (Wagner 1991). Detection of scattered quanta adds a "uniform," noisy background to the image, reduces image contrast, signal-to-noise ratio and the dynamic range available for recording useful information.

Most mammography is performed using a radiographic grid. Although the scattered radiation does not carry useful information, it does generate light from the screen which exposes the film, helping to achieve the required optical density. The loss of this scattered radiation, and inefficiency of the grid in transmitting the desired primary radiation to the screen, results in a requirement of increased radiation dose (by a factor of 2-3) to the patient compared to imaging without a grid (Wagner 1991).

Physics of Digital Mammography

In digital mammography the screen-film image receptor is replaced with a detector which provides an electronic signal proportional to the intensity of x rays transmitted by the breast. The image is digitized, stored in computer memory, then processed and displayed on a video monitor or laser-printed onto film. By separating the image acquisition from the storage and display functions, each can be optimized. Potentially this allows the limitations of screen-film mammography to be overcome and facilitates improved detection or diagnosis of breast cancer.

Technical Requirements of the Detector

Important detector properties for digital mammography are: field coverage, geometrical characteristics, quantum efficiency, sensitivity, spatial resolution, noise characteristics, dynamic range, uniformity, acquisition speed, and cost. For dynamic studies (breast angiography, tomosynthesis), the rate at which sequential images can be acquired is also important.

Field Coverage

The imaging system must be able to record the transmitted x-ray signal over the entire projected area of the breast. Mammography can be accommodated by a receptor of dimensions 18 cm × 24 cm for small and average-size breasts, however, an imaging field of 24 cm × 30 cm may be required to image larger breasts in a single exposure.

Geometric Characteristics

Some of the factors to be considered here are the "dead regions" that may exist within and around the edges of the detector. In an electronic detector used for digital radiography, these might be required for routing of wire leads or placement of auxiliary detector components such as buffers, clocks, etc. Dead regions can also result when a large area detector is produced by abutting together smaller detector units (tiling). For detectors composed of discrete detector elements or "dels" (as distinguished from displayed picture elements or pixels) elements, we define the fill-factor as the fraction of the area of each detector element that is sensitive to the incident x rays. Any dead area within the detector results in inefficient use of the radiation transmitted by the patient. In mammography, it is important that the active area of the detector extends as close to the patient's chest wall as possible to avoid excluding breast tissue from the image. Most screen-film mammography systems lose no more than 3 mm coverage at the chest wall.

Another geometrical factor which must be considered is distortion. A high quality imaging system will present a faithful spatial mapping of the input x-ray pattern to the image output. The image may be scaled spatially, however the scaling factor should be constant over the image field. Distortion will cause this mapping to become non-linear. It may become spatially or angularly dependent. This may be the case when lens, fibre or electron optics are used in the imaging system and give rise to "pin-cushion" or "barrel" distortion.

Digital detectors can be of two general types, captive sensors or replaceable cassettes. In the former, the receptor and its readout are integrated into the x-ray machine. While this requires a specially-designed machine with higher capital cost, it also eliminates the need for loading, unloading and carrying of cassettes to a separate reader and the labor costs involved. As well, the use of a single or a limited number of receptors simplifies the task of correction for non-uniformities of the receptors (see below). A reusable cassette system has the advantage of being compatible with existing mammography units.

Quantum Efficiency

In all x-ray detectors, to produce a signal, the x-ray quanta must interact with the detector material. The probability of interaction or quantum efficiency for quanta of energy $E = h\nu$ is given by:

$$\eta = 1 - e^{-\mu(E)T} \tag{1}$$

where μ is the linear attenuation coefficient of the detector material and T is the active thickness of the detector. The quantum efficiency must be specified at each energy in the spectrum or must be expressed as an "effective" value over the spectrum of x-rays incident on the detector. This spectrum will be influenced by the filtering effect of the patient which is to "harden" the beam, i.e., to make it more energetic and, hence, more penetrating. The quantum efficiency can be increased by making the detector thicker or by using materials which have higher values of μ because of increased atomic number or density. The quantum efficiency versus x-ray energy for various thicknesses of some phosphor and solid state detector materials considered for digital mammography is plotted in Figure 4. The quantum efficiency generally decreases with increasing energy. If the material has an atomic absorption edge in the energy region of interest, then quantum efficiency increases dramatically above this energy, causing a local minimum in η for energies immediately below the absorption edge.

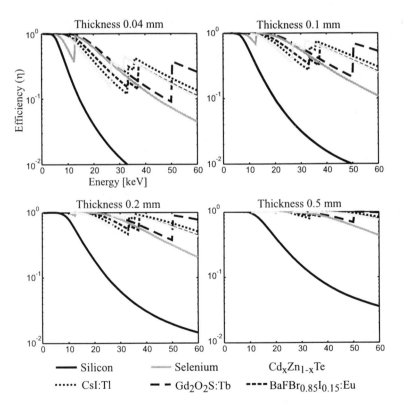

Figure 4. Quantum interaction efficiency, η, of typical detector materials.

Spatial Resolution

Spatial resolution in mammography is determined both by the receptor characteristics and by factors unrelated to the receptor such as penumbra due to the effective size of the x-ray source and the magnification between the anatomical structure of interest and the plane of the image receptor or relative motion between the x-ray source, patient and image receptor during the exposure. Detector-related factors arise from its effective aperture size, spatial sampling interval between measurements and any lateral signal spreading effects within the detector or readout.

Detectors for digital radiography are often composed of discrete dels, generally of constant size and spacing. The dimension of the active portion of each del defines an aperture. The aperture determines the spatial frequency response of the detector. For example, if the aperture is square with dimension, d, then the modulation transfer function (MTF) of the detector will be of the form sinc (f), where f is the spatial frequency along the x or y directions, and the MTF will have its first zero at the frequency $f = d^{-1}$, expressed in the plane of the detector. A detector with $d = 50$ μm will have an MTF with its first zero at $f = 20$ cycles/mm. Because of magnification, this frequency will be higher in a plane within the breast.

Also of considerable importance is the sampling interval, p, of the detector, i.e., the pitch in the detector plane between sensitive elements or measurements. The sampling theorem states that only spatial frequencies in the pattern below $(2p)^{-1}$ (the Nyquist frequency) can be faithfully imaged. If the pattern contains higher frequencies, then aliasing occurs where the frequency spectrum of the image pattern beyond the Nyquist frequency is mirrored or folded about that frequency and added to the spectrum of lower frequencies, increasing the apparent spectral content of the image at these lower frequencies (Bendat et al. 1986). In a detector composed of discrete elements, the smallest sampling interval in a single image acquisition is $p = d$, so that the Nyquist frequency is $(2d)^{-1}$ while the aperture response falls to 0 at twice that frequency (higher if the dimension of the sensitive region of the detector element is smaller than d, *e.g.,* because the fill-factor of the detector element is less than 1.0). Thus, such detectors are susceptible to aliasing. Issues of sampling in digital radiographic systems have been reviewed by (Dobbins 1995). Although there are other potential sources of image unsharpness due to the size of the focal spot and patient motion, because of the relatively large dels (40-100 μm), the detector is virtually always the main factor limiting the spatial resolution of digital mammography.

Noise

All images generated by quanta are statistical in nature, i.e., although the image pattern can be predicted by the attenuation properties of the patient, it will fluctuate randomly about the mean predicted value. The fluctuation of the x-ray intensity follows Poisson statistics, so that the variance, σ^2, about the mean number of x-ray quanta, N_0, falling on a detector element of a given area, is equal to N_0. Interaction with the detector can be represented as a binomial process with probability of success, η, yielding a Poisson distribution with standard deviation

$$\sigma = \left(N_0\, \eta\right)^{1/2} \tag{2}$$

If the detection stage is followed by a process that provides a mean gain $\bar{g}$, then the "signal" becomes:

$$q = N_0\, \eta\, \bar{g} \tag{3}$$

while the variance in the signal is:

$$\sigma_q^2 = N_0\, \eta\left(\bar{g}^2 + \sigma_g^2\right) \tag{4}$$

In general, the distribution of q is not Poisson even if g is Poisson distributed. Similarly, the effect of additional stages of gain (or loss) can be expressed by propagating this expression further (Rabbani et al. 1987, Cunningham et al. 1994). It is also possible (and likely) that other independent sources of noise will be contributed at different stages of the imaging system. These noise sources are not necessarily Poisson distributed. In some cases, their effect on the variance at that stage will be additive. The resultant fluctuation will be subject to the gain of subsequent stages of the imaging system.

A complete analysis of signal and noise propagation in a detector system must take into account the spatial frequency dependence of both signal and noise. Signal transfer can be characterised in terms of the modulation transfer function, MTF(f), where f is the spatial frequency, while noise is described by the noise power or Wiener spectrum W(f). Methods for calculating the Wiener spectral properties of a detector must correct for nonlinearities in the detector and must properly take into account the spatial correlation of signal and statistical fluctuation.

A useful quantity for characterizing the overall signal and noise performance of imaging detectors is their spatial frequency-dependent detective quantum efficiency, DQE(f). This describes the efficiency in transferring the signal-to-noise ratio (squared) contained in the incident x-ray pattern to the detector output. Ideally, DQE(f) = η for all f, however, additional noise sources will reduce this value and often cause the DQE to decrease with increasing spatial frequency. DQE(f) can be treated as a sort of quantum efficiency, in that when it is multiplied by the number of quanta incident on the detector, one obtains $SNR^2_{out}(f)$, also known as the number of noise equivalent quanta, NEQ(f), used to form the image. Typically DQE for a screen-film detector has a value on the order of 0.3 at a spatial frequency of 0 cycles/mm and this may fall to 0.05 at a few cycles/mm (Bunch et al. 1997).

It is important to ensure that the number of secondary quanta or electrons at each stage of the detector is somewhat greater than $N_0 \eta$, to avoid having the detector noise being dominated by a "secondary quantum sink."

Sensitivity

The final output from the detector is an electrical signal, so that sensitivity can be defined in terms of the charge produced by the detector (before any external amplification) per incident x-ray quantum of a specified energy. The sensitivity of any imaging system depends on η and on the the efficiency of converting the energy of the interacting x-ray to a more easily measurable form such as optical quanta or electric charge. Conversion efficiency can be expressed in terms of the energy, w, necessary to release a light photon in a phosphor, an electron-hole pair in a photoconductor (or semiconductor) or an electron-ion pair in a gaseous detector. Values of w for some typical detector materials are given in Table 1.

Table 1. Properties of phosphors and photoconductors used as x-ray detectors for digital radiography, including atomic number, Z, and K absorption energy, E_K, of the principal absorbing elements. Sensitivity is expressed as the energy, W, which must be absorbed to release a quantum of light in a phosphor or an electron-hole pair in a photoconductor. The fluorescent yield, ω_K, is the probability that when a K-shell photoelectric interaction occurs, a fluorescent (characteristic) x-ray will be emitted.

Material	Z	E_K (keV)	W (eV)	ω_K approx.
CdTe	48/52	26.7/31.8	4.4	.85-.88
High purity Si	14	1.8	3.6	< .05
Amorphous selenium	34	12.7	50 (at 10V/μm)	.6
CsI(Tl)	55/53	36.0/33.2	19	.87
Gd_2O_2S	64	50.2	13	.92
BaFBr (as photostim. phosphor)	56/35	37.4/13.5	50-100	.86

The limiting factor is related to the intrinsic band structure of the solid from which the detector is made. In Figure 5, the basic band structure of crystalline materials is shown. Normally the valence band is fully populated with electrons and the conduction band is empty. The energy gap governs the scale of energy necessary to release an electron hole pair, i.e., to promote an electron from the valence band to the conduction band. However, though this energy is the <u>minimum</u> permitted by the principle of conservation of energy, this can be accomplished only for photons of energy exactly equal to the energy gap. For charged particles releasing energy (e.g., through the slowing down of high energy electrons created by an initial x-ray interaction), requirements of conserving both energy and crystal momentum as well as the presence of competing energy loss processes require, on average, at least three times as much energy as the band gap to release an electron hole pair (Klein 1968). In Figure 5b the situation for a phosphor is shown. In this case, the first requirement is to obtain an electron hole pair. Subsequently, the electron returns to the valence band via a luminescence centre created by an activator added to the host material. This requires that the energy E_F of the fluorescence light must be less than the band gap energy E_G and therefore there are further inefficiencies in a phosphor.

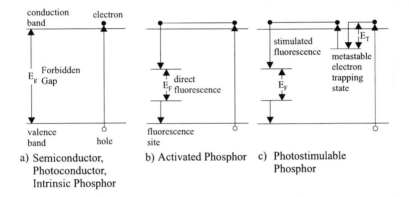

a) Semiconductor, Photoconductor, Intrinsic Phosphor

b) Activated Phosphor

c) Photostimulable Phosphor

Figure 5. Energy level structure for detector materials. a) semiconductor detector, b) activated phosphor c) photostimulable phosphor.

Dynamic Range

The dynamic range can be defined as:

$$DR = \frac{X_{max}}{X_{noise}} \tag{5}$$

where X_{max} is the x-ray fluence providing the maximum signal that the detector can accommodate and X_{noise} is the fluence that provides a signal equivalent to the quadrature sum of the detector noise and the x-ray quantum noise.

In practice, the required dynamic range for an imaging task can be decomposed into two components. The first describes the ratio between the unattenuated beam and the x-ray attenuation of the most radio-opaque path through the breast to be included on the same image. The second is the precision of x-ray signal to be measured in the most radio-opaque part of the image. In mammography, for an effective energy of 20 keV and a breast composed of 50% adipose tissue and 50% fibro-glandular tissue, 6 cm thick, the attenuation factor is approximately 42. If it is required to have 1% precision in measuring the signal in the most attenuating region, then the dynamic range requirement would be 4200.

In defining the range of operation for a detector, one must consider both the need for adequate x-ray fluence to achieve the desired quantum counting statistics at the low end of the range as well as detector phenomena such as saturation or "blooming" that can occur with large signals. The dynamic range of the detector may be reduced by flat-fielding operations to correct for nonuniformity, as discussed in the next section.

Uniformity

It is important that the radiographic imaging system provide uniformity, i.e., the sensitivity be constant over the entire area of the image. Otherwise patterns that might disrupt the effective interpretation of the image may result. These patterns are sometimes referred to as "fixed pattern noise." In a screen-film system, much effort is made to avoid such nonuniformities through manufacturing practices. In a digital system, the task is much easier, because differences in response from element to element can be corrected. This is accomplished by imaging an object of uniform x-ray transmission, recording the detector response and using this as a "correction mask." This process is called "flat fielding." If the detector has linear response to x rays, then the correction involves two masks—one with and one without radiation, to provide slope and intercept values for the correction of each element. It is often observed that slight nonlinearities exist in detectors and the degree of nonlinearity varies among dels. When such differential nonlinearity exists, flat-fielding may be effective in correcting images produced at detector signals near the intensity used for calibrating the flat field correction, however, nonuniformity over the image will become apparent for other intensity levels, depending on how much they differ from the flat-fielding condition. If the detector response is nonlinear, then measurements must be made over a range of intensities and a nonlinear function fit to the response of each element to obtain the correction coefficients.

In some detectors, non-uniformities might exist only over rows and columns of the detector rather than over individual elements. This greatly reduces the number of coefficients that must be stored.

Flat fielding causes the original detector signals to be altered. If signal values are restricted to a fixed scale, on initial acquisition, e.g., 0-4095, then the flat-fielding correction may reduce the dynamic range of the detector. A sufficient number of images must be added together to create the flat field mask so that the noise in the flat field correction does not unduly increase the noise in the final image.

X-ray Detectors for Digital Mammography

Phosphor-based Detector Systems

Most x-ray imaging detectors employ a phosphor in the initial stage to absorb the x rays and produce light which is then coupled to an optical sensor (photodetector). The use of relatively high atomic number phosphor materials causes the photoelectric effect to be the dominant type of x-ray interaction. The photoelectron produced in these inter-actions is given a substantial fraction of the energy of the x-ray. This energy is much larger than the bandgap of the crystal (Figure 5b) and, therefore, in being stopped, a single interacting x-ray has the potential to cause the excitation of many electrons in the phosphor and thereby the production of many light quanta. We describe this "quan-tum amplification" as the <u>conversion gain</u>, g_1. For example, in a Gd_2O_2S phosphor, the energy carried by a 25 keV x-ray quantum is equivalent to that of 10,400 green light quanta ($E_g = 2.4$ eV). Because of competing energy loss processes and the need to con-serve momentum, the <u>conversion efficiency</u> is only about 15%, so that, on average, it requires approximately 13 eV per light quantum created in this phosphor (Table 1). The conversion gain is then approximately 1560 light quanta per interacting x-ray quantum.

The energy loss process is stochastic and, therefore, g has a probability distribution, with standard deviation, σ_g, about its mean value as illustrated in Figure 6. Swank described this effect and the "Swank factor," A_s, characterizes this additional noise source (Swank 1973). The Swank factor is calculated in terms of the moments of the distribution of g as:

$$A = \frac{M_1^2}{M_0 M_2}$$

(6)

where M_i indicates the ith moment of the distribution.

The actual number of quanta produced by an interacting x-ray will also depend both on its incident energy and the mechanism of interaction with the phosphor crystal. The most likely type of interaction, the photoelectric effect, will result in both an energetic photoelectron and either a second (Auger) electron or a fluorescent x-ray quantum. The energy of fluorescence depends on the shell in which the photoelectric interaction took place. The threshold K-shell energy for these interactions is shown for some common radiographic phosphors in Table 1. Also in the table is the K-fluorescence yield; the probability of emission of x-ray fluorescence, given that a K-shell photoelectric inter-action has occurred. Materials produce the most intense x-ray fluorescence just below the K edge. The fluorescent quanta are either reabsorbed in the phosphor or escape. In either case, if they are not absorbed locally, the apparent energy deposited in the phosphor from the x-ray quantum is reduced, giving rise to a second peak in the dis-tribution with a lower value of g.

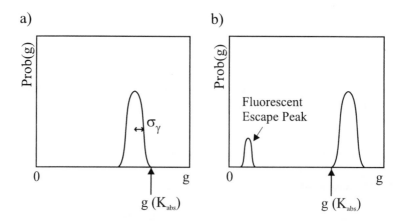

Figure 6. Probability distribution of signal produced per interacting x-ray.
a) below K absorption edge, b) above K edge with fluorescence escape

The effect of fluorescence loss is to broaden the overall distribution of g (Figure 6b), thus decreasing A_s and causing an increase in σ_g. For many detector materials (e.g., Gd_2O_2S), their K-shell interactions lie above the energy range used for mammography and therefore, K fluorescence effects are not an issue.

There are both advantages and disadvantages in imaging with an x-ray spectrum that exceeds the K edge of the phosphor. Clearly, the value of η increases, however the "Swank noise" does also. In addition, deposition of energy from the fluorescence at some distance from the point of initial x-ray interaction causes the point spread function of the detector to increase, resulting in decreased spatial resolution.

After their formation, the light quanta must successfully escape the phosphor and be effectively coupled to the next stage for conversion to an electronic signal and read-out. It is desirable to ensure that the created light quanta escape the phosphor efficiently and as near as possible to their point of formation.

Figure 7 illustrates the effect of phosphor thickness and the depth of x-ray interaction on spatial resolution of a phosphor detector. The probability of x-ray interaction is exponential so that the number of interacting quanta and the amount of light created will be proportionally greater near the x-ray entrance surface.

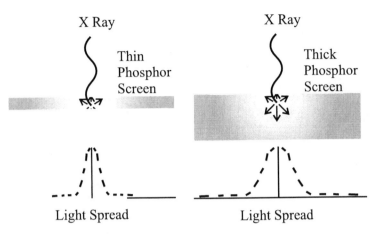

Figure 7. Effect of phosphor thickness on image blurring.

While travelling within the phosphor, the light will spread—the amount of diffusion being proportional to the path length required to escape the phosphor. X rays interacting close to the photodetector give rise to a sharper (less blurred) optical signal than those which interact more distantly. The paths of most optical quanta will be shortest if the photodetector is placed on the x-ray entrance side of the phosphor. It is usually necessary, however, to record the photons which exit on the opposite face of the phosphor screen, i.e., those which have had a greater opportunity to spread. If the phosphor layer is made thicker to improve quantum efficiency, the spreading becomes more severe. This imposes a fundamental compromise between spatial resolution and η. Methods to collect the emission from the entrance side of the phosphor or to channel the optical photons out of the phosphor without spreading can significantly improve phosphor performance.

Figure 8 illustrates the propagation of signal through the various energy conversion stages of an imaging system. In the diagram, N_0 quanta are incident on a specified area of the detector surface (Stage 0). A fraction of these, given by the quantum detection efficiency, η, interact with the detector (Stage I). In a perfect imaging system, η would be equal to 1.0. The mean number, N_1 of quanta interacting represents the "primary quantum sink" of the detector. The fluctuation about N_1 is $\sigma_{N1} = (N_1)^{1/2}$. This defines the signal to noise ratio, SNR, of the imaging system which increases as the square root of the number of quanta interacting with the detector.

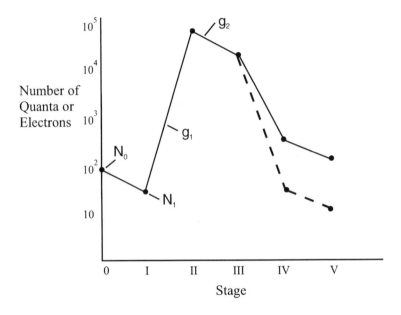

Figure 8. Propagation of signal magnitude through a detector system. Gain or efficiency of each stage must be adequate to avoid a secondary quantum sink.

Regardless of the value of η, the maximum SNR of the imaging system will occur at this point and if the SNR of the imaging system is essentially determined there, the system is said to be <u>x-ray quantum limited</u> in its performance. However, the SNR will, in general, become reduced in passage of the signal through the imaging system because of losses and additional sources of fluctuation.

To avoid losses that can occur at subsequent stages, it is important that the detector provide adequate quantum gain, g_1 directly following the initial x-ray interaction. Stages II and III illustrate the processes of creation of many light photons from a single interacting x-ray (often referred to as conversion gain) and the escape of quanta from the phosphor with mean probability g_2. Here, light absorption, scattering and reflection processes are important.

Further losses occur in the coupling of the light to the photodetector which converts light to electronic charge (Stage IV) and in the spectral sensitivity and optical quantum efficiency of the photodetector (Stage V). If the conversion gain of the phosphor is not sufficiently high to overcome these losses and the number of light quanta or electronic charges at a subsequent stage falls below that at the primary quantum sink, then a "secondary quantum sink" is formed. In this case the statistical fluctuation of the light or charge at this point becomes an additional important noise source. Even when an actual secondary sink does not exist, a low value of light or charge will cause increased noise. This becomes especially important when a spatial-frequency-dependent analysis of SNR is carried out and, as discussed earlier, its effect is to cause reduction of the detective quantum efficiency with increasing spatial frequency (Maidment et al. 1994) .

Figure 9 illustrates two approaches for coupling a phosphor to a photodetector. Traditionally, a lens (Figure 9a) is used to collect light emitted from the surface of the phosphor material.

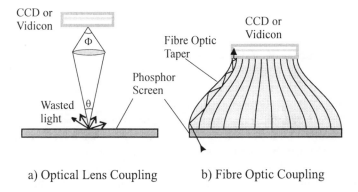

a) Optical Lens Coupling   b) Fibre Optic Coupling

Figure 9. Methods of coupling x-ray absorber to readout device a) lens, b) fibreoptic bundle

Because the size of available photodetectors such as CCDs are limited from manufacturing considerations to a maximum dimension of only 2-5 cm, it is often necessary to demagnify the image from the phosphor to allow coverage of the required field size in the patient. The efficiency of lens coupling is determined largely by the solid angle subtended by the collecting optics. For a single lens system, the coupling efficiency is given by (Miller 1991, Maidment 1996):

$$\xi = \frac{\tau}{4\,F^2\,(m+1)^2} \tag{7}$$

where τ is the optical transmission factor for the lens, F is the "f-number" of the lens (ratio of the focal length to its limiting aperture diameter) and m is the demagnification factor from the phosphor to the photodetector. For a lens with $F = 1.2$, $\tau = 0.8$ and $m = 10$, ξ will be 0.1%.

Because of this low efficiency, the SNR of systems employing lens coupling is often limited by a secondary quantum sink, especially where the demagnification factor is large and/or g_1 is small.

It is also possible to use fibre optics to effect the coupling. These can be in the form of fibreoptic bundles (Figure 9b), where optical fibres of constant diameter are fused to form a light guide. The fibres form an orderly array so that there is a one-to-one correspondence between the elements of the optical image at the exit of the phosphor and at the entrance to the photodetector. To accomplish the required demagnification, the fibre optic bundle can be tapered by drawing it under heat. While facilitating the construction of a detector to cover the required anatomy in the patient, demagnification by tapering also reduces coupling efficiency by limiting the acceptance angle at the fibre optic input. A simplified expression for the coupling efficiency of a fibre optic taper is:

$$\xi = \alpha\,\tau(\theta)\frac{NA^2}{m^2} \tag{8}$$

where α is the fraction of the entrance surface that comprises the core glass of the optical fibres, $\tau(\theta)$ is the transmission factor for the core glass, NA is the numerical aperture of the untapered fibre and m is the demagnification factor due to tapering. For example, a taper with 2 times demagnification ($m = 2$), with $\alpha = 0.8$, $\tau = 0.9$ and NA = 1.0, has an efficiency of 18%, about seven times higher than a lens with F = 1.2 with the same demagnification factor and about 2.5 times higher than a lens with F = 0.7. It should be noted that for both lenses and fibre optics, the transmission efficiency is dependent on the angle of incidence, θ of the light and, therefore, a complete analysis involves an integral of the angular distribution of emission of the phosphor over θ. A comparison of the efficiency of lens versus fibreoptic coupling is shown (Hejazi et al. 1996) in Figure 10.

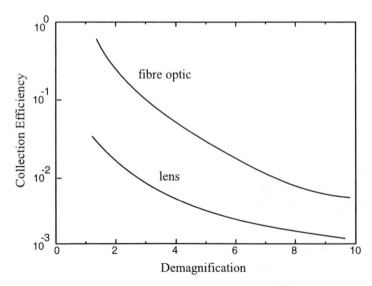

Figure 10. Comparison of lens versus fibreoptic coupling methods.
In both cases, demagnification reduces efficiency.

Both fibreoptic (Figure 11a) and lens designs are used in small field of view cameras for digital mammography to couple a phosphor to a full-frame CCD photodetector (Roehrig et al. 1994). These systems are used for guiding needle biopsy and for localization of suspicious lesions. Typically, no more than 2x demagnification is employed, resulting in acceptable coupling efficiency. The advantages of digital detectors over screen-film for such procedures was almost immediately obvious in terms of improved contrast and rapid access to images without the need to wait for film processing.

Full-area Digital Mammography Detector Systems

Demagnifying Phosphor/Fibreoptic/CCD System

Although it is possible to extend the approach described above to create a full-area detector, the large demagnification factor that would be required would result in unacceptably low coupling efficiency and a secondary quantum sink. This problem has been circumvented by one of the manufacturers, Trex, who have designed their detector as a mosaic of 3×4 smaller detector modules, each one employing a demagnification on the order of 2 x. This system produces a full size image of the breast with approximately 40 micron pixels (Figure 11b.)

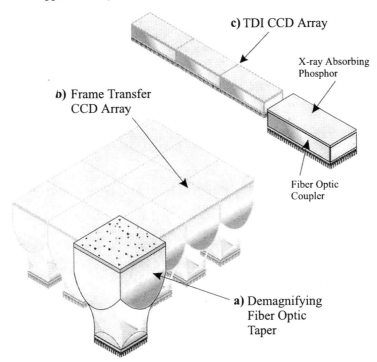

Figure 11. Phosphor/fibreoptic/CCD detectors. a) small format detector for guidance of biopsies, b) full-area detector, c) slot-scanning TDI system.

Amorphous Silicon Phosphor Flat-panel Detectors

Active matrix LCDs (AMLCDs) have been made using amorphous (hydrogenated amorphous silicon (Piper et al. 1986, Powell 1989) and these are widely used for lap top computer displays. The active matrix is a large-area integrated circuit consisting of a large number of thin-film field-effect transistors (TFTs) connected to individual photodetector elements in a matrix.

The potential advantages of such self-scanned, compact readout systems include their compactness, freedom from veiling glare, geometric uniformity and immunity to stray magnetic fields. A thallium-doped caesium iodide (CsI:Tl) phosphor layer can be evaporated directly onto the active matrix (Perez-Mendez et al. 1989, Fujieda et al. 1991).

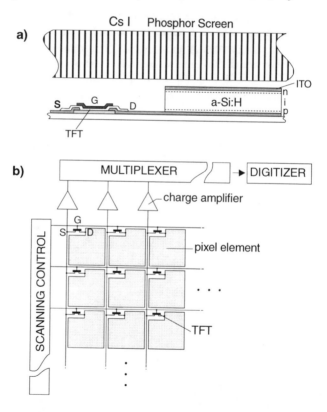

Figure 12. Amorphous silicon readout for large area detector. a) cross section with phosphor x-ray absorber, b) readout matrix with a-Si photodiodes and TFT switches.

The principle of operation of an amorphous silicon detector is shown schematically in Figure 12. The dels are configured as photodiodes (Figure 12a) which convert the optical signal from the phosphor to charge and store that charge on the capacitance of the element. Being low-noise devices, the photodiodes provide a very large dynamic range, on the order of 40,000:1. A typical thin film transistor readout array is shown in Figure 12b. The signal is read out by activation of scanning control lines for each row of the device, connected to the gates of TFTs located on each detector pixel. An entire row of the detector array is activated simultaneously and the signal is read on lines for each column in the array which connects all the TFT sources in that column to a low-noise charge amplifier. The amplified signals from the columns are then multiplexed and digitized. This allows fast detector readout and requires a number of electronic channels equal to the number of columns of the array.

Alternatively, instead of TFT readout various diode switching schemes can be used (Chabbal et al. 1996, Graeve et al. 1996). The advantage of the diode approach is that since the photodiode has to be made anyway, the switching diode can be made at the same time without increase in the number of material processing steps. The disadvantages of diode readout is a strong non-linearity and large charge injection.

The area allocated to each pixel of the array must contain the photodiode, switching device and control and signal lines so that the fill factor is less than 100%. This potential loss of x-ray utilization efficiency becomes proportionately greater as the pixel size is decreased and provides a challenge for the application of this technology to very high resolution applications. Currently dels of 100 μm have been produced and new techniques should allow sizes down to 50 or 60 μm (Rahn et al.).

The advantage of utilizing CsI as the x-ray absorber is that it can be grown in columnar crystals which act as fibre optics. When coupled to the photodiode pixels, there is little lateral spread of light and, therefore, high spatial resolution can be maintained. In addition, unlike conventional phosphors in which diffusion of light and loss of resolution become worse when the thickness is increased, CsI phosphors can be made thick enough to ensure a high value of η while maintaining high spatial resolution. General Electric has produced a system using CsI on a-Si with a del of 100 μm. The detector (Niklason et al. 1996) assembly fits onto a modified GE conventional mammography unit.

Photostimulable Phosphors

Probably the most widespread detectors for digital radiography to date have been photostimulable phosphors, also known as storage phosphors. These phosphors are commonly in the barium fluorohalide family, typically $BaFBr:Eu^{2+}$, where the atomic energy levels of the Europium activator determines the characteristics of light emission. X-ray absorption mechanisms are identical to those of conventional phosphors. They differ in that the useful optical signal is not derived from the light that is emitted in prompt response to the incident radiation, but rather from subsequent emission when electrons and holes are released from traps in the material (Takahashi et al. 1984, von Seggern et al 1988). The initial x-ray interaction with the phosphor crystal causes electrons to be excited (Figure 5c). Some of these produce light in the phosphor in the normal manner, however, the phosphor is intentionally designed to contain traps which store the charges. By stimulating the crystal by irradiation with red light, electrons are released from the traps and raised to the conduction band of the crystal, subsequently triggering the emission of shorter wavelength (blue) light. Photostimulable phosphor imaging has been reviewed by Kato (Kato 1994) and Bogucki (Bogucki 1995).

The imaging plate is positioned in a light tight cassette or enclosure, exposed and then read by raster scanning the plate with a laser to release the luminescence (Figure 13). The emitted light is collected and detected with a photomultiplier tube whose output signal is digitized to form the image.

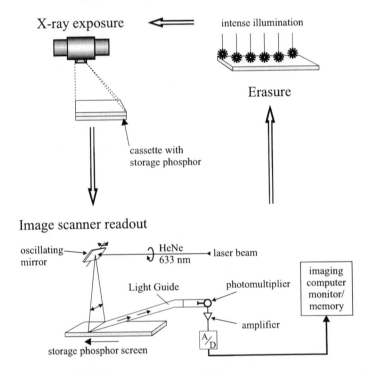

Figure 13. Photostimulable phosphor imaging system.

The energy levels in the crystal are critical to the effective operation of the detector (Figure 5c). The energy difference between the traps and the conduction band E_T must be small enough so that stimulation with laser light is possible, yet sufficiently large to prevent random thermal release of the electron from the trap. The energy levels should be such that the wavelength of the emitted light can be efficiently detected by a photomultiplier and that there is adequate wavelength separation between the stimulating and emitted light quanta to avoid contaminating the measured signal. The electrons liberated during irradiation either produce light promptly or are stored in traps. Because the "prompt" light is not of interest in this application, the efficiency of the storage function can be improved by increasing the probability of electron trapping. On the other hand, when these electrons are released by the stimulating light during readout, the probability of their being retrapped instead of producing light, would then be higher, so that the efficiency of readout would be reduced. The optimum balance occurs where the probabilities of an excited electron being retrapped or stimulating fluorescence are equal. This causes the conversion efficiency to be reduced by a factor of 4 compared to the same phosphor without traps—i.e., a factor of 2 from the prompt light given off during x-ray exposure and another factor of 2 from unwanted retrapping of the electrons during readout.

In addition, the decay characteristics of the emission must be sufficiently fast such that the image can be read in a conveniently short time while capturing an acceptable fraction of the emitted energy. In practice, depending on the laser intensity, the readout of a stimulable phosphor plate yields only a fraction of the stored signal. This is a disadvantage with respect to sensitivity and readout noise, however, it can be helpful by allowing the plate to be "pre-read"—i.e., read out with only a small part of the stored signal, to allow automatic optimization of the sensitivity of the electronic circuitry for the main readout. Fuji is currently performing clinical evaluation of a photostimulable phosphor plate system for use in digital mammography.

Scanned-beam Acquisition

In these systems, the detector is in the form of a linear or multilinear array of dels and the image is acquired by scanning the detector assembly across the breast in synchrony with a fan beam of x rays. This design limits the required number of dels, while allowing high spatial resolution (small detector aperture and pitch) to be achieved. This is an important cost factor when expensive detector technologies are employed. Another advantage is the inherent high efficiency rejection of scattered radiation afforded by slot-beam systems, where the detector can be collimated to match the pre-patient fan beam. This can be accomplished without the need for interspace material in the beam.

One disadvantage of scanning systems is the longer overall time to acquire the image. Although this may preclude some dynamic studies, it does not result in blurring because each portion of the image is acquired in a very short time. If there is significant motion in the breast, then a misregistration artifact is more likely to occur. Another disadvantage is that because most of the x-ray beam is removed by the fan-beam collimation, there is inefficient use of x-ray tube heat loading. This requires that the x-ray tube used in this application be designed with an increased heat capacity. To mitigate against both of these effects, it is preferable to use multiline detectors. The system design then involves a tradeoff between the shorter imaging time and improved use of heat loading afforded by a wide slot detector system and the improved scatter rejection and less critical mechanical alignment available with a narrower slot.

In scanning systems, it is useful to acquire the image in time delay integration (TDI) mode in which the x-ray beam is activated continuously during the image scan and charge collected in pixels of the CCDs is shifted down CCD columns at a rate equal to but in the opposite direction as the motion of the x-ray beam and detector assembly across the breast. The collected charge packets remain essentially stationary with respect to a given projection path of the x rays through the breast and the charge is integrated in the CCD column to form the resultant signal. When the charge packet has reached the final element of the CCD, it is read out on a transfer register and digitized. The CCD array can be cooled using thermoelectric devices to reduce noise and increase the dynamic range of the image receptor as necessary. In such systems the spatial resolution is dependent on accurate alignment of the signal-gathering columns of the detector with the scan direction and on correct synchronization with charge clocking in the CCDs with the scan motion. Fischer Imaging Inc. has developed a scanning digital mammography system whose detector is based on the phosphor/fiberoptic taper/CCD concept illustrated in Figure 11c. This is currently being evaluated at several clinical sites.

Solid State Electrostatic Systems

Amorphous selenium

There are several advantages in the use of solid state electrostatic systems rather than phosphors. One of these is avoiding the lateral spread of light between the point of x-ray absorption and the photodetector. X rays interacting in the photoconductor plate release electrons and holes, which, because they are charged, can be guided directly to the surfaces of the photoconductor by the applied electric field. The latent charge image on the photoconductor surface is, therefore, not blurred significantly even if the plate is made thick enough to absorb most incident x-rays (Que et al. 1995). Because a very large number of charge carriers are created per interacting x-ray and because these are collected much more efficiently than in an optical system, it is possible to completely eliminate the problem of secondary quantum sinks and also to improve the Swank factor.

Amorphous selenium (a-Se) is the most highly developed photoconductor for x ray applications. Its amorphous state makes possible the maintenance of uniform imaging characteristics to almost atomic scale (there are no grain boundaries) over large areas. The primary function of the a-Se layer is to attenuate x rays, generate free electron-hole pairs (in proportion to the intensity of the incident x rays) and collect them at the electrodes. To achieve a high value of η, the detector must be of adequate thickness (Figure 4). High conversion efficiency in converting absorbed x-ray energy into free electron-hole pairs requires high electric fields.

Each surface must have an electrode attached to permit collection of charge from the a-Se while preventing entry of charge from the electrodes into the a-Se. This is called a <u>blocking contact</u>. Finally the surface of the a-Se at which the image is formed must have a very small transverse conductivity. Otherwise the image charge could migrate laterally and destroy the resolution.

Lee et al. (Lee et al. 1996) have described a flat panel method for radiography, based on the use of an active matrix readout method for *a-* Se and a similar approach has also been advocated by Zhao and Rowlands (Zhao et al 1995). The potential features of this method are: high image quality; real-time readout rate; and compact size. The basic concept is shown in Figure 14. During x-ray exposure, energy is absorbed by the *a*-Se layer and the charge created is drawn by the internal electric field E_{Se} to the surfaces. The image charge is collected by the pixel electrode and accumulated onto the pixel capacitance (i.e., self-capacitance and an integrated storage capacitor). The pixel electrode and storage capacitor are connected to the TFT switch of each pixel. The readout device can be similar to that used with amorphous silicon (Figure 12b). The external scanning control circuit generates pulses to turn on all the TFT switches on a row of the array and transfers charge from the pixel capacitors to the readout rails (columns). The charge is then collected and amplified by an amplifier on each rail and the data for the entire row is multiplexed out. (The amplifiers and multiplexer are in another single crystal silicon integrated circuit which is wirebonded to the array.) This sequence is repeated for each row of the array. Fahrig et al. (1995) have analyzed the factors influencing DQE in *a*-Se x-ray detectors.

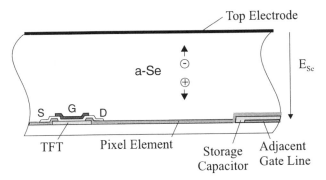

Figure 14. Amorphous selenium large area detector.

Other Direct Conversion Systems

A number of other direct conversion materials are also being considered for application in digital mammography. These include: zinc cadmium telluride, lead iodide (Street et al. 1999), mercuric iodide, or thallium bromide (Shah et al. 1989). These materials could be deposited on an amorphous silicon readout device to form a large area detector.

Alternatively, for use in a scanning system ,the detector could be formed as a hybrid between an array of photodiodes or photoconductive elements and a TDI CCD readout fabricated on a separate substrate (Figure 15) . The two matrices are joined on a

pixel-by-pixel basis by a series of microscopic indium "bumps." Thus charge liberated in the detector elements is transferred to the CCD to be collected and integrated
down CCD columns and then digitized. Detectors of this design were initially used
for imaging in the infra red spectrum and have been shown to provide very high spatial resolution and other desirable imaging characteristics when modified for use with
x rays (Henry et al. 1995).

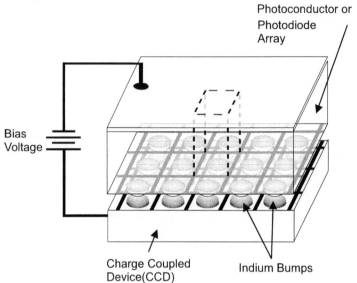

Figure 15. Hybrid direct conversion detector for slot-scanning imaging system.
X-ray absorber can be a photodiode or photoconductive material.

Practical Issues in Image Acquisition

Exposure Techniques for Digital Mammography

Unlike screen-film imaging, where the required exposure is defined by the need to
attain a specific optical density, there is much more flexibility of exposure in digital
mammography. An initial technique (exposure level and spectrum) can be selected for
a particular type of unit, based on the recommendations of the manufacturer and experience with phantom images. It is not restrictive to impose the requirement that the
images receive a passing score on the the ACR Accreditation Phantom at a dose no
greater than the Mammography Quality Standards Act (MQSA) maximum level (for
screen-film) of 3 mGy. In fact, if the phantom image were the main consideration,
much lower doses could be used. The image SNR should be evaluated for phantoms
representing the attenuation of breasts of different thicknesses and compositions and
exposure levels selected that provide an acceptable level of SNR and detectability of
phantom structures. Because of the variable display contrast of digital mammography,
there are preliminary indications that x-ray spectra that are higher in effective energy
than those used in screen-film mammography may be appropriate (Fahrig et al. 1994).

Scatter Rejection

In conventional mammography, the detection of scattered radiation at the detector reduces image contrast and a grid normally employed to reduce the detrimental effects of scatter. This improvement comes at the cost of increased radiation dose because, to maintain constant film optical density, the amount of radiation reaching the detector must be maintained. Exposure to the breast is increased when a grid is used to compensate for a) loss of primary radiation absorbed by the grid interspace material and septa and b) loss of the scattered radiation, which contributed to film darkening.

In digital mammography, scatter can be reduced either by using a narrow beam scanned acquisition technique or, in the case of an area detector, using a grid. In the latter case, it is not necessary to compensate for the loss of scatter to the detector, because the final image display brightness can be controlled independent of the radiation level used. On the other hand, it may not be desirable to use a grid at all with the area detectors. There are several effects of detected scattered radiation. Contrast is reduced, the dynamic range of the detector is somewhat reduced because part is used for recording scatter, and the signal to noise ratio is reduced because scattered radiation increases quantum noise without adding useful signal. Only the last of these issues is fundamental in influencing imaging performance. Elimination of the grid allows more of the primary transmitted signal to reach the detector, improving the SNR per patient dose. This effect may outweigh the benefit, in terms of SNR, of using a grid.

Flat Fielding Corrections

In digital systems, a flat fielding procedure is routinely used to remove stationary image noise and to compensate for non-uniformities in sensitivity. Improper flat fielding can result in noisy images, creation or amplification of artifacts, loss of data at the skin line, and various other image distortions. For some systems, because of nonlinear effects, proper flat fielding may require the acquisition of a set of calibration images at several average signal levels, or possibly with more than one type of x-ray spectrum. In addition, systems may differ in the required frequency with which calibration images must be updated in order to maintain a given level of performance.

Display of Digital Mammograms

One of the potential advantages of digital mammography is the extended dynamic range compared to screen-film. One of the challenges in making digital mammography practical is to develop an effective means for displaying the enormous amount of information contained in an image. This is a challenging problem, because of limitations of current display technology (Ascher et al. 1998). The number of image elements in a digital mammogram depends on the image field size and on the size of the displayed pixel. Systems also vary in the number of bits used to encode each image element. Table 2 summarizes these requirements.

Table 2. Number of image elements in a digital mammogram ($\times$ 106).

Image dimensions (cm)$\Downarrow$		Pixel size (μm)$\Rightarrow$	40	50	100
18	$\times$	24	27	17.28	4.32
24	$\times$	30	45	28.8	7.2

The two most practical display technologies currently available are laser film printers and cathode ray tube (CRT) monitors. Neither has sufficient latitude or dynamic range to accommodate the data available in a digital mammogram in a single display representation. High resolution laser film printers are able to provide an adequately number of pixels and a sufficiently small printing spot size such that all of the image elements of the digital mammogram can be recorded on the film, however, the single emulsion film used for printing has a lower range of optical densities than conventional mammography film. As a result, unless multiple versions of the image are printed with different display parameters, some or all of the image is likely to be displayed at reduced contrast, making it difficult to detect the extremely subtle differences between cancers and the surrounding normal tissue.

Similarly "soft copy" devices such as CRT monitors do not have sufficient dynamic range to display all of the intensity information at one setting, however they allow interactive adjustment of display while viewing the image. The radiologist can then explore the acquired information with different display settings. While this is not difficult to do, it is time consuming and not practical for routine work in a busy radiology department. If inappropriate settings are used, it is possible that a cancer will be missed.

In addition, for several of the digital mammography systems, even state-of-the-art CRT monitors are not able to display a full digital mammogram at more than half its spatial resolution. This problem can be partially overcome using a combination of image roam and local zoom features, however, once again, this is a labor-intensive process and there is the risk that the radiologist, in performing these operations will lose image context.

Therefore, unless effort is spent in developing new display technologies or improving existing technologies to create a practical method for presenting digital mammograms to radiologists, some of the advantages of digital mammography will be lost. Indeed, the clinical acceptance of digital mammography will be seriously compromised.

One way to overcome some of the limitations of display technology is to use image processing techniques to enhance lesion visibility. Current efforts in this area by various investigators include the use of wavelet transformations, image filtering, and grey-level enhancements (Clarke et al. 1994, Laine et al. 1994, Morrow et al. 1992, Pisano et al. 1991, Tachoes et al. 1992, Wei et al. 1993, Cowen et al. 1993, Freedman et al. 1994). Preliminary results from these studies have shown two important points. First, with image processing, the image lesions become more easily detectable. Secondly, these studies indicate that different types of mammographic lesions (masses, microcalcifications, architectural distortions, etc.) need different types of enhancements (either different algorithms or a different set of parameters). For this be practical, processing would have to take place with little or no intervention by the radiologist.

Peripheral Equalization

One drawback of using local enhancement is that the dynamic range of the image is still large—greater than the latitude of laser printers and CRT monitors. The large dynamic range requirement comes about because of two factors, the varying thickness of the breast and variations in tissue composition. This is illustrated in Figure 16. The thickness variations take place mainly in the periphery where it is difficult to accomplish uniform mechanical compression of the breast.

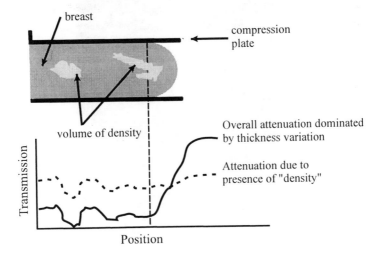

Figure 16. Dynamic range of an image is determined by thickness variations and by tissue composition.

It is possible to reduce the dynamic range requirement of the display medium by suppressing the effect of the thickness variations. This can be accomplished by traditional image processing techniques such as unsharp masking, or by using a more spatially selective peripheral equalization technique (Byng et al. 1997).

The technique involves low-pass filtering of the digital mammogram and automated identification of a transition region where the thickness of the breast decreases from the value in the region of uniform compression to zero at the edge of the breast.

A correction algorithm is then applied which does not alter the uniformly compressed region of the image, but uses the low-pass filtered image to derive a compensation function which is applied over the transition region. The correction essentially equalizes the apparent thickness of the breast in the image. Because the correction is based only on the low frequency components of the image, local variations due to composition are maintained without distortion, providing an image which preserves fine and intermediate detail, but which encompasses a lower dynamic range than the original image.

An important feature of this approach is that it has a direct physical basis, as it is sensitive to the actual anatomical variations in breast thickness in the imaging system. An example of a mammogram processed using this method is given in Figure 17.

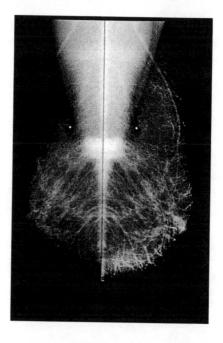

Figure 17. Example of peripheral equalization to reduce dynamic range of a digital mammogram. Left—conventional processing, Right—with peripheral equalization.

Clinical Status of Digital Mammography

Four digital mammography systems are currently being evaluated in the clinical environment. Each of the manufacturers is conducting studies to attempt to satisfy USFDA requirements on equipment performance. In addition, there are two major multi-institutional clinical studies in progress to compare the performance of digital mammography to that of screen-film mammography. The results of these studies are not yet available, however, radiologists note that while the spatial resolution of the images is not as high as in screen-film mammography, the contrast, and the ability to visualize structures surrounded by dense tissue is often better.

Integration of Digital Mammography and PACS

One of the potential benefits of digital mammography is an improvement in the efficiency and convenience of image storage, retrieval and extraction of key data for the purposes of planning, research, etc. To fully realize these benefits, the digital mammography system must be effectively integrated with a PACS.

This is indeed a challenging task because of the sheer amount of data involved in digital mammograms. The size of digital mammograms in Mbytes can be obtained from Table 2 for various values of pixel size and image dimensions. Typically, each digitized pixel is represented by 2 bytes (required dynamic range is 12-14bits).

This information must be transferred from the digital mammography system to the image database and the archiving system and must be able to be retrieved promptly for review by the radiologist. For a facility that has 4 mammography units, with 20 4-view examinations carried out on each, the daily data volume from digital mammography would be 320 times the appropriate value in Table 2 times 2 bytes/image element. For the 50 μm system and the small field size, this is 11.06 Gbytes/day or 2.7 Tbytes/year.

Typically, the radiologist needs to view the four images of the current examination and compare these with the four from the previous exam to look for changes in patterns. Obviously, an efficient means of pre-fetching and loading these large images will be required if digital mammography is to be practical for soft-copy viewing.

Applications of Digital Mammography

The most obvious benefit expected from digital mammography is an improvement in sensitivity and specificity brought about by improved quality of image acquisition and by the ability to manipulate the digital image while it is being viewed. In addition, digital mammography can facilitate the introduction of powerful imaging applications which were largely impractical until the images were available in digital form. These include computer-aided detection and diagnosis, telemammography, tomosynthesis, breast angiography, dual energy mammography and risk prediction.

Computer-aided Detection and Diagnosis

Digital mammography will greatly facilitate the use of computer-aided detection and computer-aided diagnosis (CAD), i.e., detection or diagnosis by a radiologist who considers the results of pattern analysis and statistical information performed by a computer. These serve as a "second opinion" that the radiologist can take into consideration in making his/her final interpretation. In the absence of digital mammography, performance of CAD requires the cumbersome and time-consuming step of digitization of film images.

Computer vision may detect lesions that are missed by the radiologist in order to increase detection sensitivity. After a lesion is detected, artificial intelligence could be used to estimate the likelihood of malignancy in order to reduce the number of false positive biopsies and thereby increase diagnostic specificity. Even with high quality modern mammography, some breast cancers may be missed on initial interpretation yet are visible in retrospect (Bird et al. 1997, Harvey et al. 1993). Double reading of screening mammograms by a second radiologist has been shown to improve the cancer detection rate by 9%-10% (Anderson et al. 1994, Thurfjell et al. 1994) Presumably computer-aided detection could have the same type of effect. Because computers are not subject to fatigue or distraction, CAD results for a particular algorithm should be free of intra-observer variation.

Telemammography

Telemammography refers to the transmission of mammographic images from one location to another in digital format. These locations can be within a particular facility, e.g., the mammography clinic and the operating room or separated by much longer distances, such as between a mammography unit in a remote facility, lacking a specialized trained mammographic radiologist, and a center of expertise where interpretation or consultation would be provided (Abdel-Maleck et al. 1994, Mattheus et al. 1991, Sund 1991).

A practical telemammography system requires that the images be in digital form. This can be accomplished by film digitization, but it is much more desirable and convenient if they are acquired directly on a digital system. Other likely features of a telemammography system are image compression to reduce the amount of data that must be transmitted, image management, to provide effective and convenient image retrieval, and a mechanism for remote consultation (Batnitzky et al. 1990). The telemammography system must not degrade the diagnostic quality of the mammograms. This requires that any compression and display strategies maintain the high intrinsic quality of the images and introduce no unacceptable artifacts.

Image compression can be performed to reduce transmission costs and increase speed. It can be either lossless (no information is deleted from the image) or "lossy." Although the latter can provide greater compression ratios—i.e., reduction of the amount of data in an image by a factor of 10 or more, the more moderate gains (a factor of 2-3) obtained with lossless compression may more preferable for legal reasons, and with high speed transmission, may be completely satisfactory. In either case, mechanisms for automatic correction of transmission errors will be necessary.

The transmission speed (and cost) depends on the type of network technology that is employed. The requirements for speed depend on whether the images are to be sent as a batch, perhaps overnight, or to be sent and interpreted in real time. For batch transmission, even networks of modest speed may be acceptable. For real time applications, even slight delays of several seconds may be disturbing to the radiologist.

Depending on needs and budget, image transmission could be carried out over standard T1 telephone links (up to 1.544 Mbits/s) or higher speed asynchronous transfer mode (ATM) links. For more remote locations where the infrastructure for these may not exist, satellite communication may be more appropriate, despite the higher initial setup cost, since it can provide arbitrarily high speed and can be operated virtually anywhere, including mobile van sites.

Several possible applications of telemammography can be anticipated. At present, when diagnostic mammography is performed in the absence of an on-site expert radiologist, patients may require a second appointment to receive supplementary views so that their breast problem can be adequately evaluated. Telemammography would allow radiologists to monitor and interpret problem-solving mammography on line for a nearby or even distant location. Screening studies could also be read remotely, eliminating the need to transport films from the remote fixed site or mobile van to the main facility. Clinical images could be remotely monitored for technical quality as they are performed so that patients would not have to return for repeat exposures. Telemammography could also facilitate second-opinion interpretation or consultation. Interactive teaching conferences could be conducted between different sites. Finally, mammographic images could be transmitted to the offices of referring physicians, expediting patient care and eliminating the need for patients to transport and possibly misplace their own studies.

Tomosynthesis

A significant advantage of digital imaging is that image data can be readily manipulated. This advantage is particularly apparent in tomosynthesis, which is a refinement of blurring tomography, a technique that has long been performed with screen-film technology. In blurring tomography, the x-ray source and image receptor move in a linear, circular or other more complex path during the exposure of the patient in such a manner as if they were connected to move about a fulcrum. The motion has the effect of blurring anatomical structures lying above or below the plane of the fulcrum, thereby largely obliterating their contrast. Structures in the "focal plane" are imaged sharply, giving the impression that only a slice of the patient anatomy is imaged. In digital mammographic tomosynthesis, this principle can be applied by moving the x-ray source in a pattern and obtaining a series of low dose images at different source positions. The detector remains stationary and the image data can be shifted appropriately in the computer to synthesize the tomographic image. Tomosynthesis improves the conspicuity of lesions by eliminating irrelevant contrasts and may be useful in imaging the dense breasts where fibrous tissue can obscure the visibility of a mass or other signs of cancer. Because each image can be acquired at low dose, the overall examination may not require any more radiation than does a single, high quality image. Furthermore, by increasing conspicuity of structures tomosynthesis may allow mammography to be done with less compression of the breast—in fact, reduced compression may facilitate tomosynthesis by increasing the z-axis separation of structures.

Breast Angiography

Often, it is found in surgery that the extent of the cancer exceeds that indicated by the suspicious area in the mammogram. Using intravenously administered contrast media and MRI, it has been shown that the extent of disease can be more accurately assessed. In fact, some cancers appear on MRI that cannot be seen at all on mammography. Since the major impact of this type of imaging is probably due to use of the contrast agent, it may be possible to obtain similar improvements in mammography by following the uptake of dye using serial low-dose digital mammographic images. This is currently an area under investigation in several institutions.

Risk Assessment

Following pioneering work by Wolfe (Wolfe 1976), we have been assessing whether quantitative analysis of density data and textures of digitized film mammograms of asymptomatic women can allow prediction of future risk of breast cancer. There is now good evidence that this is the case (Boyd et al. 1995) and a relative risk of a factor of four to six has been associated with high versus low density mammographic patterns. Density scores and other relevant information could be automatically extracted from digital mammograms in the future to help, for example, in defining the optimum screening interval for different risk groups or to monitor whether risk can be reduced by dietary or drug interventions.

Dual Energy Mammography

It has been suggested that even if the contrast limitations of film-screen mammography were overcome with digital mammography, some lesions would still be missed, particularly in dense breasts, because of the complexity of overlying fibroglandular structures. Unwanted contrasts caused by these structures form "clutter" noise which masks the structures of greatest interest. The availability of digital imaging facilitates the implementation of techniques to increase lesion conspicuity. One technique, is dual energy mammography (Johns et al. 1985, Johns et al. 1987). By obtaining digital images with two substantially different x-ray spectra, it is possible to combine these images to produce hybrid images in which the contrast of relevant structures is preserved while the unwanted masking contrasts are largely removed. This process could be done at the viewing station so that various structures within the image can be surveyed dynamically.

Quality Control for Digital Mammography

For digital mammography to maintain high sensitivity and specificity in detection and diagnosis of breast cancer, the equipment must operate at peak performance levels. As in conventional mammography this requires rigorous acceptance testing of the systems followed by a comprehensive program of quality control testing at regular intervals.

With conventional mammography, relatively standardized techniques have been established for acceptance testing (Hendrick et al. 1994, Gray et al. 1994, Rossi 1994, Yaffe et al. 1994, Barnes et al. 1991, Frey 1991, Kimme-Smith et al. 1996). The results of these tests help determine whether the equipment is operating in a manner suitable for use on patients. They ensure that radiation is used efficiently and also provide a set of baseline measurements to guide the QC program.

Because digital mammography is a new modality, specific testing techniques and protocols are only beginning to be established. It is reasonable to begin by basing testing protocols on those used for screen-film mammography, although, some of the tests will have to be modified and new guidelines for performance defined. As we develop a better understanding of the particularities of digital mammography, more relevant testing parameters are likely to emerge.

One fundamental difference between digital and screen-film mammography is that in screen-film mammography the functions of image acquisition and image display are inextricably linked through the sensitometric properties of the film, whereas in digital mammography they are decoupled. This may influence the exposure techniques that are chosen for imaging. In screen-film mammography these are based on two goals— attainment of a target optical density on the processed film and adequate penetration of as much of the breast as possible. The first is achieved by the use of the automatic exposure control, the second primarily by choice of the x-ray spectrum. The main objective is to achieve a certain level of image contrast in all areas of the breast. With film, this may occur at the expense of image signal-to-noise ratio (SNR), a fundamental property determining its information content.

In digital mammography, both image contrast and brightness can be controlled during image display and, therefore, there is no single image, but an enormous range of possibilities for how the image is displayed. For this reason, in digital mammography it is more appropriate to optimize the acquisition technique for SNR rather than brightness or contrast, and therefore, use a measure of SNR as an index of imaging performance. In addition, the substantially wider dynamic range of the x-ray detector reduces the concern regarding variation in penetration of different regions of the breast and may change the weighting of considerations in determining the x-ray spectrum.

Important factors in the acquisition stage that require assessment include: geometrical alignment of components of the imaging system in relation to breast positioning, spatial resolution and signal-to-noise properties. In the display stage, it is essential to monitor the performance of hardware components which are subject to deterioration and mis-calibration as well as software components such as look-up tables and enhancement algorithms which must be optimized for the imaging task.

Researchers working with digital mammography have developed a phantom (Figure 18) for evaluation of some aspects of imaging performance. This phantom is used in several of the tests to be carried out in a QC program for digital mammography described below.

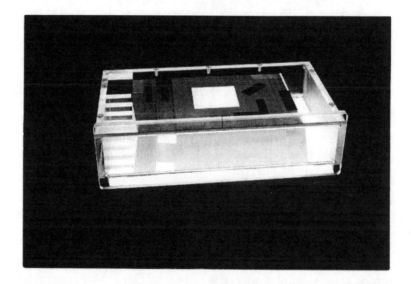

Figure 18. A quality control phantom for digital mammography. Developed by physicists in the International Digital Mammography Development Group (Yaffe et al. 1998).

a) **Geometric alignment and tissue coverage.** It is essential that as much breast tissue as possible be included in each examination. All mammography systems exclude some tissue because of geometric constraints in their design. A test incorporated in the phantom allows measurement of the amount of tissue missed at the chest wall and provide a measure of the overall image area. It also will provide an indication of the alignment of the focal spot, collimation and edges of the image receptor. The phantom has protrusions at the chest wall to limit its approach to the imaging unit in a manner similar to that of the patient's chest both at the breast support plate and at the compressor.

Slanted rulers at the chest wall on each side of the phantom make it easy to determine the amount of tissue which is missed.

b) **"Spatial fidelity and uniformity"** In digital systems there are unique potential artifacts associated with image stitching (i.e., building a complete image from physically separated but adjacent sub-images) and scanning motions. Mis-registration and individual pixel dropouts can occur both on full-field image plates and on scanning systems. Spatially nonlinear warps and image dislocations must be evaluated as they can create discontinuities in images which can disturb the perception of subtle image features. The digital phantom includes specific patterns to characterize uniformity and geometric distortion in the image acquisition system. Uniform phantoms with no structure and phantoms with regular patterns are imaged to allow assessment of the performance of the stitching and flat-fielding algorithms as well as to detect any other structural and spatial artifacts which may reveal themselves as distinct structures such as lines or as variations in image texture.

c) **X-ray dosimetry (entrance exposure, E, and mean glandular dose, MGD).** These are measured i) for regulatory compliance, ii) as a means to compare performance to conventional systems, iii) to standardize imaging between facilities and systems and iv) to enable determination of the detective quantum efficiency. Radiation output in mR/mAs is measured for phantoms representing different thicknesses and compositions of breasts using both manual and AEC (if available) modes. The standard approach as described in the ACR Mammography Quality Control Manual (Hendrick 1999) can be used for digital systems.

d) **HVL.** This is performed as in the ACR Manual.

e) **Dosimetry.** For systems that use anode/filter combinations employed in screen-film mammography, exposure-to-dose conversion tables are available [see ACR Manual (Hendrick et al 1999) or (Wu et al. 1991)]. Because of the greater range of spectral possibilities for digital mammography, it will be necessary to measure or calculate conversion values for other anode/kVp/filter combinations].

f) **Accuracy of slot collimation for scanning systems.** The use of a scanning slot geometry allows elimination of the grid and potentially a large saving in patient dose. To achieve this saving, it is important that the pre-breast beam collimation be accurately aligned with the detector collimation. Under-collimation will result in inefficient use of the detector and increased eat loading, while, exceeding the detector area will deliver wasted dose to the patient. Vibration or mis-synchronization of the beam and the detector may cause ripple in the image.

g) **AEC functioning/thickness tracking.** In digital mammography it is important that the image SNR is adequate. At this point the algorithms that will be used in the digital systems are still being defined although the method used should evaluate the SNR of the image for a region of interest for a prescribed range of thicknesses of phantom material for the various AEC modes available with each system.

h) **Effective resolution and MTF.** This measurement reflects both the intrinsic resolution associated with the detector and focal spot as well as effects caused by focal spot "wobble" and mechanical vibrations. The isotropy and isoplanaticity of resolution should also be assessed by measuring in different positions in the image field and at different orientations. The definitive measurement of spatial resolution uses the modulation transfer function (MTF) (ICRU 1986). To assess the role of the detector aperture, focal spot effects and motion, the presampled MTF is meaured, using a slanted radiation-opaque edge at a number of angular orientations (perpendicular to, parallel to and at 45° to the chest wall). In addition, as an overall measurement including the effect of detector sampling, the MTF is measured without the artificial oversampling provided by the slanted edge technique. In addition, it may be useful to measure the limiting spatial resolution with high resolution bar-patterns located at a position corresponding to the upper surface of the breast (e.g., 4.5 cm above breast support) so that both the effects of detector unsharpness and focal spot/magnification blurring on spatial resolution are included. MTF should be measured using high and medium contrast edges (Critten et al. 1996) to test for signal-dependent variations (e.g., due to response of amplifiers, etc.)

i) **Dynamic range.** For a digital system, the dynamic range of image acquisition should be much higher than in film-based mammography. Dynamic range assesses the maximum and minimum exposure levels that can be handled by the imaging system and how accurately the detector signal reflects the x-ray attenuation of the breast. Dynamic range is measured by producing an image with a standard technique of a phantom containing regions of varying x-ray attenuation from 100% to near 0 transmission, and by measuring the SNR versus material thickness

j) **Noise Power Spectrum (NPS).** Among the important characteristics in mammography, and especially with digital detectors are the noise properties. Ideally, noise will be dominated by the Poisson quantum fluctuations of the absorbed x rays, however, additional noise sources may be significant and must be quantified. The noise power spectrum can be used to characterize system noise and to determine the extent to which imaging is x-ray quantum limited, and as well, whether the image contains periodic disturbances due to interference from power sources, clock frequencies, etc.

k) **Noise Equivalent Quanta [NEQ(f,E)].** This is the signal-to-noise ratio of the output image and when expressed versus the spatial frequency, f, provides possibly the most useful indication of image quality. NEQ is calculated from the MTF and the NPS measurements. It should be evaluated over a range of exposure levels to evaluate the extent to which the system is Poisson noise limited.

l) **Detective quantum efficiency [DQE(f,E)].** While NEQ gives a measure of image quality, DQE provides an indication of the efficiency of the imaging system in utilizing the information carried by the x-ray beam. Calculation of DQE(f,E) requires the MTF and NPS results as well as knowledge of the entrance exposure and the measured x-ray spectrum incident on the detector.

m) **Video monitor brightness and contrast.** Digital mammograms may be recorded on laser-printed films, but will also be viewed on CRT display either for interpretation or just for initial quality verification. For this reason, it is important that proper QC is carried out on these displays. In general, the QC procedure should adhere to the ACR/NEMA display function standard guidelines for measurement and standardization of digital image display (Roehrig et al. 1996, Hemminger et al. 1996). A digital test pattern is useful in evaluating geometric fidelity, contrast, brightness, spatial resolution of the display, etc. Output brightness and contrast should be monitored in specific locations on the display device using an external calibrated photometer. Visual interpretation of resolution and spatial linearity should also be done.

n) **The quality control of the hard copy laser film printing is clearly of key importance.** Regular photographic quality control should be performed on the processor, and the printer internal calibration film checked regularly. A SMPTE pattern printed routinely will verify that the contrast or uniformity has not changed drastically. Uniform fields at a range of densities should be printed to verify proper focus across the scanning field, and rule out the presence of roller marks or other processor artefacts. A magnifying glass must be used to examine both edges and centre of the image. Dimensional accuracy (aspect ratio) and pixel jitter should be evaluated with a pattern formed of 1pixel wide lines in orthogonal as well as 45 deg angles. This should be done for both white lines on black as well as black lines on white. Please see the chapter by Seibert for more information on laser printers.

o) **Contrast-to-noise ratio.** A contrast-detail phantom can be used to determine the overall subjective low contrast performance of the systems.

Although a large number of test measures have been described, these are greatly simplified and facilitated by the fact that all of the image data are already in digital form. It is feasible to develop a computer program to automatically analyze appropriate sections of the digital phantom image and produce the results with a minimum of user input

Cooperation from Manufacturers

Because digital mammography is a new mammography and technical changes will be continuously occurring, it is important to obtain close cooperation from the manufacturer so that the medical physicist understands the function of the equipment and the software for flat-fielding, image correction, and calibration. The manufacturer also benefits from this interaction as the medical physics community is likely to provide the standards for acceptance testing and QC and their understanding of the issues is likely to facilitate meaningful standards and test techniques.

Computerized QC Package

Because the data from digital mammography are in convenient digital form, it is reasonable that computer methods should be used to carry out QC testing, and to gather and analyze data. Following a defined protocol, a sequence of test images can be produced using a standard set of phantoms. The phantoms can include fiducial registration marks that will appear on the images. Analysis algorithms can then "read" the acquired image data and use the registration marks to select the region of interest for each test and to establish proper spatial alignment. The algorithms could automatically analyze the selected parts of each image to calculate image quality measures, e.g., MTF, DQE following the general strategy described by Chakraborty (Chakraborty 1996). Additional data, such as measurements of exposure, HVL, etc. can be entered into the computer and the results stored in a database. Standards can be established for each measure with limits indicating a warning level as well as a level at which imaging will not be permitted. This approach could make the quality control procedure automatic, reproducible and efficient.

Table 3. Quality control responsibilities of personnel.

Activity	Interval	Performed by	Result
acquire digital phantom image	Daily	tech	automatic analysis of geometric factors, linearity, dynamic range, resolution/MTF NEQ, distortion, etc.
CRT display performance	Weekly	tech	enter measurements
acquire ACR	Daily	tech	visual inspection
exposure measurement	Monthly	physicist	dose calculation
HVL	semi-annual	physicist	

Acknowledgment

Portions of the material in this chapter have been previously published in an article entitled: "X-ray detectors for digital radiography" by Martin J. Yaffe and John A. Rowlands, Physics in Medicine and Biology 42, 1-39, 1997 and are reprinted with permission of IOP Publishing Ltd. I am also grateful for the advice of John Rowlands and Gordon Mawdsley. The physicists of the International Digital Mammography Development Group, including Mark Williams, Andrew Maidment, Loren Niklason, Carolyn Kimme-Smith and Dev Chakraborty have all contributed to the development of lthe QC program for digital mammography. Parts of the research supporting the work described were funded by the Canadian Breast Cancer Research Initiative, The National Cancer Institute and The Office of Women's Health (HHS).

References

Abdel-Malek, A., Kopans, D., Moore, R., et al. "Telemammographic System Development Issues and Possible Solutions." In: *Digital Mammography.* Gale, A.G. (Ed.) Bristol, IOP Publications, 1994.

Anderson, E.D.C., Muir, B.B., Walsh, J.S. et al. "The efficacy of double reading mammograms in breast screening." *Clinical Radiology* 49:248; 1994.

Ascher, S., Shtern, F., Winfield, D. et al. "Final report of the technology transfer workshop on breast cancer detection, diagnosis and treatment." *Academic Radiology,* Nov. 1998 (in press).

Barnes, G.T., Frey, G.D., (Eds.) *Screen Film Mammography Imaging Considerations and Medical Physics Responsibilities.* Madison: Medical Physics Publishing 115-134; 1991.

Barnes, G.T. and Frey, G.D. "Mammography Acceptance Testing and Quality Control Documentation and Reports." In Barnes, G.T., Frey, G.D. (Eds): *Screen Film Mammography Imaging Considerations and Medical Physics Responsibilities.* Madison: Medical Physics Publishing 203-220; 1991.

Batnitzky, S., Rosenthal, S.J., Siegal, E.L., et al. "Teleradiology: an assessment." *Radiology* 177:11; 1990.

Bendat, J.S., Piersol, A.G. *Random Data Analysis and Measurement Techniques,* 2nd Edition. Wiley, New York 338; 1986.

Bird, R.E., Wallace, T.W., Yankaskas, B.C. "Analysis of cancers missed at screening mammography." *Radiology* 184:613; 1992.

Bogucki, T.M., Trauernicht, D.P. and Kocher, T.E. "Characteristics of a storage phosphor system for medical imaging." *Technical and Scientific Monograph No. 6,* Eastman Kodak Health Sciences Division, 1995.

Boyd, N.F., Byng, J.W., Jong, R.A., et al. "Quantitative classification of mammographic densities and breast cancer risk: results from the Canadian National Breast Screening Study." *J. Natl. Cancer Inst.* 87:670; 1995.

Bunch, P.C., "The effects of reduced film granularity on mammographic image quality" in *Medical Imaging 1997: Physics of Medical Imaging,* R.Van Metter and J Beutel, (Eds.) *Proc. SPIE* 3032: 302-317; 1997.

Byng, J.W., Critten, J.P. and Yaffe, M.J. "Thickness equalization processing for mammographic images." *Radiology* 203:564-568; 1997.

Chabbal, J., Chaussat, C., Ducourant, T., Fritsch, L., Michailos, V., Spinnler, V., Vieux, G., Arques, M., Hahm, G., Hoheisel, M., Horbaschek, H., Schulz, R., Spahn, M. "Amorphous silicon x-ray sensor. Medical Imaging; 1996." *Physics of Medical Imaging,* R. Van Metter and J. Beutel (Eds.) *Proc SPIE* 2708: 499-510; 1996.

Chakraborty, D.P. "Physical measures of image quality in mammography." *Proc. SPIE* 2708: 179-193; 1996.

Clarke, L.P., Kallergi, M., Qian, W., Li, H.D., Clark, R.A., Silbiger, M.L. "Tree-structured non-linear filter and wavelet transform for microcalcification segmentation in digital mammography." *Cancer Letters* 77:173-181; 1994.

Cowen, A.R., Giles, A., Davies, A.G., Workman, A. "An image processing algorithm for PPCR imaging." *Proc. SPIE* 1898:833-841; 1993.

Critten, J.P., Emde, K.A., Mawdsley, G.E. and Yaffe, M.J. "Digital mammography image correction and evaluation" In *Digital Mammography 96.* Doi, K., Giger, M.L., Nishikawa, R.M. and Schmidt, R.A. (Eds.) Excerpta Medica International Congress, Series 1119: 455-458; 1996.

Cunningham, I.A., Westmore, M.S. and Fenster, A. "A spatial frequency dependent quantum accounting diagram and detective quantum efficiency model of signal and noise propagation in cascaded imaging systems." *Medical Physics* 21(3):417-427; 1994.

Dobbins, J.T. III. "Effects of undersampling on the proper interpretation of modulation transfer function, noise power spectra, and noise equivalent quanta of digital imaging systems." *Medical Physics* 22:171-181; 1995.

Fahrig, R., Rowlands, J.A., Yaffe, M.J. "X-ray imaging with amorphous selenium: Detective quantum efficiency of photoconductive receptors for digital mammography." *Medical Physics* 22:153-160; 1995.

Fahrig, R., Yaffe, M.J. "A model for optimization of spectral shape in digital mammography." *Medical Physics* 21:1463-1471; 1994.

Freedman, M., Pe E., Zuurbier, R., Katial, R., Jafroudi, H., Nelson, M., Lo, S-CB, Mun, S.K. "Image processing in digital mammography." *Proc. SPIE* 2164:57-554; 1994.

Frey, G.D. "Screen-film mammography: equipment acceptance testing and quality control." In: *Screen Film Mammography Imaging Considerations and Medical Physics Responsibilities.* Barnes, G., Frey, G.D. (Eds.) Madison: Medical Physics Publishing 177-202; 1991.

Fujieda, I., Cho, G., Drewery, J., Gee, T., Jing, T., Kaplan, S.N., Perez-Mendez, V., Wildermuth, D. "X-ray and charged particle detection with CsI(Tl) layer coupled to a-Si:H photodiode layer." *IEEE Transactions in Nuclear Science* 38:255-262; 1991.

Graeve, T., Li, S., Alexander, S.M., Huang, W. "High-resolution amorphous silicon image sensor." In: *Medical Imaging: Physics of Medical Imaging,* R. Van Metter and J. Beutel (Eds.). Proc SPIE 2708:494-498; 1996.

Gray, J.E. and Stears, J.G. "Acceptance testing of diagnostic x-ray imaging equipment: consideration and rationale equipment requirements and quality control for mammography." In: *Specification, Acceptance Testing and Quality Control of Diagnostic X-ray Imaging Equipment.* J.A. Seibert, G.T Barnes and R.G. Gould, (Eds.) American Institute of Physics, Woodbury New York. (American Association of Physicists in Medicine Monograph #20), 1-9; 1994.

Harvey, J.A., Fajardo, L.L., Innis, C.A. "Previous mammograms in patients with impalpable breast carcinoma: retrospective vs blinded interpretation." *American Journal of Roentgenology* 161:1167; 1993.

Hejazi, S., Trauernicht, D.P. "Potential image quality in scintillator CCD-based imaging systems for digital radiography and digital mammography." In: *Medical Imaging 1996: Physics of Medical Imaging,* R. Van Metter and J Beutel, (Eds.) Proceedings of the Society of Photo-Optical Instrumentation Engineers 2708:440-449; 1996.

Hemminger, B.M., Blume, H., Roehrig, H., Johnston, R.E. "Demonstration of display system measurement and conformance to the proposed ACR/NEMA working group 11 display function standard." RSNA Inforad Exhibit. Supplement to *Radiology* 201:553; 1996.

Hendrick, R.E. et al. American College of Radiology Committee on Quality Assurance in Mammography. Mammography Quality Control Manual; 1999.

Henry, J.M., Yaffe, M. J., Pi, B., Venzon, J.E., Augustine, F. and Tumer, T.O. "Solid state x-ray detectors for digital mammography." In: *Medical Imaging : Physics of Medical Imaging,* R. Van Metter and J. Beutel (Eds.) Proceedings of the Society of Photo-Optical Instrumentation Engineers 2432:392-401; 1995.

International Commission on Radiation Units and Measurements. Modulation Transfer Function of Screen-Film Systems, Report No. 41. International Commission on Radiation Units and Measurements, Bethesda MD; 1986.

Johns, P.C. and Yaffe, M.J "X-ray characterization of normal and neoplastic breast tissues." *Physics in Medicine and Biology* 32:675-695; 1987.

Johns, P.C., Yaffe, M.J. "Theoretical optimization of dual-energy x-ray imaging with application to mammography." *Medical Physics* 12:289; 1985.

Johns, P.C., Yaffe, M.J. "X-ray characterization of normal and neoplastic breast tissues." *Physics in Medicine and Biology* 32:675; 1987.

Kato, K. "Photostimulable phosphor radiography design considerations." In: *Specification, Acceptance Testing and Quality Control of Diagnostic X-ray Imaging Equipment.* J.A. Seibert, G.T. Barnes and R.G. Gould, (Eds.). American Institute of Physics. Woodbury New York. (American Association of Physicists in Medicine Monograph #20), 731-769; 1994.

Kimme-Smith, C.M., Williams, M.B., Fajardo, L.L., Bassett, L.W., Valentino, D.J. "Correspondence of quality control failures and clinical image failures in digital mammography." (RSNA Inforad Exhibit). Supplement to *Radiology* 201:555; 1996.

Klein, C.A. *Journal of Applied Physics* 39:2029; 1968.

Laine, A., Fan, J., Schuler, S. "A framework for contrast enhancement by dyadic wavelet analysis." In: *Digital Mammography.* Gale, A.G., Astley, S.M., Dance, D.R., Cairns, A.Y. (Eds.). Elsevier Publishing, Amsterdam, 91-100; 1994.

Landis, S.H., Murray, T., Bolden, S., Wingo, P.A. "Cancer statistics, 1998." *CA Cancer J. Clin.* 48:6-29; 1998.

Lee, D.L.Y., Cheung, L.K., Palecki, E.F. and Jeromin, L.S. "A discussion on resolution, sensitivity, S/N ratio and dynamic range of Se-TFT direct digital radiographic detector." Proceedings of the Society of Photo-Optical Instrumentation Engineers 2708:511-522; 1996.

Maidment, A.D.A. and Yaffe, M.J. "Analysis of signal propagation in optically coupled detectors for digital mammography: II lens and fibre optics." *Phys. Med. Biol.* 41:475-493; 1996.

Maidment, A.D.A. and Yaffe, M.J. "Analysis of the spatial-frequency dependent DQE of optically coupled digital mammography detectors." *Medical Physics* 21:721-729; 1994.

Mattheus, R.A., Temmerman, Y. Verhellen P, et al. "Management system for a PACS network in a hospital environment." *Proc SPIE;* 1991.

Miller, L.D. "Transfer characteristics and spectral response of television camera tubes" In: *Photoelectronic Imaging Devices,* Vol. 1, Biberman, L.M. and Nudelman, S. (Eds.). Plenum New York, 267-290; 1991.

Morrow, M.W., Paranjape, R.B., Rangayyan, R.M., Desautels, J.E.L. "Region-based contrast enhancement of mammograms." *IEEE Transactions on Medical Image Processing* 11:392-406; 1992.

Niklason, L.T., Christian, B.T., Whitman, G.J., Kopans, D.B., Rougeot, H.M., Opsahl-Ong, B. "Full-field digital mammographic imaging." (RSNA Scientific Exhibit). Supplement to *Radiology* 201: 446; 1996.

Perez-Mendez, V., Cho, G., Fujieda, I., Kaplan, S.N., Qureshi, S., Street, R.A. "The application of thick hydrogenated amorphous silicon layers to charged particle and x-ray detection." *Mat. Res. Soc. Symp. Proc.* 149 621-630 (also Lawrence Berkeley Laboratories Report LBL-26998, April 1989).

Piper, W., Bigelow, J.E., Castleberry, D.E. and Possin, G.E. "The demands on the *a*-Si FET as a pixel switch for liquid crystal displays." In: *Amorphous Semiconductors for Microelectronics,* SPIE, 617:10-15; 1986.

Pisano, E., Johnston, R.E., Pizer, S., McLelland, R. "Computer enhancement of digitized mammograms." *Radiology* 181:5-15; 1991.

Powell, M. "The physics of amorphous-silicon thin-film transistors." *IEEE Trans. Electron Devices,* 36:2753-2763; 1989.

Que, W. and Rowlands, J. A. "X-ray imaging using amorphous selenium: Inherent resolution." *Med. Phys.* 22:365-374; 1995.

Rabbani, M., Shaw, R., Van Metter, R. "Detective quantum efficiency of imaging systems with amplifying and scattering mechanisms." *J. Optical Soc. Am.* A 4, 895-901; 1987.

Rahn, J.T., Lemmi, F., Weisfeield, R.L., et al. "High resolution, high fill factor a-Si:H sensor arrays for medical imaging." *Proc. SPIE* 3659, Medical Imaging 99 (in press).

Roehrig, H., Blume, H., Hemminger, B.M. "Image quality control and image quality measurements for display systems." (RSNA Inforad Exhibit). Supplement to *Radiology* 201:553; 1996.

Roehrig, H., Yu, T., Schempp, W.V. "Performance of x-ray imaging systems with optical coupling for demagnification between scintillator and CCD readout." *Proc. SPIE* 2279 388-401; 1994.

Rossi, R. "X-ray generator and automatic exposure control device acceptance testing." In: *Specification, Acceptance Testing and Quality Control of Diagnostic X-ray Imaging Equipment.* J.A. Seibert, G.T. Barnes and R.G. Gould, (Eds.). American Institute of Physics. Woodbury New York. (American Association of Physicists in Medicine Monograph #20), 267-301, 1994.

Shah, K.S., Lund, J.C., Olschner, F., Moy, L. and Squillante, M.R. "Thallium bromide radiation detectors." *IEEE Trans. Nuclear Science* 36: 199-202; 1989.

Smart, C.R., Hendrick, R.E., Rutledge, J.H. III, et al. "Benefit of mammographic screening in women ages 40-49 years." *Cancer* 75:1619; 1995

Street, R.A., Rahn, J.T., Shah, K., et al. "X-ray imaging using lead iodide as a semi-conductor detector." *Proc. SPIE Medical Imaging* 99, 3659 (in press) 1999.

Sund, T. "Full-scale replacement of a visiting radiologist service with teleradiology." Proc International Symposium, Canadian Assoc Radiol, Berlin: Springer-Verlag, 811; 1991.

Swank, R.K. "Absorption and noise in x-ray phosphors." *J. Appl. Phys.* 44:4199-4203; 1973.

Tabar, L., Fagerberg, G., Chen, H-H, et al. "Efficacy of breast cancer screening by age: new results from the Swedish Two-County Trial." *Cancer* 75:2507, 1995.

Tachoes, P.G., Correa, J., Souto, M., Gonzalez, C., Gomez, L., Vidal, J. "Enhancement of chest and breast radiographs by automatic spatial filtering." *IEEE Transactions on Medical Imaging* MI-10: 330-335, 1992.

Takahashi, K., Kohda, K., Miyahara, J. "Mechanism of photostimulated luminescence in BaFX:Eu2+ (X = Cl,Br)" *J. Luminescence* 266; 1984.

Thurfjell, E.L., Lernevall, K.A., Taube, A.A.S. "Benefit of independent double reading in a population-based mammography screening program." *Radiology* 191:241; 1994.

von Seggern, H., Voigt, T., Knupfer, W. and Lange, G. "Physical model of photostimulated luminescence of x-ray irradiated BaFBr:Eu^{2+}" *J. Appl. Phys.* 64 1405-1412; 1988.

Wagner, A.J. "Contrast and grid performance in mammography." In: *Screen-film mammography imaging considerations and medical physics responsibilities.* Barnes, G.T., Frey, G.D., (Eds.). Madison: Medical Physics Publishing, 115-134; 1991.

Wei, Q., Clarke, L.P., Kallergi, M, Li, G-D, Velthuizen, R.P, Clark R.A., Silbiger, M.L. "Tree-structured nonlinear filter and wavelet transform for microcalcification segmentation in mammography." *Proc SPIE* 1905: 509-520; 1993.

Wolfe, J.N. "Breast patterns as an index of risk for developing breast cancer." *American Journal of Radiology* 126:1130-1139; 1976.

Wolfe, J.N. "Risk for breast cancer development determined by mammographic parenchymal pattern." *Cancer* 37:2486; 1976.

Wu, X., Barnes, G.T, Tucker, D.M. "Spectral dependence of glandular tissue dose in screen-film mammography." *Radiology* 179:143-148; 1991.

Yaffe, M.J., Williams, M.B., Niklason, L.T., Mawdsley, G.E., Maidment, A.D.A. "Development of a quality control system for full-field digital mammography." (abstract) *Radiology* 209 (P): 160; 1998.

Yaffe, M.J. and Mawdsley, G.E. "Equipment Requirements and Quality Control for Mammography." In: *Specification, Acceptance Testing and Quality Control of Diagnostic X-ray Imaging Equipment.* J.A. Seibert, G.T. Barnes and R.G. Gould (Eds.). American Institute of Physics, Woodbury New York. (American Association of Physicists in Medicine Monograph #20), 303-357; 1994.

Zhao, W. and Rowlands, J.A. "X-ray imaging using amorphous selenium: Feasibility of a flat panel self-scanned detector for digital radiology." *Medical Physics* 22:1595-1604; 1995.

Image Quality and Dose

Ian A. Cunningham, Ph.D.
Imaging Research Laboratory, The John P. Robarts Research Institute
Department of Diagnostic Radiology, London Health Sciences Centre
Department of Diagnostic Radiology and Nuclear Medicine,
University of Western Ontario, London, Ontario, Canada

Introduction

The development and application of new digital x-ray imaging technologies has altered the traditional trade-offs between image quality and patient dose familiar to users of film-screen systems. With film-based technologies, image spatial resolution, patient dose and image noise are generally dictated by the choice of beam kVp and film-screen combination. These choices are made by the policy-makers of medical facilities and particular film-screen combinations are made available for each radiographic procedure. For instance, high-resolution, lower-speed (less sensitive to radiation) combinations may be used for orthopedic and extremity work while medium-resolution, higher-speed (more sensitive to radiation) combinations may be used for general or chest radiography. With digital technologies, the operator often has greater control over the radiographic parameters of kVp and mAs due to the large dynamic range of many systems.

The ability of digital systems to operate over a range of low- and high-dose levels can be a mixed blessing. For instance, the wide latitude may increase the tolerance of these systems to unintentional errors in exposure control, resulting in high-quality images over a wider range of exposures than could be obtained with film-screen systems, and therefore a reduced re-take rate. However, with digital systems (e.g. computed radiography systems), re-takes may be necessary only when exposures are unacceptably low, when quantum noise or system noise compromises image quality, and may not be necessary when exposures are unnecessarily high. This may result in an increased tendency for operators to err on the side of greater-than-necessary patient exposures, requiring an increased awareness and vigilance on the part of the operator to ensure that an appropriate trade-off between image quality and patient dose is being achieved. Part of that awareness is the ability to quantify image noise and to compare it with the minimum theoretical noise expected for a specified radiation exposure.

Figure 1 shows four images of an anthropomorphic skull phantom obtained on a typical digital angiographic suite using an x-ray image intensifier (XRII)

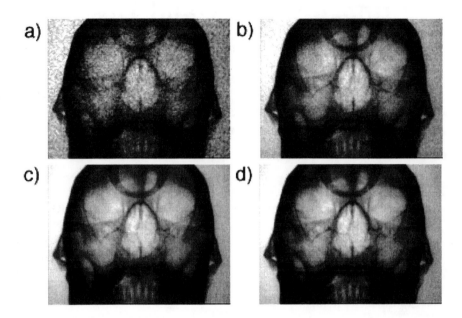

Figure 1: Image quality is dependent on the number of quanta used to create the image as illustrated in this example. The average XRII exposure per image is approximately: a) 0.16 μR, b) 1.6 μR, c) 16 μR, and d) 24 μR.

and video camera. The XRII input exposure for each image as measured by an ionization chamber placed behind the phantom forehead, and corresponding number of x-ray quanta per mm^2, are summarized in Table 1. All images were acquired using a 60 kVp beam hardened with 2 cm of Al and 3 mm of Cu. The exposures in a) and b) are typical of a single frame of fluoroscopy while the exposures in c) and d) are typical of a single cine or digital angiogram frame. It is clear that increasing the exposure to the detector - and therefore exposure to the patient - reduces image noise and increases image quality. In

	XRII Exposure	Quanta per mm^2
a)	0.16 μR	45
b)	1.6 μR	450
c)	16 μR	4,500
d)	24 μR	6,720

Table 1: Summary of incident XRII exposure and number of quanta per mm^2 per frame used to create images in Figure 1.

particular, an increased exposure is necessary to see smaller objects (more detail) and/or lower contrasts. However, there reaches a point where additional exposure to the patient does not show an appreciable improvement as illustrated by the change from c) to d).

The relationship between image noise and the number of quanta used to create the image was first recognized by Rose in the late 1940's.[1-4] While the "Rose SNR" (described below) is considered by many to be too simplistic to have much practical value, it is still useful as a conceptual tool for developing an understanding of fundamental relationships. However, the view that an imaging system must faithfully *transfer* the input image signal and noise from the input to the output suggested the use of foundations laid out by scientists and engineers studying communications theory, and in particular, use of the Fourier-transform (see the appendix) linear-systems approach was found to be particularly important.[5]

Fourier-based methods were initially applied in the imaging sciences by Rossmann and co-workers,[6,7] including use of the modulation-transfer function (MTF) and related concepts. General works have subsequently been published by Dainty & Shaw,[8] Gaskill,[9] Papoulis,[10] Doi, Rossmann and Haus,[11] Barrett and Swindell,[12] Metz and Doi,[13] and many others.

In this chapter, methods of measuring, quantifying, comparing and understanding image noise are described. Emphasis is placed on representing imaging problems equally in the spatial and spatial-frequency domains, and to solve many problems by fluently moving between the two. In particular, use is made of the modulation-transfer function (MTF), noise-power spectrum (NPS), quantum sinks, noise-equivalent number of quanta (NEQ), and detective quantum efficiency (DQE) in the description of image noise. The Fourier transform is described in the appendix, but read Bracewell[14] for an excellent description of applications of the Fourier transform, and Brigham[15] for a clear description of the discrete Fourier transform. Excellent references for a description of stochastic processes are Bendat and Piersol[16] or Papoulis.[17]

Background Concepts

Images and their Units

In this chapter, an image will correspond to three different types of quantities: 1) an *analog image*, $d(r)$; 2) a *digital image*, d_n; and, 3) a *distribution of quanta*, $q(r)$. For instance, the input to an x-ray imaging system is always a distribution of x-ray quanta, $q(\boldsymbol{r})$, and the output will generally be either an analog image $d(\boldsymbol{r})$ or a digital image d_n. These names and distinctions are just the author's preference, but are important as they have different units and physical meanings, and must therefore be treated differently mathematically. In this section, these three types of images and their physical bases are described.

Analog Image

The term *analog image* will be used to describe a spatially-varying signal $d(\boldsymbol{r})$. It can be expressed as a function of a continuous variable such as $\boldsymbol{r}$, representing a two-dimensional position in the image, or x, representing a position along a line in one dimension. Units of $d(\boldsymbol{r})$ may be relative or arbitrary. Examples include the voltage from a video camera as a function of position along a trace, optical density in a radiographic film, or emitted intensity from a CRT monitor.

Digital Image

A *digital image* is generally a two-dimensional array of discrete numerical values, d_n, representing image intensity where n identifies a particular pixel (picture element) in the image. The numerical values in a digital image are dimensionless, such as the digital value produced by an analog-to-digital converter (ADC).

Quantum Image

A *quantum image* $q(\boldsymbol{r})$ is a distribution of quanta. X rays transmitted through a patient and incident on an imaging detector form an x-ray image. Each x-ray quantum has negligible spatial extent, and is considered to be a point or impulse object represented as a single Dirac delta function $\delta(\boldsymbol{r} - \boldsymbol{r}_o)$ where $\boldsymbol{r}_o$ is a vector describing the location of the quantum.

There are two important reasons why manipulating quantum images is slightly more complicated than manipulating analog or digital images. The first is that they must be interpreted as *distributions* in the mathematical sense, having dimension area^{-1}. The implications of this are described in more detail below. The second reason is that image quanta have fundamental statistical properties that cannot be ignored. It is therefore necessary to describe images in terms of random variables. For instance, we describe the position of each quantum in an image using the random vector variable $\tilde{\boldsymbol{r}}$ which has the set of values $\{r_i\}$ and where each value describes the position of one quantum. The quantum image $q(r)$ is a particular realization of these random variables, and can be expressed as

$$q(r) = \sum_{i=1}^{N_q} \delta(r - r_i) \tag{1}$$

where N_q, the total number of quanta in the image, is given by

$$N_q = \int_{-\infty}^{\infty} q(r)\mathrm{d}^2 r. \tag{2}$$

While it is not possible to know *precisely* where the x-ray quanta are in a particular distribution due to the uncertainty principle, $q(r)$ represents a particular *possible* distribution, that is a sample image, where the quanta may be statistically correlated - or not - in some specified way. The expectation value (i.e. an ensemble average of many such realizations) of $q(r)$ will be written as $\mathrm{E}\{q(r)\}$, and describes the expectation distribution of quanta per unit area at position r. If the image consists only of a Poisson distribution of quanta, $\tilde{r}$ is randomly distributed and uncorrelated over the image area, and $\mathrm{E}\{q(r)\}$ is a constant independent of position.

Quantum images are generally two dimensional. However, it will be convenient, particularly for illustrations, to consider a one-dimensional quantum image consisting of a distribution of quanta along a line, $q(x)$, having dimension length^{-1}.

Image Contrast

Contrast is a measure of the relative brightness difference between two locations in an image. Relative brightness is often a more important parameter than absolute brightness since absolute brightness is often dependent on display hardware (e.g. video monitor brightness setting or viewbox intensity), and may therefore have no particular significance in an absolute sense. The contrast between locations 1 and 2 having image signals d_1 and d_2 is C where

$$C = \frac{<d_2> - <d_1>}{\frac{1}{2}[<d_2> + <d_1>]} \tag{3}$$

and where $<>$ indicates an expectation value. For small contrasts, $d_2 \approx d_1$ and

$$C \approx \frac{<d_2> - <d_1>}{<d_2>}. \tag{4}$$

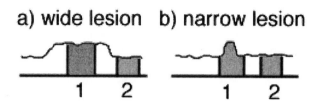

Figure 2: Profiles through an image containing: a) a wide lesion relative to the measurement area (shaded region); and b) a narrow lesion. The measured contrast will be accurate for the wide lesion but inaccurate for the narrow lesion. In general, measured contrast depends on both the size and shape of the lesion relative to the size and shape of the measurement area.

Noise Variance

Image noise is defined here as random variations in image signals. For instance, an image of a uniform object might have a uniform intensity over a specified region of interest if not for these random variations. Therefore, one way of describing noise is to calculate the variance in measurements of the image signal over a specific region of interest which has a uniform mean. This noise variance, equal to the mean squared deviation from the mean, can therefore be written as σ_d^2 where

$$\sigma_d^2 = \frac{1}{N-1} \sum_{n=0}^{N-1} \left(d_n - \overline{d} \right)^2 \tag{5}$$

where the mean $\overline{d}$ is given by

$$\overline{d} = \frac{1}{N} \sum_{n=0}^{N-1} d_n \tag{6}$$

and is calculated using N measurements of signal d_n. Units of the variance σ_d^2 are the same as the units of the squared signal d_n^2.

The Need for the Fourier Domain

The simplistic concepts of contrast and noise variance are not really very useful in practice. The sensitivity of a particular system to image contrast depends on the size and shape of structures in the input image in addition to

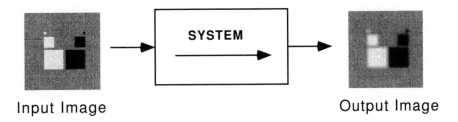

Input Image   Output Image

Figure 3: A system with poor spatial resolution transfers large-area contrast better than small-area contrast. As a result, the contrast of fine detail is reduced and the transferred image appears "blurred".

the size and shape of measurement areas (which are directly related to the spatial resolution of the system). This is illustrated in Fig. 2 where profiles through two lesions are shown. Measurements of the image signal requires use of a detector having finite physical size (even if it is one "pixel") as indicated by the shaded region of each profile. Thus, contrast measured using regions 1 and 2 near the wide lesion will be much greater than contrast measured using regions 1 and 2 near the narrow lesion. The manufacturer of an imaging system could boast excellent contrast sensitivity according to a particular test using large lesions, even if the system is close to useless for imaging small lesions. The concept of contrast sensitivity is therefore related to the spatial resolution of a system. This is illustrated in Fig. 3 where the input-output relationship is shown for a system that transfers large-area (relative to the measurement area) contrast fairly well, but small-area contrast poorly. The result is an output image in which the contrast of fine details (small lesions and edges) is reduced, giving rise to an image which appears to be "blurred" by the system.

The simplistic concept of noise variance also has limited value in practice, as illustrated in Fig. 4. The two profiles each have unity noise variance; however, they look very different because the noise in a) is correlated over only a very short distance while noise in b) is correlated over a much greater distance. Thus, concepts of image noise must also be tied to concepts of object size and system spatial resolution.

One way of doing this would be to describe spatial-resolution characteristics in terms of how a sharp line appears in the image - the line-spread function (LSF), and to describe image noise in terms of statistical correlations in image signals - the autocovariance function. However, it is more convenient to to express these same concepts in the spatial-frequency domain using the Fourier transform. The uniqueness of the Fourier transform means that any

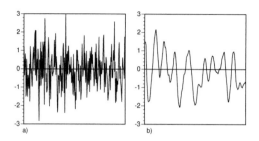

Figure 4: These one-dimensional profiles have the same noise variance but look very different. Noise in b) is correlated over a greater distance than noise in a).

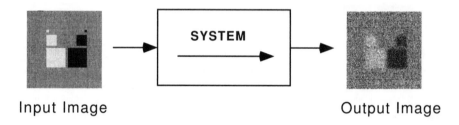

Input Image   Output Image

Figure 5: A system which degrades spatial resolution and also increases noise will severely compromise image quality as illustrated here, particularly for the visualization of small details.

problem can be solved equivalently in either the spatial (x) or the spatial-frequency (u) domain. It is often easier to find a solution in one domain than in the other, and so every imaging problem should be examined in both.

Figure 5 illustrates the input-output relationship of a system which passes contrast in a manner identical to that in Fig. 3, but increases noise as well. The resulting image is severely compromised, and small structures are barely detectable, if at all.

The concepts of image signal-to-noise ratio (SNR) and the ability to visualize image structures are therefore tied to: 1) input image structure sizes; 2) input image noise; 3) system spatial resolution ("measurement area"); and, 4) the extent of noise correlations and additional noise sources added by the system. The first two concepts are dependent on the input signal and thus are not system-dependent parameters. The second two can be described in terms of the spatial-frequency-dependent signal- and noise-transfer characteristics of the system as described in this chapter.

Particle-Based Metrics of System Performance

The stochastic nature of image quanta imposes a fundamental limitation on the performance of photon-based imaging systems, and gives rise to stochastic fluctuations in the image signals contributing to image formation. In this section, metrics developed to describe image quality in terms of signal and noise are described.

Photon Counting Signal-to-Noise Ratio

The signal from a simple photon-counting x-ray detector is proportional to the number of quanta interacting in the detector. Thus, the signal d is given by

$$d = k\alpha N_q \qquad (7)$$

where N_q is the number of incident quanta, α is the detector quantum efficiency, and k is a constant relating the number of interacting quanta to the detector signal. X-ray quanta are Poisson distributed, and so the variance in the number of incident quanta is $\sigma_q^2 = \overline{N}_q$ resulting in a detector signal-to-noise ratio SNR_d of

$$\mathrm{SNR}_d = \frac{\overline{d}}{\sigma_d} = \frac{k\alpha \overline{N}_q}{\sqrt{k^2 \alpha \overline{N}_q}} = \sqrt{\alpha \overline{N}_q} \qquad (8)$$

where σ_d could be measured using Eq. (5). This result is applicable only to a single isolated detector. It shows that the SNR is equal to the square root of the number of interacting quanta. As a consequence, with all other factors constant, image SNR is proportional to the square root of the patient dose.

Noise-Equivalent Number of Quanta, NEQ

Equation (8) gives the output SNR of this simple detector that would be measured in practice. One way of specifying the information content in this signal is to determine the number of Poisson-distributed quanta incident on an ideal detector that would give the same SNR. This is called the noise-equivalent number of quanta, NEQ. Since these quanta are Poisson distributed,

$$\mathrm{SNR}_{ideal} = \sqrt{\mathrm{NEQ}} \qquad (9)$$

and

$$\mathrm{NEQ}_d = \mathrm{SNR}_d^2 = \alpha \overline{N}_q. \qquad (10)$$

It should be becoming clear that the SNR has fundamental importance in specifying the performance of an x-ray detector.

Detective Quantum Efficiency, DQE

The NEQ describes the "information content" in a detector signal. The corresponding performance of the detector is called the detective quantum efficiency, DQE, equal to the NEQ as a fraction of the total number of incident quanta. Thus, the DQE of this simple photon-counting detector is given by

$$\text{DQE} = \frac{\text{NEQ}_d}{\overline{N}_q} = \alpha. \tag{11}$$

In this form, the DQE is the ratio of the squared actual SNR to the squared ideal SNR:

$$\text{DQE} = \frac{\text{SNR}_d^2}{\text{SNR}_{ideal}^2} \tag{12}$$

where $\text{SNR}_{ideal}^2 = \overline{N}_q$. It is a measure of the ability of the imaging system to take full advantage of the information content of the incident x-ray beam in terms of the SNR.

DQE of a Cascaded Particle Detector

When an x ray interacts in a radiographic screen, it produces a small flash of light. This flash consists of a large number of light quanta (typically 500 - 1000) which are subsequently detected by a light detector. The combination of a screen and light detector can be represented as a cascaded system as illustrated in Fig. 6. Spreading of light in the screen is ignored in this simple model, but is addressed later in the Fourier-based model.

The concept of noise transfer through cascaded multi-stage systems has been known for some time. Notably, Zweig[18] described the effect of multi-stage gains in terms of the DQE in the nineteen-sixties. Using this approach, an x-ray detector is represented as a cascade of amplification-only stages, and from the binomial theorem it is known that the DQE for an N-stage Zweig-type cascaded model can be written approximately as

$$\text{DQE} = \cfrac{1}{1 + \cfrac{1}{\overline{g}_1} + \cfrac{1}{\overline{g}_1\overline{g}_2} + ... + \cfrac{1}{\overline{g}_1\overline{g}_2\cdots\overline{g}_N}} \tag{13}$$

where $\overline{g}_j$ is the mean quantum gain of the j-th amplification stage. The product $P_j = \overline{g}_1\overline{g}_2...\overline{g}_j$ gives the normalized number of quanta at the j-th

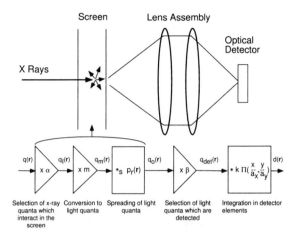

Figure 6: Schematic illustration of a cascaded system consisting of a radiographic screen, lens assembly and light detector.

stage. If P_j is always much greater than unity, the output SNR is determined only by the number of input quanta. However, if P_j falls to less than unity at any stage, a bottleneck occurs that will degrade the output SNR and reduce the DQE. When this happens, this stage is sometimes referred to as the "quantum sink" of the system. It is important that any imaging system be designed to ensure the quantum sink exists at the input to the system. If it happens at a later stage, the patient is being exposed to more radiation than would be necessary with a properly designed system.

Figure 7 shows the product P_j as a function of stage number, called a "quantum accounting diagram" (QAD). In this example, the quantum sink is at stage 1 corresponding to the number of interacting x rays, emphasizing again the need for a detector quantum efficiency to be close to unity. Any stage with a product less than unity is a quantum sink, degrades the system DQE, and results in extra dose to the patient. There is almost a secondary quantum sink in the number of light quanta detected by the optical detector.

This type of analysis has been performed routinely for many medical imaging systems.[19-21] It has great utility for "back-of-the-envelope" type calculations of the DQE, but it is now known this analysis is too simplistic and was responsible for much wasted effort in the development of some new designs by failing to predict quantum sinks at non-zero spatial frequencies.

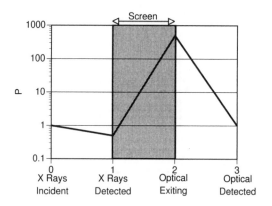

Figure 7: Particle-based QAD analysis of the cascaded detector in Fig. 6.

Rose Model Signal-to-Noise Ratio

The importance of the statistical nature of image quanta was first recognized by Rose and their work forms the basis of many introductory texts on the nature of signal and noise in radiography.[2,3,22-24] The relationship between the number of image quanta and perception of detail is embodied in the "Rose Model," as it has come to be known, that describes the SNR for the detection of a uniform object of area A in a uniform background having a mean $\bar{q}_b$ quanta per unit area. If $\bar{q}_o$ is the mean number of quanta per unit area in the region of the object, the resulting contrast C can be written as

$$C = (\bar{q}_b - \bar{q}_o)/\bar{q}_b. \tag{14}$$

Rose defined the signal to be the incremental change in the number of image quanta due to the object. Note that this is a different to the definition of signal used in Eq. (7). Thus, S_{Rose} is given by

$$S_{Rose} = (\bar{q}_b - \bar{q}_o)A = CA\bar{q}_b. \tag{15}$$

Rose defined noise to be the standard deviation in the number of quanta in an equal area of uniform background, σ_b. For the special case of uncorrelated background quanta, noise is described by Poisson statistics and, similar to the above reasoning, $\sigma_b = \sqrt{A\bar{q}_b}$ so that the Rose SNR, SNR_{Rose}, is given by

$$\text{SNR}_{Rose} = \frac{A(\bar{q}_b - \bar{q}_o)}{\sqrt{A\bar{q}_b}} = C\sqrt{A\bar{q}_b}. \tag{16}$$

Rose showed that SNR_{Rose} must have a value of approximately five or greater for reliable detection of an object. At this limit, detectability is proportional to contrast C and the square root of the object's area, $\sqrt{A}$. This relationship forms the basis of "contrast-detail" phantoms for testing imaging systems, consisting of circular objects having various contrasts and diameters (the word detail refers to the size, and therefore area, of the circular objects). Further implications and limitations of the Rose model are described in terms of modern detection theory by Burgess.[25]

Fourier-Based Metrics of System Performance

The Rose model played an essential role in establishing the fact that image quality is ultimately limited by the statistical nature of image quanta. However, its limitations quickly become apparent when used to assess image quality in many practical situations. The primary restriction is the definition of noise used by Rose in Eq. (16) that is valid for statistically uncorrelated image quanta, but not for estimates of noise based on measured image data. The problems include additive system noise (e.g. electronic or film noise) and correlations in the image data caused by scatter of x rays or secondary quanta in the detector system (e.g. light in a radiographic screen). For these reasons, the original Rose model needs appropriate extension to be of practical value in the analysis of most modern medical imaging systems. This is accomplished with the use of Fourier-based metrics of system performance.

Noise-Power Spectrum (NPS)

One way of describing noise in the presence of correlations in a real image signal $d(x)$ is with the autocovariance, $K_d(x)$, given by

$$K_d(x) = \lim_{X \to \infty} \frac{1}{X} \int_X \Delta d(x' + x) \Delta d(x') \mathrm{d}x' \tag{17}$$

where $\Delta d(x) = d(x) - \mathrm{E}\{d(x)\}$. Technically, this definition is valid only for wide-sense stationary (WSS) random processes[17] which means that the mean and autocorrelation of $d(x)$ are independent of x. In practice, this means that it is often necessary to restrict a measurement of image noise to the central region of a uniform image. In addition, this result is only valid for ergodic systems, which means that expectation values can be estimated from either time averages or space averages. Many systems are ergodic in practice. The variance of $d(x)$, σ_d^2, is related to the autocovariance by

$$\sigma_d^2 = \lim_{X \to \infty} \frac{1}{X} \int_X \Delta d^2(x) \mathrm{d}x \tag{18}$$

$$= \lim_{X\to\infty} \frac{1}{X} \int_X \Delta d(x'+x)\Delta d(x')\mathrm{d}x' \bigg|_{x=0} \tag{19}$$

$$= \mathrm{K}_d(x)|_{x=0}. \tag{20}$$

It is generally more convenient to view noise in the spatial-frequency domain. The Fourier transform of $\mathrm{K}_d(x)$ is the noise-power spectrum (NPS) of $d(x)$ given by

$$\mathrm{NPS}_d(u) = \mathrm{F}\{\mathrm{K}_d(x)\} \tag{21}$$

$$= \lim_{X\to\infty} \frac{1}{X} \mathrm{E}\left\{\left|\int_X \Delta d(x)e^{-i2\pi ux}\mathrm{d}x\right|^2\right\}. \tag{22}$$

The units of $\mathrm{NPS}_d(u)$ are equal to those of $d^2(x) \times x$. The variance and NPS are therefore related by

$$\sigma_d^2 = \mathrm{K}_d(x)|_{x=0} = \int_{-\infty}^{\infty} \mathrm{NPS}_d(u)\mathrm{d}u \tag{23}$$

and the zero-frequency value of the NPS is given by

$$\mathrm{NPS}_d(u)|_{u=0} = \int_{-\infty}^{\infty} \mathrm{K}_d(x)\mathrm{d}x. \tag{24}$$

NPS in One and Two Dimensions

While a two-dimensional analysis of the NPS is sometimes necessary,[26] visualization in two dimensions can be problematic. In many situations it is adequate to examine the two-dimensional NPS in only one specified direction at a time (which we will call the x direction with corresponding spatial frequency u), where the dependence of the NPS in the perpendicular direction has been removed by integration. For instance, if we define $d_Y(x)$ as

$$d_Y(x) = \int_Y d(x,y)\mathrm{d}y, \tag{25}$$

the NPS of $d_Y(x)$, $\mathrm{NPS}_{d_Y}(u)$, is given by

$$\mathrm{NPS}_{d_Y}(u) \tag{26}$$

$$= \lim_{X,Y\to\infty,\infty} \mathrm{E}\left\{\frac{1}{XY}\left|\int_X \Delta d_Y(x)e^{-i2\pi ux}\mathrm{d}x\right|^2\right\} \tag{27}$$

$$= \lim_{X,Y\to\infty,\infty} \mathrm{E}\left\{\frac{1}{XY}\left|\int_X\left[\int_Y \Delta d(x,y)e^{-i2\pi(ux+vy)}\mathrm{d}y\right]_{v=0}\mathrm{d}x\right|^2\right\} \tag{28}$$

which is the two-dimensional NPS of $d(x, y)$ evaluated along the $v = 0$ axis and therefore

$$\text{NPS}_{d_Y}(u) = \text{NPS}_d(u, v)|_{v=0}. \tag{29}$$

The NPS of a two-dimensional random process, $d(x, y)$, whether expressed as a one-dimensional or two-dimensional NPS, will have the units of $d^2(x, y) \times x^2$. The NPS of an analog image is generally expressed in units of mm^2.

NPS of a Quantum Image

A two-dimensional random distribution of uncorrelated x-ray quanta has a uniform expectation value of $\text{E}\{q\}$ quanta/mm^2, and the two-dimensional NPS is given by[8]

$$\text{NPS}_q(u, v) = \text{E}\{q\}. \tag{30}$$

It has an unlimited bandwidth and hence the variance in this distribution is

$$\sigma_q^2 = \int_{-\infty}^{\infty} \int_{-\infty}^{\infty} \text{NPS}_q(u, v) du dv = \int_{-\infty}^{\infty} \int_{-\infty}^{\infty} \text{E}\{q\} du dv \tag{31}$$

which is undefined.

Noise-Equivalent Number of Quanta (NEQ)

As indicated above, units of the NPS depend on the physical basis of the image signal $d(x)$, and may be arbitrary or specific to a particular imaging system. By expressing image noise in terms of the number of Poisson-distributed input photons per unit area at each spatial frequency, Shaw obtained a common *absolute* scale of noise - the noise-equivalent number of quanta (NEQ).[8,27] For a system with an average output $\bar{d}$ corresponding to an average input of $\bar{q}$ quanta per unit area, the NEQ is perhaps best defined as[28]

$$\text{NEQ}(\bar{q}, u) = \frac{\bar{q}^2 \left| \frac{\partial \bar{d}}{\partial \bar{q}} \right|^2 \text{MTF}^2(u)}{\text{NPS}_d(u)} \tag{32}$$

where $\partial \bar{d}/\partial \bar{q}$ is the incremental change in average output signal $\bar{d}$ due to an incremental change in the average input signal $\bar{q}$ at an average input level $\bar{q}$. For a linear imaging system where $\bar{d}$ is proportional to $\bar{q}$, this corresponds to

$$\text{NEQ}(\bar{q}, u) = \frac{\bar{q}^2 \bar{G}^2 \text{MTF}^2(u)}{\text{NPS}_d(u)} \tag{33}$$

$$= \frac{\text{MTF}^2(u)}{\text{NPS}_d(u)/\bar{d}^2} \tag{34}$$

where $\bar{q}$ is the (uniform) average number of incident quanta per unit area, $\overline{G}$ is the scaling factor relating $\bar{q}$ to $\bar{d}$, and $NPS_d(u)$ is the output NPS. The units of NEQ are determined by the units of the NPS. For a two-dimensional random process such as a quantum image, the NEQ will have dimension quanta per unit area.

Equation (34) is particularly convenient to use in many practical situations as it only requires $MTF^2(u)$ and the NPS normalized by the mean signal squared, $NPS_d(u)/\bar{d}^2$, both of which are readily determined experimentally from measured image data. Further detail, including the NEQ of non-linear systems, is described elsewhere.[5] A more detailed description of the NEQ and modern detection theory is available as an ICRU report.[28]

Detective Quantum Efficiency (DQE)

In the Fourier-based approach, the DQE is given by

$$DQE(\bar{q}, u) \quad = \quad \frac{NEQ(\bar{q}, u)}{\bar{q}} \tag{35}$$

$$= \quad \frac{\bar{q} \left| \frac{\partial \bar{d}}{\partial \bar{q}} \right|^2 MTF^2(u)}{NPS_d(u)}. \tag{36}$$

A practical expression for use when measuring the DQE of a linear system is given by

$$DQE(\bar{q}, u) \quad = \quad \frac{\bar{q}\overline{G}^2 MTF^2(u)}{NPS_d(u)} \tag{37}$$

$$= \quad \frac{\bar{d}^2 MTF^2(u)}{\bar{q} NPS_d(u)} \tag{38}$$

In the absence of additive noise, the DQE is independent of $\bar{q}$ for a linear imaging system. The DQE is always dimensionless, and can be no greater than unity.

The term $\bar{q}$ is the total number of incident quanta per unit area, independent of the energy of the quanta. It can be determined from a measurement of the actual exposure X at the detector input (excluding backscatter) with the expression

$$\bar{q} = X \left(\frac{\Phi}{X} \right) \tag{39}$$

where X is the measured exposure (in roentgens), and (Φ/X) is the x-ray fluence per R for the particular spectrum used. Approximate values of (Φ/X)

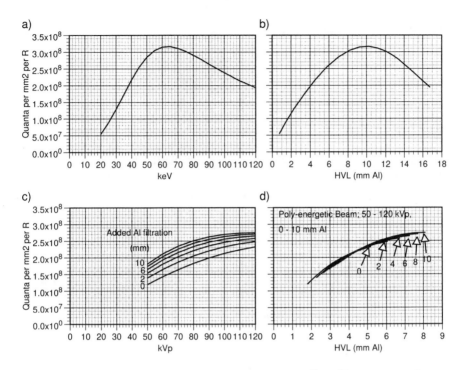

Figure 8: The conversion factor Φ/X (quanta mm^{-2} R^{-1}) is shown: a) as a function of mono-energetic keV; b) as a function of beam HVL for a mono-energetic beam; c) as a function of kVp for a poly-energetic beam with various thicknesses of added aluminum; and d) as a function of HVL for the same poly-energetic beams with added aluminum

have been calculated[29] and are shown in Fig. 8a for mono-energetic beams with energies between 20 and 120 keV, and in 8b as a function of half-value layer (HVL) in mm of Al for the same beams. Figure 8c shows values of (Φ/X) as a function of kVp for various thicknesses of added aluminum and spectra generated using the method of Tucker.[30] It is clear that the actual value of (Φ/X) is specific to details of the spectrum used, but *insensitive* to both kVp and thickness of added aluminum when expressed as a function of the beam HVL (Fig. 8d). Thus, an estimate of (Φ/X) with sufficient accuracy can often be obtained using Fig. 8d if the HVL can be measured for the particular test conditions.

The DQE is sometimes written as[31]

$$DQE(u) = \frac{SNR_{out}^2(u)}{SNR_{in}^2(u)} \tag{40}$$

where $SNR_{out}^2(u) = \bar{d}^2 MTF^2(u)/NPS_d(u)$ is the output signal-to-noise ratio (SNR) squared and $SNR_{in}^2(u) = \bar{q}$ is the input or ideal SNR squared. This interpretation is sometimes appealing as it presents the DQE in terms of a transfer relationship (transfer of the squared SNR). However, it does not clearly specify what is meant by signal and noise, giving rise to ambiguous and sometimes incorrect interpretations. It should be avoided.

Fourier-Based DQE of Cascaded System

The Zweig-type DQE model of a cascaded system has been generalized to include second-order statistics[32] using the noise-transfer relationships of Rabbani et al.[33] It was shown that the frequency-dependent DQE of a cascaded system consisting of amplification and scattering stages is described by

$$DQE(u) = \frac{1}{1 + \dfrac{1 + \epsilon_{g_1} MTF_1^2(u)}{\bar{g}_1 MTF_1^2(u)} + ... + \dfrac{1 + \epsilon_{g_N} MTF_N^2(u)}{\bar{g}_1...\bar{g}_N MTF_1^2(u)...MTF_N^2(u)}} \tag{41}$$

where ϵ_{g_j} is the gain Poisson excess of the j-th stage given by

$$\epsilon_{g_j} = \frac{\sigma_{g_j}^2}{\bar{g}_j} - 1. \tag{42}$$

Poisson gain corresponds to a variance $\sigma_{g_j}^2 = \bar{g}_j$ and excess $\epsilon_{g_j} = 0$. Deterministic gain (a gain with no random variability) corresponds to a variance $\sigma_{g_j}^2 = 0$ and excess $\epsilon_{g_j} = -1$. $MTF_j(u)$ is the MTF of the scattering process at the j-th stage. Each stage can represent only an amplification or scattering process, but not both. For amplification at the j-th stage, $MTF_j(u) = 1$. For a scattering j-th stage, $\bar{g}_j = 1$ and $\epsilon_{g_j} = -1$. In practice, the excess terms are often small enough to be neglected and Eq. (41) then simplifies to

$$DQE(u) \approx \frac{1}{1 + \dfrac{1}{\bar{g}_1 MTF_1^2(u)} + ... + \dfrac{1}{\bar{g}_1...\bar{g}_N MTF_1^2(u)...MTF_N^2(u)}} \tag{43}$$

which has a pleasing symmetry with Eq. (13) and is often sufficiently accurate for "back-of-the-envelope"-type calculations.

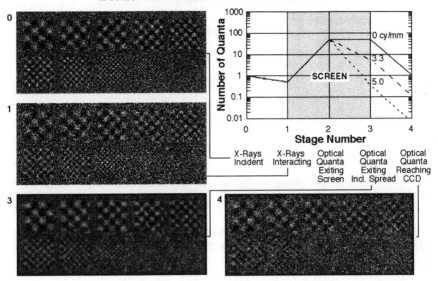

Figure 9: The "quantum accounting diagram" analysis of the system in Fig. 6 shows that a secondary quantum sink exists in the number of optical quanta at spatial frequencies greater than approximately 2.5 cycles/mm. A Monte Carlo calculation was used to generate images composed of the distribution of image quanta at each stage of the cascade, illustrating the degradation in image quality.

The Fourier-based Eq. (41) differs to the particle-based Eq. (13) in several respects. It shows that scattering stages can degrade the DQE dramatically when the MTF value drops with increasing spatial frequency. In fact, where Eq. (13) might predict that a minimum of approximately 10 quanta at each stage will easily prevent a secondary quantum sink, Eq. (41) shows that approximately 10 times that number is required at the frequency for which the MTF has a value of 0.3. Specific values will depend on system particulars, but it is clear that the frequency dependence of this type of analysis can have critical importance.

The Fourier-based QAD analysis provides a theoretical estimate of the DQE based only on the mean gain, gain variance, and scattering MTF of each stage - parameters that can generally by estimated or measured from an analysis of each stage independently. Equation (41) also establishes a direct theoretical relation between the frequency-dependent DQE and the number of primary

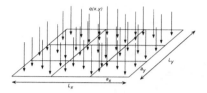

Figure 10: Integration of quanta in detector elements of width a_x is represented as convolution of $q(x)$ with $\Pi(-x/a_x)$ in the spatial domain, and multiplication with an aperture OTF, $\mathrm{OTF}_{a_x}(u)$, in the frequency domain.

or secondary image quanta at each stage. If any of the product terms of gains and squared scatter MTFs in the denominator of Eq. (41) are less than unity at any specified frequency, the DQE will be degraded. This result forms the basis for interpretation of a Fourier-based quantum sink concept that can be used to ensure that a sufficient number of quanta are present at each stage to adequately transfer the SNR for all spatial frequencies of interest.[32]

The visual appearance of a secondary quantum sink at non-zero frequencies is illustrated in Fig. 9 with a Monte Carlo calculation for the hypothetical imaging system illustrated in Fig. 6 including scattering of light. Figure 9 shows the corresponding QAD analysis with simulated images corresponding to each stage in the cascaded model, demonstrating the deteriorating image quality.[34] In this example, a secondary quantum sink exists in the detected optical quanta at spatial frequencies greater than approximately 2.5 cycles/mm causing a loss of image SNR for the high-frequency patterns.

Fourier-Based Metrics of Digital-System Performance

An analysis of noise in digital imaging systems is more complex system. The Fourier-based approach is almost always required (exceptions are few). In this section, concepts of the digital MTF and digital NPS are introduced. These are then used to describe one way in which the NEQ and DQE of digital systems might be expressed.

We will view a digital-imaging detector as a two-dimensional array of discrete detector elements.* The detector produces a signal that is proportional to the number of incident quanta interacting in each detector element (Fig. 10). Thus, each element functions as a spatial integrator of image quanta.

---

* Physical detector elements are called "dels" by Dr. Martin Yaffe to make a distinction from picture elements - "pixels" - as they need not be the same thing.

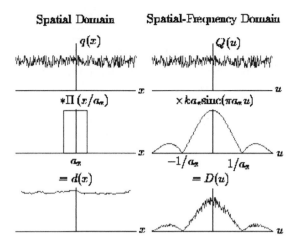

Figure 11: Integration of quanta in detector elements of width a_x is represented as convolution of $q(x)$ with $\Pi(-x/a_x)$ in the spatial domain, and multiplication with the OTF, $ka_x\mathrm{sinc}(\pi a_x u)$, in the frequency domain.

Detector-Element Size and the Aperture MTF

Integration of quanta in each detector element can be represented as convolution with an aperture function in the spatial domain, giving rise to a corresponding "aperture MTF" in the spatial-frequency domain. This is illustrated in Fig. 11, where a distribution of x-ray quanta $q(x)$ are incident on a detector. The left column shows $q(x)$ in one dimension, and the right column shows $|Q(u)|$ where $Q(u)$ is the Fourier transform of $q(x)$.

In the following it is assumed that each detector element has unity quantum efficiency and a width of a_x. The signal from the nth element centered at $x = nx_o$, d_n, is therefore given by the integral

$$d_n = k \int_{nx_o - a_x/2}^{nx_o + a_x/2} q(x)\mathrm{d}x \tag{44}$$

where k is a constant relating the number of interacting quanta to the detector output as a digital value. This integral can also be written as

$$d_n = k \int_{-\infty}^{\infty} q(x)\Pi\left(\frac{x - nx_o}{a_x}\right)\mathrm{d}x \tag{45}$$

where

$$\Pi\left(\frac{x}{a_x}\right) = \begin{cases} 1 & \text{for } -a_x/2 \le x \le a_x/2 \\ 0 & \text{otherwise} \end{cases}. \tag{46}$$

Equation (45) is recognized as being a correlation integral evaluated at the center of the element, $x = nx_o$, and hence

$$d_n = k\, q(x) \star \Pi\left(\frac{x}{a_x}\right)\Big|_{x=nx_o} \tag{47}$$

or similarly as the convolution of $q(x)$ with $\Pi(-x/a_x)$,

$$d_n = k\, q(x) * \Pi\left(\frac{-x}{a_x}\right)\Big|_{x=nx_o} = d(x)|_{x=nx_o} \tag{48}$$

where

$$d(x) = kq(x) * \Pi(-x/a_x). \tag{49}$$

The function $d(x)$ is called the *detector presampling signal*. It is a function that, when sampled at positions corresponding to the center of each element, gives the detector output values for each element. Thus, $d(x)$ describes the detector signal for all possible detector element positions, physical and non-physical.

This is a general result, showing that the effect of integrating quanta in a detector element can be represented as a convolution integral. The function $\Pi(-x/a_x)$ is the sampling function in the sense of distribution theory (see appendix), describing the measurement of $q(x)$. Convolution in the spatial domain corresponds to multiplication in the spatial-frequency domain, and Eq. (49) can therefore be expressed in the spatial-frequency domain as

$$D(u) = ka_x Q(u)\mathrm{OTF}_{a_x}(u) \tag{50}$$

where $D(u)$ is the Fourier transform of $d(x)$ and $\mathrm{OTF}_{a_x}(u)$, the Fourier transform of the aperture function $\Pi(-x/a_x)$, is called the optical-transfer function. The aperture MTF, or "del" MTF, is given by the magnitude of the OTF after normalization to unity area. The aperture MTF provides a spatial-frequency description of spatially integrating quanta in each detector element. When quanta are integrated in elements of width a_x, the aperture MTF is given by

$$\mathrm{MTF}_{a_x}(u) = |\mathrm{OTF}_{a_x}(u)| = |\mathrm{sinc}(\pi a_x u)|. \tag{51}$$

As the widths of detector elements are increased, the bandwidth of the aperture MTF is reduced. As would be expected, high-resolution imaging detectors require the use of narrow detector elements.

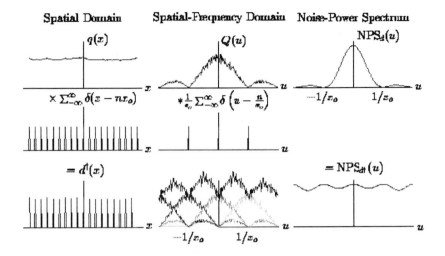

Figure 12: Sampling a function at uniform spacing x_o results in spectral aliasing if the presampling signal $d(x)$ has frequency components above the sampling cut-off frequency $1/x_o$.

Digital MTF: Presampling MTF and Aliasing

The quantity $d(x)$ is the presampling detector signal as described in the previous section, and evaluation of $d(x)$ at the centers of each detector element gives the detector signal for each element. The process of evaluating a function is called sampling (see appendix). Evaluating $d(x)$ at positions $x = nx_o$ for all n can be represented as multiplication with a comb function $\sum \delta(x - nx_o)$ giving $d^\dagger(x)$, where

$$d^\dagger(x) = d(x) \sum_{n=-\infty}^{\infty} \delta(x - nx_o) = \sum_{n=-\infty}^{\infty} d_n \delta(x - nx_o) \tag{52}$$

which consists of an infinite train of δ-functions scaled by the detector values d_n. This process is illustrated in the two domains in Fig. 12. Multiplication with $\sum_{n=-\infty}^{\infty} \delta(x - nx_o)$ in the spatial domain corresponds to convolution with $\frac{1}{x_o} \sum_{n=-\infty}^{\infty} \delta(u - 1/nx_o)$ in the spatial-frequency domain. Therefore, the Fourier transform of $d^\dagger(x)$ is given by

$$F\{d^\dagger(x)\} = D(u) * \frac{1}{x_o} \sum_{n=-\infty}^{\infty} \delta(u - 1/nx_o) \tag{53}$$

as illustrated in Fig. 12 where $D(u)$ is the Fourier transform of $d(x)$. This illustration shows that sampling of $d(x)$ at uniform spacings of x_o corresponds to the production of aliases of $D(u)$ at spacings of $u = 1/x_o$. If the aliases overlap, aliasing occurs. Excellent descriptions of sampling and aliasing in medical imaging systems are given elsewhere by Barrett & Swindell,[12] and Metz & Doi[13] among others.

The performance of a digital system can therefore be expressed as the pre-sampling MTF, $\mathrm{MTF}_{pre}(u)$, consisting of the aperture MTF and any other MTF factor resulting from blurring effects in the detector,

$$\mathrm{MTF}_{pre}(u) = \mathrm{MTF}_{detector}(u)\mathrm{MTF}_{x_o}(u), \qquad (54)$$

and aliasing determined by the sample spacing x_o. The overall effect of the detector in the Fourier domain is to attenuate spatial frequencies by the presampling MTF and to introduce aliasing if there remain frequencies greater than the sampling cut-off frequency given by $u_c = 1/2x_o$. Both steps are required for the description of digital detectors. The presampling MTF can be measured on real systems using techniques such as the slanted-edge method.[26,35,36] Dobbins et al.[37] describe the effects of aliasing and Fourier-domain phase errors due to an inadequate sampling frequency that may be encountered in digital imaging.

Digital NPS: Presampling NPS and Noise Aliasing

When the DFT is defined as used in Eq. (88), the NPS estimated from digital data is given as

$$\mathrm{NPS}_{dig}(u) = \frac{x_o}{N}\mathrm{E}\left\{|\mathrm{DFT}\{d_n - \mathrm{E}\{d_n\}\}|^2\right\} \qquad (55)$$

for $u = m/Nx_o$ and $-N/2 \leq m \leq N/2 - 1$, and is called here the *digital NPS*. If d_n are samples of the detector presampling signal $d(x)$, represented as $d^\dagger(x)$, an array of δ-functions scaled by the values d_n. The NPS of $d^\dagger(x)$ is given by

$$\mathrm{NPS}_{d^\dagger}(u) = \frac{1}{x_o^2}\mathrm{NPS}_d(u) * \sum_{n=-\infty}^{\infty} \delta\left(u - \frac{n}{x_o}\right) \qquad (56)$$

$$= \frac{1}{x_o^2}\left[\mathrm{NPS}_d(u) + \sum_{n=1}^{\infty} \mathrm{NPS}_d\left(u \pm \frac{n}{x_o}\right)\right] \qquad (57)$$

with units of $d^2(x) \times x^{-1}$. It is clear from Eq. (57) that the NPS of $d^\dagger(x)$ consists of a fundamental presampling NPS, $\mathrm{NPS}_d(u)$, plus aliases centered at the frequencies $u = n/x_o$, and scaled by the factor $1/x_o^2$. If the aliases overlap, noise aliasing takes place, potentially increasing image noise at all frequencies below the sampling cut-off frequency.

The sampling theorem states that frequencies above the cut-off frequency $u_c = 1/2x_o$ cannot be represented with samples obtained with a uniform sampling frequency of $u_s = 1/x_o$. We therefore introduce $\text{NPS}_{est}(u)$ which is truncated to this frequency range, and is the NPS of $d_{est}(x)$, an estimate of $d(x)$ interpolated using the digital values d_n and given by

$$d_{est}(x) = \sum_{n=-\infty}^{\infty} d_n \text{sinc}\left(\pi \frac{x - nx_o}{x_o}\right) \tag{58}$$

$$= d^\dagger(x) * \text{sinc}(\pi x_o u) \tag{59}$$

and

$$\text{NPS}_{est}(u) = \text{NPS}_{d^\dagger}(u) \, x_o^2 \Pi(x_o u). \tag{60}$$

The functions $d(x)$ and $d_{est}(x)$ are equal if there is no aliasing.

The digital NPS, $\text{NPS}_{dig}(u)$, given by Eq. (55) and based on the digital data d_n, is defined only for the frequencies evaluated by the DFT, which are $u = m/Nx_o$ for $-N/2 \le m \le N/2 - 1$. At those frequencies, it is also equal to $\text{NPS}_{est}(u)$, and therefore $\text{NPS}_{dig}(u)$ is related to the presampling NPS, $\text{NPS}_d(u)$, by

$$\text{NPS}_{dig}(u) = \text{NPS}_{est}(u) \tag{61}$$

$$= x_o^2 \text{NPS}_{d^\dagger}(u) \tag{62}$$

$$= \text{NPS}_d(u) + \sum_{n=1}^{\infty} \text{NPS}_d\left(u \pm \frac{n}{x_o}\right) \tag{63}$$

for $u = m/Nx_o$ and $-N/2 \le m \le N/2 - 1$, explicitly stating the undesirable effects of noise aliasing with the second term. This expression of the digital NPS was first described to the medical imaging community by Giger.[38] The noise variance in $d(x)$ is conserved by the process of noise aliasing, so that

$$\sigma_d^2 = \int_{-\infty}^{\infty} \text{NPS}_d(u) du \tag{64}$$

$$= x_o^2 \int_{-1/2x_o}^{1/2x_o} \text{NPS}_{d^\dagger}(u) du \tag{65}$$

$$= \int_{-1/2x_o}^{1/2x_o} \text{NPS}_d(u) + \sum_{n=1}^{\infty} \text{NPS}_d\left(u \pm \frac{n}{x_o}\right) du. \tag{66}$$

Noise aliasing cannot be undone once it has occurred. It can be prevented only by implementing a spatial anti-aliasing filter which would reduce the bandwidth of the presampling NPS, $\text{NPS}_d(u)$, such that negligible noise power exists at frequencies above the sampling cut-off frequency.

Digital NEQ

The NEQ as given by Eq. (32) applies to digital systems although made more complicated by the potential presence of signal and noise aliasing. The numerator describes the system transfer of signals from the input to the output, and thus the MTF for digital systems is the presampling MTF which includes the aperture MTF. Noise in a digital image is given by Eq. (63) and so the digital NEQ can be given by

$$
\text{NEQ}_{dig}(\overline{q}, u) = \frac{\overline{q}^2 \left| \dfrac{\partial \overline{d}}{\partial \overline{q}} \right|^2 \text{MTF}_{pre}^2(u)}{\text{NPS}_{dig}(u)} \tag{67}
$$

for $u = m/Nx_o$ and $-N/2 \le m \le N/2 - 1$ where x_o is the center-to-center spacing of detector elements. For linear digital systems, the NEQ can be calculated using

$$
\text{NEQ}_{dig}(\overline{q}, u) = \frac{\text{MTF}_{pre}^2(u)}{\text{NPS}_{dig}(u)/\overline{d}^2} \tag{68}
$$

$$
= \frac{\text{MTF}_{pre}^2(u)}{\dfrac{x_o}{\overline{d}^2 N} \text{E}\left\{ |\text{DFT}\{d_n - \text{E}\{d_n\}\}|^2 \right\}} \tag{69}
$$

for $u = m/Nx_o$ and $-N/2 \le m \le N/2 - 1$ when using a DFT given by Eq. (88). Interpretation of the digital NEQ is possibly easier when expressed in the form

$$
\text{NEQ}_{dig}(\overline{q}, u) = \frac{\text{MTF}_{pre}^2(u)}{\dfrac{1}{\overline{d}^2}\left[\text{NPS}_d(u) + \displaystyle\sum_{n=1}^{\infty} \text{NPS}_d\left(u \pm \dfrac{n}{x_o} \right) \right]} \tag{70}
$$

for $u = m/Nx_o$ and $-N/2 \le m \le N/2 - 1$. The NEQ is decreased by the effects of noise aliasing. It is defined only for frequencies less than the sampling cut-off frequency, $u_c = 1/2x_o$.

Digital DQE

Similar to the digital NEQ, the digital DQE is defined here as

$$\text{DQE}_{dig}(\bar{q}, u) = \frac{\text{NEQ}_{dig}(\bar{q}, u)}{\bar{q}} \tag{71}$$

$$= \frac{\text{MTF}^2_{pre}(u)}{\dfrac{\bar{q}}{\bar{d}^2}\left[\text{NPS}_d(u) + \displaystyle\sum_{n=1}^{\infty}\text{NPS}_d\left(u \pm \dfrac{n}{x_o}\right)\right]} \tag{72}$$

where $\bar{q}$ is the average number of x-ray quanta incident on the detector per unit area. Similar to the digital NEQ, the digital DQE is reduced by the effects of noise aliasing.

Appendix

Quantifying image noise requires some familiarity with the Fourier transform and other mathematical relationships as summarized in this appendix

The Dirac δ-Function, Sampling, and the Sifting Property

The Dirac δ-function, or impulse function, is important both for the representation of quantum images and the analysis of digital systems. The symbol $\delta(x - x_o)$ represents an impulse at position x_o with the property that

$$\delta(x - x_o) = \begin{cases} 0 & \text{for } x \neq x_o \\ \text{undefined} & \text{for } x = x_o \end{cases} \tag{73}$$

and with the constraint that

$$\int_{-\infty}^{\infty} \delta(x - x_o)\mathrm{d}x = 1. \tag{74}$$

The δ-function always has dimension inverse to that of its argument (i.e. x^{-1} in this case). In addition, for any function $f(x)$ which is continuous at $x = x_o$,

$$\int_{a}^{b} f(x)\delta(x - x_o)\mathrm{d}x = \begin{cases} f(x_o) & \text{if } a < x_o < b \\ 0 & \text{otherwise} \end{cases} \tag{75}$$

and from which comes the *sifting* property:

$$\int_{-\infty}^{\infty} f(x)\delta(x - x_o)\mathrm{d}x = f(x_o)\int_{-\infty}^{\infty} \delta(x - x_o)\mathrm{d}x = f(x_o) = f(x)|_{x=x_o}. \tag{76}$$

The sifting property provides a mechanism whereby the process of *sampling*, that is, evaluating a function at a specified position $x = x_o$, can be expressed in terms of the linear operation of multiplication with a δ-function:

$$f(x)\delta(x - x_o) = f(x_o)\delta(x - x_o). \tag{77}$$

It is important to note that multiplication with the δ-function does not result in the sample value alone - it results in a δ-function *scaled* by the sample value $f(x_o)$. The sample value may be dimensionless, but the δ-function is not.

The δ-function is a *generalized* function in the mathematical sense as opposed to a "well-behaved" function. For this reason it is sometimes referred to as the δ-symbol rather than the δ-function. While it is tempting to manipulate the δ-function as if it were well behaved, it is really defined only in terms of its properties, such as those described by Eqs. (73) to (76), and must be treated accordingly and with great care.

In addition to the sifting property, other important properties of the δ-function include:[9,12,14]

$$\delta(ax) = \frac{1}{|a|}\delta(x) \tag{78}$$

$$\delta(-x) = \delta(x) \tag{79}$$

$$x\delta(x) = 0. \tag{80}$$

$$F\left\{\sum_n \delta(x - na)\right\} = \frac{1}{a}\sum_n \delta\left(u - \frac{n}{a}\right) \tag{81}$$

where F{ } represents the Fourier transform. The Dirac δ-function should not be confused with the Kronecker δ-function, defined as

$$\delta_m = \begin{cases} 1 & \text{for } m = 0 \\ 0 & \text{for } m \neq 0, \end{cases} \tag{82}$$

often used in the description of discrete systems.

Generalized Functions

Use of the δ-function is often convenient, but it must be emphasized again that it is a *generalized* function, and must be treated with care. The class of generalized functions used here can be defined as the limit of a sequence of well-behaved functions. The one-dimensional δ-function can be expressed in terms of many such limits, two being

$$\delta(x) = \lim_{\tau \to \infty} \frac{\sin(\pi\tau x)}{\pi x} = \lim_{\tau \to \infty} \tau \text{sinc}(\pi\tau x) \tag{83}$$

and

$$\delta(x) = \lim_{\tau \to \infty} \frac{\sin^2(\pi\tau x)}{\pi^2 x^2} = \lim_{\tau \to \infty} \tau\,\mathrm{sinc}^2(\pi\tau x). \tag{84}$$

Refer to Bracewell[14] or Gaskill[9] for a description of δ-functions, distributions and generalized functions in linear-systems theory.

Distribution Theory

Images consisting of a distribution of quanta *must* be interpreted using distribution theory. A distribution can be measured only through the use of a *sampling function,*† $\phi(x)$, which describes the measurement process. For example, if a measure of the one-dimensional quantum image $q(x)$ is obtained with a detector of width a, producing a signal proportional to the number of interacting quanta, the result d may be expressed as the integral

$$d = k \int_{x_o-a/2}^{x_o+a/2} q(x)\mathrm{d}x = k \int_{-\infty}^{\infty} q(x)\Pi\left(\frac{x-x_o}{a}\right)\mathrm{d}x \tag{85}$$

where the detector is centered at $x = x_o$ and k is a constant relating the number of interacting quanta to the detector output signal that might be a voltage, or an analog-to-digital converter value. In this example, the sampling function is $\phi(x) = \Pi(x/a)$ which is a rectangle of unity value and width a.

Fourier Transform

There are several excellent texts describing the Fourier transform including Bracewell[14] and Brigham.[15] See Peters and Williams[39] for a description of the Fourier transform as applied in medical imaging.

The Fourier transform of $d(x)$ is $D(u)$, and the inverse Fourier transform of $D(u)$ is again $d(x)$. This reciprocal relationship is expressed by

$$D(u) = \int_{-\infty}^{\infty} d(x)e^{-i2\pi ux}\mathrm{d}x \tag{86}$$

$$d(x) = \int_{-\infty}^{\infty} D(u)e^{i2\pi ux}\mathrm{d}u \tag{87}$$

where u is the spatial frequency along the x axis. It is seen that the units of $D(u)$ will always be those of $d(x) \times x$. In general, both $d(x)$ and $D(u)$ are complex.

---

† The sampling function is sometimes called an *aperture function* when used to describe the sensitivity profile of a detector. Do not confuse it with the sampling operation where a waveform is multiplied with a δ-function.

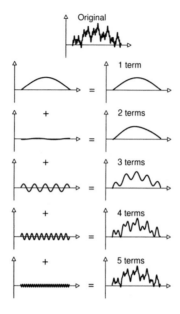

Figure 13: The sum of the Fourier components of a function looks more and more like the original function (top) as more components are added with increasing frequencies. Five such components of a real-only function are shown in the left-hand column, and the accumulated sums in the right.

The Fourier transform expresses the fact that $d(x)$ can be written as the sum of a distribution of sinusoidal components (Fig. 13). As more components are included, the sum looks more and more like the original function.

Discrete Fourier Transform

A numerical implementation of the Fourier transform is called a discrete Fourier transform (DFT), and differs from the Fourier transform in subtle ways. The fast Fourier transform (FFT) refers to a number of implementations of the DFT which make use of clever programming to increase computational efficiency.

One commonly used form for the DFT of a sequence of N digital values d_n for $0 \le n \le N - 1$ is given by

$$D_m = \text{DFT}\{d_n\} = \sum_{n=0}^{N-1} d_n e^{-i2\pi nm/N} \tag{88}$$

which consists of a sequence of the N digital values D_m for $0 \leq m \leq N - 1$. The inverse DFT is given by

$$d_n = \text{DFT}^{-1}\{D_m\} = \frac{1}{N} \sum_{m=0}^{N-1} D_m e^{i2\pi nm/N}. \tag{89}$$

Other forms of the DFT exist, differing primarily by a scaler constant of N or $\sqrt{N}$. The user of any DFT should be aware of what DFT algorithm is being used before attempting any quantitative work. We shall use Eqs. (88) and (89) as definitions of the DFT.

Both d_n and D_m are dimensionless (i.e. just numbers). This is one way in which the Fourier transform and the discrete Fourier transform differ. Another important consideration is to know which index value (which value of n or m) corresponds to the zero positions $x = 0$ and $u = 0$. In many DFT implementations, the central position $x = 0$ corresponds to $n = \frac{N}{2} - 1$, while the central frequency $u = 0$ corresponds to $m = 0$. Erroneous placement of the zero position in one domain results in errors in the phase angle of the complex value in the conjugate domain as known from the shift theorem.

When the sequence d_n represents the function $d(x)$ evaluated at uniform spacings x_o, it is sometimes written as $d(nx_o)$ to retain this spatial relevance. However, this relationship is not as simple in the spatial-frequency domain, as the sequence D_m is *not* equivalent to samples of $D(u)$ at uniform spatial-frequency spacings of $1/Nx_o$, $D(m/Nx_o)$. While it may be tempting to view the DFT as a numerical implementation of the Fourier integral in Eq. (87) and write

$$D\left(\frac{m}{Nx_o}\right) = D(u)|_{u=\frac{m}{Nx_o}} \approx x_o D_m \tag{90}$$

or

$$D_m \approx \frac{1}{x_o} D\left(\frac{m}{Nx_o}\right), \tag{91}$$

extreme care must be used as the DFT is really a separate transform in its own right. The practical problems associated with this interpretation become clear when the DFT is viewed as a special case of the Fourier transform and is understood in the two domains (Brigham[15]). The problems include: a) aliasing; b) spectral leakage and side lobes; c) truncation and windowing; d) zero-position and phase errors; e) frequency wrap-around; and, f) scaling factors and units (particularly in the frequency domain).

References

1. A. Rose, "A unified approach to the performance of photographic film, television pick- up tubes, and the human eye," J Soc Motion Pict Telev Eng 47, 273-294 (1946).

2. A. Rose, "Sensitivity performance of the human eye on an absolute scale," J Opt Soc Am 38, 196-208 (1948).

3. A. Rose, "Television pickup tubes and the problem of vision," in Advances in Electronics and Electron Physics, edited by Marston (Academic Press, New York, 1948), pp. 131-166.

4. A. Rose, "Quantum and noise limitations of the visual process," J Opt Soc Am 43, 715- 716 (1953).

5. I.A. Cunningham and R. Shaw, "Signal-to-Noise Optimization of Medical Imaging Systems," J Opt Soc Am A (March 1999) [in press].

6. K. Rossmann, "Measurement of the modulation transfer function of radiographic systems containing fluoroscent screens," Phys Med Biol 9, 551-557 (1964).

7. K. Rossmann, "The spatial frequency spectrum: A means for studying the quality of radiographic imaging systems," Radiology 90, 1-13 (1968).

8. J.C. Dainty and R. Shaw, Image Science, (Academic Press, New York, 1974).

9. J.D. Gaskill, Linear Systems, Fourier Transforms, and Optics, (John Wiley & Sons, New York, 1978).

10. A. Papoulis, Systems and Transforms with Applications in Optics, (McGraw-Hill, New York, 1968).

11. K. Doi, K. Rossmann and A.G. Haus, "Image quality and patient exposure in diagnostic radiology," Photographic Science and Engineering 21, 269-277 (1977).

12. H.H. Barrett and W. Swindell, Radiological Imaging - The Theory of Image Formation, Detection, and Processing, (Academic Press, New York, 1981).

13. C.E. Metz and K. Doi, "Transfer function analysis of radiographic imaging systems," Phys Med Biol 24, 1079-1106 (1979).

14. R.N. Bracewell, The Fourier Transform and its Applications, 2 Ed. (McGraw-Hill Book Company, New York, 1978).

15. E.O. Brigham, The Fast Fourier Transform, (Prentice-Hall, Englewood Cliffs, N.J., 1974).

16. J.S. Bendat and A.G. Piersol, Random Data - Analysis and Measurement Procedures, 2 Ed. (John Wiley & Sons, New York, 1986).

17. A. Papoulis, Probability, random variables, and stochastic processes, 3 Ed. (McGraw Hill, New York, 1991).

18. H.J. Zweig, "Detective quantum efficiency of photodetectors with some amplifying mechanism," J Opt Soc Am 55, 525-528 (1965).

19. M.M. Ter-Pogossian, The physical aspects of diagnostic radiology, (Harper & Row, New York, 1967).

20. C.A. Mistretta, "X-ray image intensifiers," in AAPM No 3 The physics of medical imaging: recording system measurements and techniques, edited by A.G. Haus (American Institute of Physics, New York, 1979), pp. 182-205.

21. A. Macovski, Medical Imaging Systems, T Kailath editor, (Prentice-Hall, Inc., Englewood Cliffs, N.J., 1983).

22. P.B. Fellgett, "On the ultimate sensitivity and practical performance of radiation detectors," J Opt Soc Am 39, 970 (1949).

23. H.J. Zweig, "Performance criteria for photo-detectors - concepts in evolution," Photo Sc Eng 8, 305-311 (1964).

24. R.C. Jones, "A new classification system for radiation detectors," J Opt Soc Am 39, 327 (1949).

25. A.E. Burgess, "The Rose Model - Revisited," J Opt Soc Am A (March 1999) [In Press].

26. J.T. Dobbins, D.L. Ergun, L. Rutz, D.A. Hinshaw, H. Blume and D.C. Clark, "DQE(f) of four generations of computed radiography acquisition devices," Med Phys 22, 1581-1593 (1995).

27. R. Shaw, "The equivalent quantum efficiency of the photographic process," J Photogr Sc 11, 199-204 (1963).

28. "Medical Imaging - The Assessment of Image Quality", ICRU Report 54 (International Commission of Radiation Units and Measurements, Bethesda, 1995).

29. I.A. Cunningham, "Analyzing System Performance," in The Expanding Role of Medical Physics in Diagnostic Imaging, edited by G.D. Frey and P. Sprawls (Advanced Medical Publishing for American Association of Physicists in Medicine, Madison, Wisconsin, 1997), pp. 231-263.

30. D.M. Tucker, G.T. Barnes and D.P. Chakraborty, "Semiempirical model for generating tungsten target x-ray spectra," Med Phys 18, 211-218 (1991).

31. M.J. Tapiovaara and R.F. Wagner, "A generalized detective quantum efficiency (DQE) approach to the analysis of x-ray imaging," in Application of Optical Instrumentation in Medicine XII, edited by R.H. Schneider and S.J. Dwyer, Proc SPIE 454:540-549 (1984).

32. I.A. Cunningham, M.S. Westmore and A. Fenster, "A spatial-frequency dependent quantum accounting diagram and detective quantum efficiency model of signal and noise propagation in cascaded imaging systems," Med Phys 21, 417-427 (1994).

33. M. Rabbani, R. Shaw and R.L. Van Metter, "Detective quantum efficiency of imaging systems with amplifying and scattering mechanisms," J Opt Soc Am A 4, 895-901 (1987).

34. I.A. Cunningham, M.S. Westmore and A. Fenster, "Visual impact of the non-zero spatial frequency quantum sink," in Medical Imaging 1994: Physics of Medical Imaging, edited by R. Shaw, Proc SPIE 2163:274-283 (1994).

35. H. Fujita, K. Doi and M.L. Giger, "Investigation of basic imaging properties in digital radiography. 6. MTFs of II-TV digital imaging systems," Med Phys 12, 713-720 (1985).

36. D.W. Holdsworth, R.K. Gerson and A. Fenster, "A time-delay integration charge- coupled device camera for slot-scanned digital radiography," Med Phys 17, 876-886 (1990).

37. J.T. Dobbins, "Effects of undersampling on the proper interpretation of modulation transfer function, noise power spectra, and noise equivalent quanta of digital imaging systems," Med Phys 22, 171-181 (1995).

38. M.L. Giger, K. Doi and C.E. Metz, "Investigation of basic imaging properties in digital radiography. 2. Noise Wiener spectrum," Med Phys 11, 797-805 (1984).

39. The Fourier Transform in Biomedical Engineering, TM Peters and J Williams editors, (Birkhauser, Boston, 1998).

Networks, Pipes, and Connectivity

Brent K. Stewart, Ph.D., DABMP
Professor of Radiology, Bioengineering and Medical Education
University of Washington School of Medicine
Seattle, WA 98195-7115
bstewart@u.washington.edu

Introduction

Visit any bookstore or technical library and you will find shelves filled with books devoted to the topic of computer communications, networks, and internetworking. Each of these books contains thousands of details for specific network architectures. What then, of this enormous and exponentially increasing knowledge of network technology, is essential to the medical physicist?

The medical physicist is usually the chief technology vanguard in a Radiology department; proficient with complex computer technology as applied to medical imaging and usually tasked with the specification, selection, and the quality assurance/quality control (QA/QC) of this equipment. Thus, the medical physicist is typically requested to apply his/her technical aptitudes and understanding of complex systems toward the specification, selection, and oversight of QA/QC for teleradiology and Picture Archiving and Communication Systems (PACS) within his/her institutions. This may require the medical physicist to expand his repertoire of technical knowledge of radiological modalities into the realms of networking, telecommunications, protocol standards, computer and database architectures, and display technologies as well as image compression and data encryption. Sufficient base knowledge in all of these areas is required of the medical physicist to successfully complete this task.

Many of these topics are covered in greater depth elsewhere in this volume. It is the goal of this article to provide a basic, high-level overview of networking and digital connectivity, current trends and requirements, and how the elements tie together in the guise of networks developed for the radiological environment. It is hoped that this informatics domain knowledge will allow medical physicists to not only fulfill a limited obligation to assist in the implementation of networks for teleradiology and PACS at their institutions, but also eventually to become an essential element in the transformation of Radiology departments from somewhat passive purveyors of diagnostic radiological information to proactive participants in the evolution of medical informatics at their institutions.

Important Factors

What then are the most salient factors that form a high-level view regarding networks for the medical physicist? Among them are: network architecture and protocol stacks,

unit (PDU). An example of a PDU is an Ethernet packet. The PDU headers are used by the peer entities to enact their peer protocol. They identify which PDUs contain data and which contain control information, provide sequence numbers, etc. The layer N PDUs are then sent, with any layer N ICI to a specific SAP between layers N and N-1, and so the process continues until data are sent across the physical medium to the other network device. At this device, the PDUs at each layer are passed upwards through the appropriate SAPs between layers until the uppermost layer is reached.

ISO Reference Model for Open Systems Interconnection

The International Standards Organization (ISO) is an international agency for the development of standards in many technical fields of interest. The open systems inter-connection (OSI) model establishes a framework for defining standards for linking heterogeneous computer networks and provides a basis for connecting open systems for distributed applications processing. The OSI standard uses a partitioned basic reference model (ISO 7498-1) with seven layers (Figure 2). Each of the seven layers performs a specific set of orthogonal services, with well-defined linkages at the interface of each layer [Day 1995]. The seven layers are, from bottom to top, the physical, data link, network, transport, session, presentation, and application layers.

The physical layer (layer 1) is concerned with the transmission of an unstructured bit stream over the physical medium. Layer 1 specifies the physical, electrical, and, if applicable, optical characteristics of the connections constituting a network and encompasses such details as media, connectors, and repeaters. One may consider this as the hardware layer.

The data link layer (layer 2) provides for the reliable transfer of data across the physical medium. This layer is concerned with how electrical signals enter and exit the medium and deals with elements such as error detection, encoding methods, and tokens. Because of its complexity, the data link layer is typically broken down into two separate sub-layers: the medium access control (MAC) sub-layer and the logical link control (LLC) sub-layer. The MAC sub-layer manages network access (e.g., collision detection or token passing) and network control. The LLC sub-layer, operating at a higher level, sends and receives the data messages or packets.

The network layer (layer 3) is responsible for the establishment, maintenance, and termination of network connections and enables layers 4 through 7 to be independent from the data transmission and switching technologies used to connect systems. Layer 3 is also responsible for addressing and routing messages to their destinations.

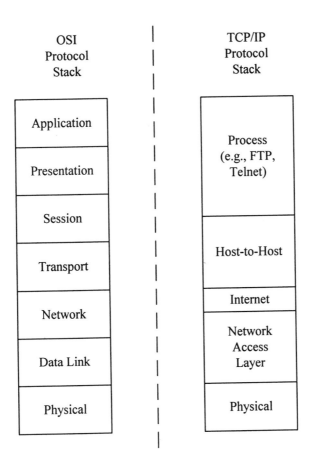

Figure 2. The seven-layer ISO Basic Reference Model for Open Systems Interconnection (OSI) and five-layer TCP/IP protocol stacks and their relationship to one another.

The transport layer (layer 4) is concerned with the reliable, transparent transfer of data between endpoints, providing end-to-end error recovery and flow control. It controls the sequencing of message components and regulates incoming traffic flow. The session layer (layer 5) deals with the control structure between applications. It allows applications running on different workstations to coordinate their communications into a single session.

The presentation layer (layer 6) performs transformations on data to provide a standardized application interface and common communication services like encryption, compression, and reformatting. If one computer is a big-endian (most significant byte of a word at the lowest address, e.g., Sun UNIX computer) and another is a little-endian (least significant byte of a word at the lowest address, e.g., PC), then the presentation layer reorders the bytes into the native internal numeric format of the host computer [Ward 1991].

The uppermost layer, the application layer (layer 7) provides services to users of the OSI environment (e.g., file transfer, electronic mail, and network management services). This is the layer an end-user interacts with.

The OSI seven-layer stack can be viewed from two different perspectives. In the first, the stack is viewed as three super layers. The bottom three layers (physical, data link, and network) contain the protocols necessary for a computer to interact with a network. The middle, or transport, layer provides a reliable, end-to-end connection, regardless of the intervening network facilities. The top three layers (session, presentation, and application) are involved in the exchange of data between users and applications, making use of the transport service for reliable data transfer.

The OSI stack may also be viewed as a different grouping of three super layers. From this perspective, the bottom two layers provide a point-to-point, link-oriented connection to the LAN. The middle three layers (layers 3 through 5) provide an end-to-end, connection-oriented service and are involved in the transfer of data from one computer to another, no matter what intervening networks are present. The top two layers form a user-oriented service concerned with the application to be performed and with any pertinent formatting issues.

TCP/IP Protocol Architecture

The development of the network messaging protocols for the U.S. Department of Defense (DOD) ARPANET occurred long before the OSI Basic Reference Model was devised. The technical requirements to be met were that computers and terminals must share a common set of communication protocols to interoperate, and the resulting suite of protocols must support an internetworking capability in a heterogeneous environment. To meet these requirements, the communication task was decomposed (as with the OSI model) into a modular architecture of several layers (Figure 2). However, this decomposition and documentation process was not as formal as that used for the OSI model, but had much of the functionality that was later used in the development of the OSI model [Stallings 1996]. Relevant documents are RFC 791 covering Internet Protocol (IP) and RFC 793 covering Transmission Control Protocol (TCP). Although encompassing more than just the network and transport layers, this model is widely known as the TCP/IP protocol architecture [Leiner 1985]. The development of the TCP/IP protocol architecture enabled the standardization of networking equipment and computers that initiated the avalanche of computer networking in the 1980's, not only in the United States but worldwide.

As in the OSI model, the lowest layer is the physical layer concerned with the physical interface between the data transmission device and the transmission medium. Next is the network access layer, which is concerned with the exchange of data between a computer and the network to which it is attached. The specific protocol used at this layer depends, of course, on the type of network used [e.g., Ethernet or Fiber Distributed Data Interface (FDDI)]. At the next layer (internet) are the procedures (internet protocol—IP) required to allow data to move between multiple networks, for example, an Ethernet network and an FDDI network. The host-to-host (or transport) layer ensures the reliable exchange of data so that all data arrive at the destination computer in the correct order of transmission. This function is embodied in the TCP. The last and uppermost layer is the process layer, containing the protocols necessary to support such well known user applications as file transfer (file transfer protocol—FTP), electronic mail (simple mail transfer protocol—SMTP), and remote terminal access (Telnet). The process layer roughly corresponds to the user-oriented service of OSI layers 6 (presentation) and 7 (application), the host-to-host and internet layers correspond to the end-to-end connection-oriented service of OSI layers 3 through 5 (session, transport and network), and the network access layer roughly corresponds to the point-to-point link-oriented service of OSI layer 2 (data link).

From the foregoing discussion of protocol stacks, it should be clear that each computer contains hardware and software at the network access layer and software at the internet, host-to-host, and process layers for one or more application processes [Stallings 1990b]. Each entity on the Internet must have a unique address, which consists of two components. Each computer or network device (host) must have a unique global network address and each application (process) running on a computer must have an address that is unique within the host. The first component allows for correct addressing to each host (e.g., IP address); the second allows data to be directed to the correct destination address (e.g., port) within the receiving host. In UNIX the combination of 32-bit IP address plus 16-bit port number is called a socket.

A brief example will illustrate these principles [Stewart 1992a]. For instance, an application process X at port 1 in computer A on LAN 1 wishes to transmit data to application process Y at port 2 in computer B on LAN 2 (Figure 3). Process X on computer A passes a block of data (message) through port 1 to the host-to-host layer. Port 1 acts as the host-to-host layer SAP. The host-to-host layer breaks the block of data into smaller pieces (segmentation) with TCP and appends a TCP header to the beginning of the data fragment. This combination of TCP header and data fragment is called a TCP segment. The TCP header contains information such as the destination port (in this case, port 2) the sequence number (to ensure that the arriving TCP segments are in the correct order for reassembly), and a checksum (i.e., a summation of digits to verify that no transmission errors occurred).

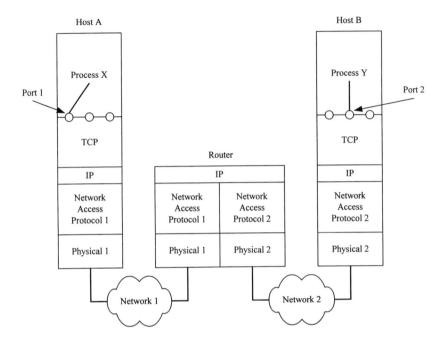

Figure 3. How two subnetworks can be connected. A router may be necessary
if the network access protocols are not equivalent.

Next, the TCP segments are forwarded to the internet layer where an IP header, which
contains the destination computer address (IP address consisting of four octets, e.g.,
128.95.xxx.yyy), is appended to the beginning of each TCP segment received from
the host-to-host layer, creating an IP datagram. This IP datagram is in turn forwarded
from the internet layer to the network access layer where another header (packet
header) is appended to the datagram, creating a packet or frame. The packet header
includes the address of the destination subnetwork. Host A connects to LAN 1 with a
unique MAC address (e.g., Ethernet 48-bit address).

If the destination computer resides on the same LAN as the source computer, the packet
arrives at the destination computer with the MAC protocol for that particular network.
If not, however, the source computer must address the packet to an internetworking
device such as a bridge or router that connects LAN 1 to the rest of the internetworking "universe," part of which includes LAN 2, the destination LAN. The
internet-working device looks at the destination address for the packet and converts
the network access protocol if the other LAN or WAN does not share the same MAC
protocol as LAN 1 (e.g., Ethernet and FDDI). This describes the first network "hop"

for the packet. Many such hops may be required before the packet eventually arrives at an internetworking device on the destination LAN (in this case, LAN 2). Depending on the loading on intervening networks, successive packets may not pass through the same series of networks. This is why it is important that the sequence number be written in the TCP segment header for reassembly at the destination computer.

The entire process, from user message at the process layer to packets at the network access protocol layer with the insertion of the various headers, is called encapsulation. When the packet arrives at the LAN where destination computer B resides, the reverse process occurs. The headers are stripped from the packets, datagrams, and segments; the TCP segments are reassembled; and the reassembled message is routed to port 2 on computer B where application Y accepts it.

DICOM Communications

The American College of Radiology (ACR) and the National Electrical Manufacturers Association (NEMA) formed a joint committee to develop a standard for Digital Imaging and Communications in Medicine (DICOM). This DICOM Standard was developed according to the NEMA procedures. This standard is developed in liaison with other standardization organizations including CEN TC251 in Europe and JIRA in Japan, with review also by other organizations including IEEE, HL7 and ANSI in the United States.

An early motivation for ACR-NEMA standards development was to develop a method that would allow users to extract digital image data and associated information from medical imaging equipment in a well described manner using extant networking practices [Bidgood 1992, Horii 1992]. Version 1.0 of the ACR-NEMA Standard, published in 1985, initiated this process with a high-speed parallel ("50-pin") interface, designed primarily for point-to-point application between medical imaging devices, not unlike a SCSI cable. As LANs proliferated in the late 1980's, version 2.0 of the ACR-NEMA Standard, published in 1988 added upper level protocol layers to the 50-pin interface so that it could provide peer-to-peer messaging capabilities over existing networks (e.g., TCP/IP) through the use of network interface unit (NIU) gateways.

The networked nature of a PACS makes it essential to describe a standard interface that can make direct use of *de facto* computer network interfaces without the need for the NIU gateways. The current version (3.0) of the ACR-NEMA standard, known more widely as DICOM addresses this through specification of the details necessary to interface to networks that support both the ISO Reference Model for Open Systems Interconnection as well as the TCP/IP Protocol Architecture. There is also backward compatible support for the point-to-point parallel interface of ACR-NEMA version 1.0, but it has passed into obscurity.

The DICOM Standard is structured as a multi-part document. Each DICOM document is identified by title and standard number, taking the form 'PS 3.x' where 'x' signifies the part number. PS 3.8 specifies the Network Support for Message Exchange. Message Exchange is described in PS 3.7. PS 3.9 specifies the Point to Point Communication Support for Message Exchange using the 50-pin interface. The OSI Basic Reference Model is used to model the interconnection of medical imaging equipment in the DICOM documents (Figure 4).

Part 8 of the DICOM Standard (PS 3.8) specifies the services and the upper layer protocols necessary to support the efficient and coordinated communication of DICOM Application Entities (AEs) in a networked environment. DICOM AEs are the software applications that exchange DICOM service object pair (SOP) instance messages [e.g., storage of a computed tomography (CT) image object instance to an archive]. In order to exchange information between the service class user (SCU) and service class provider (SCP) AEs, a logical communication channel, called an association, is set up using a simple request/response message exchange. Once the association has been opened, the two AEs trade transfer syntax information that defines what services and information objects each can support. Providing there is an overlap of requested and offered SOP classes, the specific SOP instances are transmitted. Once this has been completed, the association is terminated.

There are two additions in DICOM to the protocol stacks described above. The first is the DICOM Upper Layer (UL) Service boundary which acts to insulate the AE DICOM message exchange at the application layer from the various network protocol stacks that may be used: OSI, TCP/IP or 50-pin interface. To enable this boundary, DICOM has adopted the OSI Presentation Service (ISO 8822) augmented by the Association Control Service Element (ACSE) which together are called the OSI UL Profile. The ACSE (ISO 8649) augments the Presentation Layer Service with Association establishment and termination services. This definition of the UL Service allows the use of a fully conformant stack of OSI protocols (layers 1 through 6 plus layer 7 ACSE) to achieve robust and efficient communication.

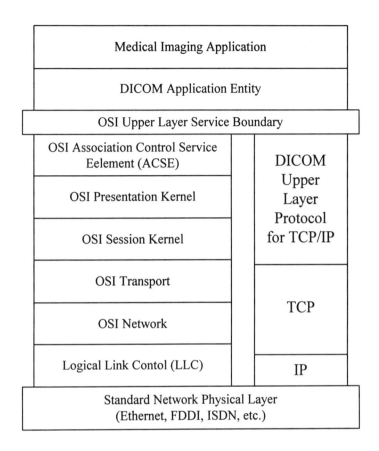

Figure 4. DICOM v3.0 protocol architecture with OSI and TCP/IP stacks.

The second addition is the UL Protocol for TCP/IP. As the TCP/IP protocol architecture was not developed with the rigor of the OSI Basic Reference Model, with the application, presentation, and session OSI layers lumped into the session layer, the UL Protocol provides the "glue" between TCP and the UL Service boundary when TCP/IP networks are used. In the case of TCP/IP, the UL Profile provides the full equivalent of ACSE. When the UL Service is provided by the UL Protocol for TCP/IP, a broad range of existing networking environments can be used for DICOM-based medical imaging communication. There is a one-to-one correspondence between a TCP transport connection and an Upper Layer Association.

The UL Service is described by a number of service primitives. They each model one of the functional interactions between the service user in the layer above and the service provider. In the context of DICOM, the service user is called the DICOM Application Service Element. The service provider is called the Upper Layer and performs the UL Protocol. The OSI UL Services defined in DICOM can be provided either by the DICOM OSI UL Profile or the DICOM UL Protocol for TCP/IP. These service primitives cross the UL Service boundary at a SAP. In most cases, a direct relationship exists between service primitives in two AEs.

The definition of a UL Service common to both OSI and TCP/IP environments allows migration from a TCP/IP to an OSI environment without impacting the DICOM Application Service Elements. It also enables the support of a wide variety of international standards-based networking technologies using the broadest choice of physical networks such as Ethernet (ISO 8802-3) CSMA/CD, FDDI, ISDN, X.25, dedicated digital circuits and many other LAN and WAN network technologies.

Parts of the association information passed between AEs are the called and calling AE titles and the called and calling presentation addresses. The AE title (AET) is a 16-character DICOM application name for the AE. A DICOM application name is often a set of acronyms or abbreviations, which may convey some meaning to a user (e.g., ALI_STORE_SCP). Application names identify a unique service or application on a specific device on the network. The calling presentation address is a structured destination address unambiguous within the global network address structure: either an OSI presentation address or an IP address. Application names are independent of network location so that the device can be physically moved while its corresponding application name(s) remain the same, even though the calling presentation address (e.g., IP address) might. The method of mapping application names to OSI or TCP/IP addresses is implementation specific (e.g., static definition, name server, etc.).

For use with TCP/IP networks a DICOM AE is identified on a given device on the network by a port number unique within the scope of said device. The port number of a DICOM AE must be configurable and either use the "well known port" registered for the DICOM UL Protocol for TCP/IP (port 104) or an alternate. If an alternate port number is used, it is assigned well out of range of other well known port numbers; that is, above 1000 (decimal). Other port numbers typically used are 3004 and 4006.

Thus, in order to get one DICOM device to communicate with another three pieces of information are required to uniquely identify the service on the remote device: AET, IP address, and port number. It is the responsibility of the called AE that received the association request to verify whether the calling AET is one of its known remote DICOM application names. Although this adds a modest element of security, most commercial AEs do not and are said to be running in promiscuous mode. It is also the responsibility of the called AE that received the association request to verify whether the called AET is its DICOM application name. This checking is not necessarily performed either.

Protocol Data Units (PDUs) are the message formats exchanged between peer entities within a layer. A PDU shall consist of protocol control information and user data. PDUs are constructed by mandatory fixed fields followed by optional variable fields, which contain one or more items and/or sub-items. The encoding of the DICOM UL PDUs is defined using big endian byte order, chosen for consistency within the OSI and TCP/IP environment and pertains to the DICOM UL PDU headers only. The encoding of the PDU message fragments is defined by the transfer syntax negotiated at association establishment. Please also see the expanded article by Richard L. Kennedy in this volume for further discussion of DICOM.

Wide Area Networks

WANs have traditionally been considered networks that cross or cover a large geographic area and in most cases rely on circuits provided by a common carrier (telco). WANs are currently used predominantly to provide long-range connectivity between LANs. A WAN typically consists of a number of interconnected switched nodes. Transmissions between LANs are routed through these nodes (internal and boundary nodes). The nodes are not concerned with the content of the data, but simply provide a switching matrix for the data to reach its final destination. In this sense, they can be thought of as inert, yet infinitely configurable data plumbing (pipes). WANs have been implemented primarily through circuit switching and packet switching. However, more recently, frame relay and cell switching [asynchronous transfer mode (ATM)] technologies have assumed increasingly important roles.

Circuit Switching

Circuit switching involves the permanent or temporary establishment of a dedicated communications path between two communications entities (phone hand set, solitary computer or LAN). In a circuit switched network, that path is a connected sequence of physical links between switching nodes. Each link provides a logical channel to the connection, each node switching incoming data to the outgoing link without delay. DS-1 and ISDN are examples of circuit switching WANs.

Packet Switching

Circuit switching requires dedicated bandwidth allocation for the duration of the logical link. With packet switching, dedicating bandwidth to the links is not necessary. Data are transmitted in a packet switched network in small quanta termed packets. These packets are passed along through the nodes of the switching fabric via non-determined paths. Contiguous packets of a larger message may pass through entirely different paths depending on congestion and node availability. At each node, the entire packet is received, stored briefly, and then retransmitted to the next node. The Internet is an example of a packet-switched WAN, where e-mail sent from coast-to-coast may pass through many routers and a few mailservers before arriving at its final destination.

Frame Relay

Frame relay [Smith 1993] is basically a high data rate version of previous packet switching networks. Frame relay uses variable length packets called frames. Due to the low bit error rates of current common carrier networks, the large protocol overhead developed for less reliable networks of previous decades is not required. The streamlined error control protocols of frame relay allow efficient operation at user data rates up to 1.5 Mbps (megabits per second).

Asynchronous Transfer Mode (ATM)

Whereas frame relay uses variable length packets, ATM [Kyas 1995] uses short, fixed length packets called cells. Due to the low bit error rate inherent in fiber optic networks, ATM provides little overhead for error control, shifting error correction to higher levels in the protocol stack. Through the use of small (53 byte) fixed length cells, the ATM switching nodes process and transmit the cells at data rates in the hundreds and thousands of megabits per second. ATM also allows the definition of multiple virtual channels with data rates dynamically defined at the time of creation. Through the use of small, full, and fixed size cells, ATM is so efficient that it can offer a constant data rate channel even though it is in actuality packet switching. Thus, ATM extends circuit switching to allow multiple channels with the data rate of each channel dynamically set on demand.

ATM is a connection-oriented network technology. In a connectionless, shared media network (e.g., Ethernet), each frame must have sufficient information in its header for the packet or frame to arrive successfully at its destination. With ATM, a virtual channel is established first between the sender and receiver followed by transmission of data through the channel. In effect, there is no need to repeat complex routing information in each cell. Logical connections between two end users in ATM are referred to as virtual channel connections (VCC). It is the basic unit of switching in an ATM network. A virtual path connection (VPC) is a bundle of VCCs that have the same endpoints. Thus all of the cells flowing over all of the VCCs in a single VPC are switched together. The use of virtual paths has several advantages: simplified network architecture, increased network performance and reliability, and reduced processing and short connection setup times.

Public Switched Telecommunications Network (PSTN)

The public switched telecommunications network (PSTN) can be decomposed into four basic architectural components: subscribers, local loops, exchanges, and trunks. Local loops are the links between the subscriber and the PSTN and predominantly use twisted-pair copper wiring. The length of a local loop is typically between one to three miles in cities, but may be several tens of miles in rural areas. It is estimated that there are over 600,000,000 local loops in the United States. Exchanges are the switching centers of the PSTN. An exchange that directly serves end users is called a central office and supports tens of thousands of users. There are over 19,000 central offices in the United States. As the number of direct links required to connect each central office to all others in the network would be greater than 200,000,000, a hierarchical mesh of switching offices has been established to interconnect all central offices. Trunks are the branches between exchanges and utilize a highly standardized carrier system using synchronous time division multiplexing to transmit multiple voice-frequency circuits. Most of the trunks have been converted to fiber optic cable, but a few still utilize microwave antenna.

PSTN Synchronous Time Division Multiplexing (STDM) Hierarchy

Synchronous time division multiplexing (STDM) is possible when the achievable data rate of the medium exceeds the data rate of the digital signals to be transmitted, as is the case with the PSTN trunk lines. For example, the voice-grade phone circuits (plain old telephone system or POTS) used for most local loop subscribers limit the frequency to around 4000 Hz. The capacity of fiber optic cabling is at least 2 GHz, so many voice circuits can be switched onto the fiber if a multiplexing scheme is used. A hierarchy of STDM structures of various capacities was devised as part of the evolution of the PSTN toward digital technology [Bellamy 1991]. The basis for the STDM hierarchy is the DS-1 transmission format, which multiplexes 24 channels (Note: the signal used for the DS-1 format is called the T-1 carrier, a subtle distinction causing some confusion). Each DS-1 frame contains 8 bits/channel plus one framing bit for a total of 193 bits/frame. Each analog voice channel is digitized using pulse code modulation (PCM) at 8 kHz, yielding a bit rate of 1.544 Mbps. The same DS-1 format is used to provide digital data service and the same 1.544 Mbps rate is used for compatibility with voice. Within each channel, seven bits can be used for user data yielding a payload rate of 56 kbps (called DS-0). Above the basic data rate of 1.544 Mbps, higher level multiplexing is achieved by interleaving bits from multiple DS-1 circuits. For example, the DS-3 format combines 28 DS-1 circuits into a 44.736 Mbps stream. Note that 28 times 1.544 equals 43.232 and not 44.736. The remaining 1.504 Mbps is utilized for framing and control bits.

Narrowband-ISDN (N-ISDN)

N-ISDN [Kessler 1993] provides end-to-end customer services whose access is through a limited number of standard digital network interfaces (e.g., Basic and Primary Rate Interfaces, below). N-ISDN makes use of the current narrowband capacity of analog voice local loops, conditioning voice grade lines into digital lines through the removal of echo suppressors and loading coils, providing 64 kbps channels, seemingly the equivalent of DS-0 dial-up service. N-ISDN, however, utilizes out-of-band signaling so that the entire 64 kbps, rather than 56 kbps, for each channel can be used. These 64 kbps channels are termed "B-channels," which are used for either data, compressed video or digitized voice. The out-of-band signaling is assigned another channel termed a "D-channel," with a bandwidth of either 16 or 64 kbps. N-ISDN provides a Basic Rate Interface (BRI): two B-channels for 128 kbps payload data rate and a 16 kbps D-channel for out-of-band signaling (total 144 kbps). For higher transfer rates, a Primary Rate Interface (PRI) is provided (akin to DS-1): 23 B-channels for 1.472 Mbps payload data rate and one D-channel at 64 kbps for out-of-band signaling (total 1.536 Mbps). A network termination device (NT-1) is required at the user premises which provides functions associated with the physical and electrical termination of the IDSN circuit and may include and interface for a phone and a PC via a multidrop line.

Synchronous Optical Network (SONET)

SONET is an optical transmission interface standardized by ANSI. The ITU-T has published a compatible version referred to as the Synchronous Digital Hierarchy (SDH) in Recommendations G.707, G.708 and G.709. SONET specifies a hierarchy of standardized digital data rates specified for both electrical (synchronous transport signal—STS) and optical (optical carrier—OC) signals [Omidyar 1993]. The signaling rate of the lowest level of the hierarchy, or STS-1 (OC-1) is 51.84 Mbps. Multiple STS-1 (OC-1) signals can be combined to form an STS-N (OC-N) signal and the data rate is simply $N \times 51.84$ Mbps. The ITU-T definition for SDH defines a minimum rate of 155.22 Mbps (SDH-1), corresponding to SONET STS-3 (OC-3). SONET rates up to OC-768 (40 Gbps) are defined. SONET at rates above OC-48 make use of wave division multiplexing (WDM) and dense WDM as described in the LAN section on fiber optic media. SONET is the predominant physical layer for fiber optic WANs.

Broadband ISDN (B-ISDN)

B-ISDN differs from N-ISDN in several ways [Kim 1994]. In order to meet requirements for high-resolution video transmission, an upper channel rate of 150 Mbps might be required. In order to support multiple concurrent interactive or distributive multimedia services, a total subscriber rate of over 600 Mbps might be required. This would obviously require fiber optics to your office or home from the PSTN central office, so these services for most subscribers are off in the not too near future. Three transmission services are defined. The first two are full-duplex services at 155.52 Mbps and 622.08 Mbps, respectively. The last is an asymmetrical service with a downstream rate to the subscriber of 622.08 Mbps and upstream rate to the central office at 155.52 Mbps. ITU-T Recommendations I.113 and I.121 for B-ISDN specify ATM as the transfer mode for B-ISDN and is independent of the means of transport at the physical layer (e.g., SONET). It is interesting that the ITU chose ATM for B-ISDN, as it is a cell (small packet)-based network. Thus, ISDN, which began as a circuit-switched entity of the PSTN, will evolve into a packet-switched network as it takes on broadband digital services.

Local Area Networks

Although LANs have traditionally made use of a broadcasting approach to communication amongst nodes, switched LANs are the most recent implementation. Examples of broadcasting include shared Ethernet and FDDI. Ethernet equipment purchased today uses switching and full-duplex operation to provide full link signaling bandwidth to and from the host computer. Another major example of a switched LAN is the use of ATM. In the case of ATM, cell switching, rather than Ethernet packet switching, is used. Among the features that differentiate various LAN technologies are the topology, transmission medium, and the medium access control technique utilized [Stewart 1992b].

LAN Topologies

Basic topologies are the bus, tree, ring, and star. These can be connected by various means to create complex topologies called meshes. An example of a bus topology is shared Ethernet (IEEE 802.3) [Stallings 1990a] with CSMA/CD (carrier-sense multiple access with collision detection). This broaches the subject of contention resolution. The ring topology is typified by FDDI (fiber distributed data interface—IEEE 802.5) with token passing. Ring topology networks consist of a number of repeaters, each connected to two others by unidirectional transmission links to form a closed loop. In a star topology network, all nodes are connected to a single, central exchange or hub, typically through half-duplex or full duplex connections. The primary function of the hub is that of a network-switching element, which broadcasts or switches network communications among the various peripheral nodes. An example of a star topology network is switched 100BaseT Ethernet (see below). The star topology is currently the most predominant as it can easily accommodate twisted-pair wiring infrastructures. The tree topology can be thought of as a special case of the star topology (hierarchical star) with a switching hub at the root and vertex of each branch (tree without branches), and as such is only of historical significance.

LAN Transmission Media

Twisted-pair wiring is the most common network physical medium, often found pre-wired in office buildings. Although easy to use for LANs, twisted-pair wire produces and absorbs a large amount of electromagnetic interference (EMI), and is thus limited in distance, bandwidth and data rate. Twisted-pair wire may be either shielded (STP) or unshielded (UTP). Shielded twisted-pair (STP) wire can sustain higher data rates over longer distances than can unshielded twisted-pair (UTP) wire, since the former is more immune to EMI. However, as UTP is less expensive, easier to work with, and simple to install, it is much more widely used than STP. There are two major categories of UTP (100 Ω used for LANs as specified by the Electronic Industries Association (EIA 568A). Category 3 corresponds to the voice-grade twisted-pair cable (3-4 twists/foot) found in abundance in most older office buildings and has transmission characteristics specified up to 16 MHz. Category 5 corresponds to data-grade twisted-pair cable (3-4 twists/inch) with transmission characteristics specified up to 100 MHz, which is increasingly common for pre-installation in new buildings. Due to attenuation losses, both are limited to a 100-meter distance. With proper design and few patches, 100 Mbps is achievable using Category 5 UTP. STP runs may be as long as 300 meters.

Fiber optic cable comes in two varieties: single-mode and multi-mode. The principle of fiber optic transmission is that of total internal reflection as a function of incidence angle. As light propagates along a thin, cylindrical glass or plastic core, rays at shallow angles along multiple paths are reflected along the fiber, while the surrounding material (cladding) absorbs rays at more oblique angles. Such is the case with multi-mode optical fiber, for which the core diameter ranges from 50 to 125 μm, but the 62.5 μm-diameter fiber has found widest acceptance. If the radius of the core is reduced to the order of a wavelength, however, only a single mode—that propagating along the central ray of the fiber cylinder—can pass through. This is the case with single-mode fiber optic cable, for which the core diameter ranges from 2 to 12 μm, but the 9 μm-diameter is most commonly used.

Fiber optic cable has a bandwidth of about 25,000 GHz and provides the greatest immunity to EMI. However, throughput using a single channel is limited to a few GHz due to current limitations in converting electrical and optical signals. It is possible through a technique termed wave division multiplexing to impress multiple non-overlapping frequency channels on the same fiber through the use of diffraction gratings. In this way 2, 4, and 8 channels can be used to transmit data simultaneously, providing approximate bandwidths of 5, 10, and 20 Gbps. A technique called dense WDM (DWDM) has been announced quite recently that purports 400 channels per fiber (1000 Gbps)!

Although fiber optic cable itself is relatively inexpensive, costs of installation and end connection (termination and fusion splicing) are relatively high (about $50-$100 per fiber). Equipment for termination and splicing is readily available, and end connectors have been standardized. Attenuation losses due to the fiber optic media and any patching limit segment length although optical repeaters can be used to extend to longer distances if necessary.

LAN Devices

The components used for LANs include network interface cards (NICs), hubs, switches, and routers. NICs are predominantly Ethernet cards that insert into your host computer. Software drivers are loaded into the host operating system to allow the NIC to operate. Hubs are the center of a star topology network, responsible for broadcasting packets amongst all of the individual connections (hub ports) to host systems. With shared Ethernet, the hub acts as level 2 repeaters, wherein all packets were copied (repeated) to each active hub port. With the advent of 100 Mbps switched Ethernet, hubs have been re-engineered into switches as they switch packets between individual host computers. The only traffic on each switched port is that inbound or outbound for that specific host computer.

A router is a device used to connect two networks that may or may not be similar. The router employs a solitary internet protocol (e.g., the IP of TCP/IP) present in each router and computer in the network, but that may use different medium access control (MAC) protocols. Routers route packets by using network layer protocols (OSI layer 3) and are responsible for identifying upper-layer protocols, routing packets, and fragmenting and reassembling user data, as well as detecting faults and updating network topology table look-ups. Routers are sophisticated hardware and software devices that connect LANs and interconnect LANs and WANs (e.g., Ethernet and Frame Relay networks). Because routers are more complex than bridges, they are also typically slower. However, new router architectures have increased throughput rates so that these new routers effectively service high-speed LANs. Multi-protocol routers can deal with heterogeneous network environments (e.g., TCP/IP and IPX) by simultaneously using multiple protocols and have hardware connections for WAN and LAN interconnection.

TCP/IP Networking Implementations

Up until about five years ago, the major TCP/IP LAN network infrastructures consisted of shared 10 Mbps Ethernet in its various flavors (10Base5, 10Base2, and 10BaseT) and 100 Mbps FDDI. Now, 100 Mbps and Gigabit switched Ethernet have become commonplace for PACS installations. The use of TCP/IP tunneling through ATM LANs has also been used for PACS, but to a much more limited extent. Both shared Ethernet and FDDI have fallen into disfavor due to low bandwidth, bandwidth contention, and, in the case of FDDI, the additional cost of fiber optic cabling. There is a copper version of FDDI (CDDI), but it has not been widely implemented.

Medium Access Control

As LANs consist of collections of nodes (e.g., computers and network devices) that must contend for transmission capacity, a means of controlling access to the network transmission medium is required and is called the medium access control (MAC). The MAC forms a sub-layer of the OSI Layer 2 (Data Link) and the Network Access Layer of the TCP/IP stack. As such, the MAC protocol is responsible for assembling data at the source computer into frames (IEEE 802 packets) with addresses and error-detection fields, managing communication over the physical link, and disassembling the transmitted frame and performing address recognition and error detection at the destination computer. There are many types of MAC protocols; however, the key distinguishing parameters are where and how network control is established. Control can be established in either a centralized or distributed manner. How control is established depends on the network topology (e.g., bus or ring) and is divided into synchronous and asynchronous techniques. Asynchronous techniques are preferred and can themselves be divided into contention, reservation, and round-robin categories.

Shared 10 Mbps Ethernet

An example of a distributed asynchronous contention network is the IEEE 802.3 (ISO 8802-3) standard carrier sense multiple access with collision detection (CSMA/CD) for bus or tree topologies [Stallings 1990a]. This type of network is also referred to as "listen while talk." While a node on the bus broadcasts its message to another node, it is listening to the medium as well. When a node has a message to broadcast, it first senses whether there is a signal on the medium. If the node senses no signal, it will begin transmitting. Obviously, if several nodes transmit messages either simultaneously or nearly so, contention for the single 10 Mbps channel results. This can be a problem especially when the network is of large geographic scope, involves a large number of nodes or experiences heavy traffic volume. The following contention arbitration rules, embedded into each node on the network, are applicable. In the event a collision is detected, the nodes immediately cease transmitting and issue brief jamming signals to advise all nodes on the network that a collision has occurred. After transmission of the jamming signal, each node backs off for a short random period of time before attempting to retransmit its message.

Shared 10 Mbps Ethernet has come in a variety of flavors over the years that used different physical media, evolving from very thick, special purpose cables to twisted pair. 10Base5 ("thicknet") used a 10 mm diameter coaxial cable, providing a maximum segment length of 500 meters, hence the "5" in 10Base5. The "10" in 10Base5 signifies the signaling rate, while the "Base" signifies that fact that a baseband signal is impressed on the cabling. 10Base2 ("thinnet") made use of a thin coaxial cable (RG-58), thus yielding a maximum segment length of 185 meters. 10BaseT, as mentioned above, uses either Category 3 or Category 5 UTP wiring. 10BaseT has been implemented using both hubs (shared) and switches (switched).

Switched 100 Mbps and Gigabit Ethernet

Fast Ethernet (100BaseT) refers to a set of specifications developed by the IEEE 802.3 committee to provide a low cost, Ethernet-compatible LAN operating at 100 Mbps [Johnson 1996]. There are three flavors: 100BaseFX that uses optical fiber, and 100BaseT and 100BaseTX that use either STP or Category 5 UTP. All use the IEEE 802.3 MAC protocol and use Ethernet switches rather than the Ethernet multiport repeater hubs used for shared 10BaseT. As 100BaseT uses only a solitary physical link between a switch port and host, even though the port only receives and transmits packets destined for that specific host IP, contention for the port can still occur when the port and host transmit simultaneously. The possibility for contention is eliminated using 100BaseTX and 100BaseFX by utilizing separate physical links for transmission and reception between the switch and host. Recently, gigabit versions using Ethernet are being deployed (1000BaseTX and 1000BaseFX) and 10 Gbps switched Ethernet specifications are being drafted.

The significance of raising Ethernet signaling rates to that typically associated with ATM and SONET is that the current investment in the Ethernet infrastructure is preserved and backward compatible with older NICs. Host link bandwidth can scale from 10 Mbps to 10 Gbps depending on end-user requirements. However, this will require new investment in high-speed Ethernet switches that support the higher rates and new investment in either fiber optic cabling or enhanced Category 5 or the soon to be ratified Category 6 copper wiring standard.

FDDI

FDDI is an example of a round-robin-distributed MAC protocol that uses a token mechanism for channel bandwidth allocation [Jain 1994]. It is based on the ANSI ASC (Accredited Standards Committee) X3T9.5 specification. FDDI has a signaling rate of 100 Mbps and is specified with dual, counter-rotating rings and 62.5 μm multi-mode fiber optic cable. The dual rings provide for fault tolerance in the case of either link or node failure. The FDDI MAC protocol uses a token that circulates around the ring when all stations are idle. The token is a small-frame bit pattern, and it is similar to the IEEE 802.5, known generically as the IBM token-ring network. FDDI uses a complex, capacity-allocation scheme that accommodates support for a mixture of steady and intermittent traffic and multiframe dialogue. Both synchronous (for continuous traffic like video or voice) and asynchronous (for intermittent traffic like image files) transmission are defined.

ATM LAN Emulation

ATM has been applied to LANs in order to satisfy the following requirements: increasing need for guaranteed classes of service (CoS) for real-time multimedia data like video and voice, the desire for scalable throughput, and to facilitate the internetworking between LANs and WANs. ATM is suited to this purpose. Through the use of virtual channels (VCC) and virtual paths (VPC), multiple CoS are accommodated. ATM is scalable through the addition of more ATM switching nodes or higher (or lower) data rates for attached nodes. Also, as ATM is also being used for WAN implementation, it can provide relatively seamless integration of LANs and WANs.

ATM can be used in the implementation of LANs by various means. An ATM switch can be used as a high-speed LAN switch between high-performance multimedia workstations and servers. A local network of ATM switches can act as a backbone to interconnect other LANs. Lastly, an ATM switch can act as a router and traffic concentrator for impressing LAN traffic onto a WAN. In practice, two or all three of these means are used. To function in the LAN environment, the ATM switch must perform protocol conversion from the LAN MAC to the ATM cell stream. In this way, the ATM switch acts as a router, meaning that the LAN MAC (e.g., Ethernet) is being encapsulated or "tunneled" through the ATM network. This is called using the ATM switch in LAN emulation mode or LANE [Minoli 1996]. Link rates between ATM switches or the ATM switch and an ATM NIC are typically 155 Mbps or 622 Mbps. The ATM switch to LAN hub/switch or LAN NIC are at the standard LAN rates (e.g., 10 and 100 Mbps for Ethernet).

Advanced Topics

IP the Next Generation

The current foundation of the Internet and a majority of multivendor intranets is IP (Internet Protocol). A next generation protocol (IPv6 or IPng) has been developed to succeed the current IP (IPv4). A driving motivation for the development of IPv6 has been the limited addressing capability afforded by the four octet (32-bit) IP address. Four octets only allow 2^{32} or approximately four billion unique addresses and while that is seemingly enough, this is less than one address per person on the planet. There are approximately 100 microprocessors in your home. In the future, it is anticipated that everything from the toaster to the lighting and heating control in your home will be on the Net. This plus the need for multiple IP addresses per host and the inefficiencies of the two-level structure of IP addressing have led to IPv6. IPv6 uses 128-bit addressing which allows for on the order of Avogadro's number (6×10^{23}) unique addresses per square meter on the planet [Hinden 1996]! Other motivations include new requirements in the areas of security, routing flexibility and traffic support. The security aspects of IPv6 are discussed in the Network Security section below.

Network Service Guarantees

In a packet-switched network, it is possible for packets to be relayed through multiple routes and, due to congestion on the many routes, packets can be delayed and arrive at the destination out of order, or due to switch element (e.g., router) buffer overflow, may be lost. While this may be tolerable for data transmissions such as e-mail and image files, it plays havoc with real-time applications like video and voice. Even though the current Internet is congested in many places, real-time streaming video (albeit at low resolution) or audio are affected though use of a buffering time long enough to account for a majority of anticipated delays. This is, however, not an effected method for Internet telephony. For these real-time applications that currently use PSTN circuit-switched capabilities, for example POTS and ISDN, assigning a priority to certain packets to enable a quality or class of service is required.

The ATM standard allows for the concept of network quality of service (QoS). This is important, as the 'A' in ATM stands for asynchronous. A variety of traffic control functions have been defined to maintain the QoS for ATM connections. These include network resource management, connection admission control, usage parameter control, priority control, and fast resource management. The network resource management allows the allocation of network resources to separate traffic flows according to service characteristics using virtual paths (VPC or VCC). With connection admission control, the user selects traffic characteristics by selecting a QoS from among the QoS classes that the network provides, essentially creating a network traffic contract. Traffic characteristics include the peak cell rate, cell delay variation, sustainable cell rate, and the burst tolerance. The ATM network accepts the connection only if it can commit resources to the connection and still maintain active connections. The usage parameter control, priority control and fast resource management control are real-time protocols to police the VPC or VCC for network traffic contract violations by the user.

IP is well behind ATM in terms of QoS provision. IPv4 does have a type-of-service field, but it is little used by current Internet devices. Several high-level protocols, like resource reservation protocol (RSVP), have been developed to support real-time multimedia delivery and QoS specifiers for multicast and unicast network services. IPv6 allows for the labeling of packets belonging to a particular traffic flow for which the sender requests special handing by intervening routers. A flow is a sequence of packets sharing attributes that affect how those packets are handled by the router, including path, resource allocation, discard requirements, and security. The router may service packets from manifold flows differently through allocation of dissimilar buffer sizes, differing forwarding precedence, and requesting disparate QoS from downstream subnetworks. However, routers employing RSVP-like or IPv6 capabilities have yet to be deployed. Thus, the only currently effective, albeit simple, mechanism to ensure a certain bandwidth is available to an application is the gross over design of network capacity so that there are absolutely no potential bottlenecks. This is a rather expensive and inelegant solution however.

Network Security

Computer and network security addresses three requirements: secrecy, integrity, and availability. Four general categories of attack are interruption, interception, modification, and fabrication. The universal technique for providing privacy for transmitted data is encryption. Encryption algorithms can be dichotomized into two general types: symmetric private key encryption and asymmetric public key encryption. With symmetric private key encryption the same key is used to encrypt and decrypt the message. Examples are DES (data encryption standard) and Triple DES. Secure key management is an obvious problem with private-key encryption schemes. Asymmetric public key encryption uses both a private encryption key and a public decryption key. Examples are the RSA scheme which is the only widely accepted and implemented approach to public-key encryption. This is what web browsers employ. Other relevant topics include authentication and digital signatures. Please also see the expanded article by Nickolas J. Hangiandreou in this volume for further discussion of encryption.

As part of the feature set for IPv6 the following capabilities have been published: an overall security architecture, packet authentication, and packet encryption. To enable backward compatibility with current IPv4 network components, these new security features are implemented as extension headers that follow the main IP header. The extension header for authentication is the Authentication header and the one for encryption is the Encapsulating Security Payload (ESP) header. Much like the associations used in DICOM messaging, a unique, unidirectional security association is set up between sending and receiving hosts consisting of the destination IP address and the security parameter index (authentication header plus ESP header). The Authentication header provides support for data integrity and authentication of IP packets. ESP provides support for privacy and data integrity of IP packets using encryption at the transport layer segment (transport mode ESP) or an entire IP packet (tunnel-mode ESP).

Firewalls are a modern equivalent of the medieval moat, where all data traffic to or from a subnetwork or distributed intranet is forced through an electronic drawbridge (firewall). For the firewall to work effectively, no other route to the protected network exists, i.e., there is no backdoor. All messages entering or leaving the protected intranet pass through the firewall, which examines each message and blocks those that do not meet specified security criteria. There are several types of firewall techniques: packet filters, application gateways, circuit-level gateways, and proxy servers. Packet filters look at each packet entering or leaving the network and accept or reject them based on user-defined rules. Packet filtering is fairly effective and transparent to users, but it is difficult to configure. In addition, it is susceptible to IP spoofing. Application gateways apply security mechanisms to specific applications, such as FTP and telnet servers. This is very effective, but can impose performance degradation. Circuit-level gateways apply security mechanisms when a TCP or UDP connection is established. Once the connection has been made, packets can flow between the hosts without afurther checking. Proxy servers intercept all messages entering and leaving the network. The proxy server, in effect, hides the true intranet network addresses from those outside. In practice, many firewalls use two or more of these techniques in concert.

PACS and Teleradiology Networking Issues

Important networking issues applied to medical imaging are the sizing of the network, network modeling and simulation, centralized versus distributed PACS architectures, last mile solutions for teleradiology, and ATM versus Fast and Gigabit Ethernet. There are a host of others, but space limitations preclude their discussion in this article.

The design of networking infrastructure systems for medical imaging applications can be complex, entailing a multitude of hard and soft variables. Careful characterization of the static image and video sources, workflow patterns, and institutional organization should precede system design [Blaine 1996]. This analysis plus thorough assessment of specific networking requirements and selection of appropriate technologies form the boundary conditions for network design. Important variables to consider include network channel capacity, throughput, latency, and end-to-end delay time. Computer modeling and simulation of the proposed network design can be very helpful in performing trade-off analysis of various architectures (e.g., centralized versus distributed PACS) [Stewart 1993a] and where the bottlenecks occur [Stewart 1993b].

A recent contested topic regarding PACS network planning concerns the relative merits of using ATM or Gigabit Ethernet for the network backbone and ATM or Fast Ethernet to the display workstation. As mentioned earlier, ATM has some very attractive capabilities: it is scalable, was designed to handle real-time application traffic like video and voice well, has QoS definitions and dynamic bandwidth allocation. However, ATM has some deficiencies as well. The segmentation and reassembly (SAR) process implemented in silicon has a signaling limit at OC-48 rates (2.5 Gbps). There is a large (10%) overhead using the small (53 byte) ATM cell structure and for LAN usage. TCP/IP tunneling must be utilized unless ATM NICs are used. ATM NICs are very expensive compared with Fast Ethernet NICs. Also, since most carrier networks are already SONET-based and ATM networks require SONET interfaces, it seems more reasonable to run IP directly over SONET and dispense with ATM LAN emulation altogether. With the wide deployment of Fast and Gigabit Ethernet and an emerging standard for 10 Gbps Ethernet, the emergence of data over voice as the most profitable telecommunications commodity and the SAR limitations of ATM, most of the new fiber optic networks being deployed nationwide (e.g., Qwest, Level 3) have bypassed the use of ATM and are utilizing IP over SONET at OC-192 rates. By transporting frames directly into the SONET payload, the overhead required in ATM cell header, IP over ATM encapsulation, and SAR functionality is eliminated. The jury is still out on this topic and both camps have defendable arguments to justify their positions.

Last Mile Solutions for Teleradiology

For DICOM-based teleradiology, hard IP addressing is used. As most Internet Service Providers (ISPs) assign IP addresses dynamically for dial-up modem connections and these modem connections are limited to 56 kbps, cable modems and digital subscriber lines (DSL) are rapidly being used for teleradiology applications. Both services provide a hard IP address and direct connection of the Ethernet NIC into the end user termination device (e.g., cable modem).

Cable Modem

As the name implies, cable modems use a converter box (the cable modem) to impress Ethernet traffic (TCP/IP) onto the cable video infrastructure where it is eventually tied into the Internet. The network interface card (NIC) sends Ethernet packets to the cable modem. The cable modem modulates the data and transmits radio frequency (RF) signals over coaxial cable to the receiving modem at the other end of the connection that is tied into the Internet. In the opposite direction, your modem converts the RF signals it receives back into Ethernet packets before sending them to the Ethernet card in your computer. Cable modems generally use about a 30-Mbps channel swath of the video cable service. This bandwidth is shared with others using cable modems in your neighborhood, so depending on their usage, your bandwidth will vary in time. Depending on your local cable infrastructure, the downstream (to your location) data rate is usually many times faster than the upstream (from your location) rate. This is of course fine for teleradiology if one is only receiving images. Typically, a hard IP address is given for use by the NIC which makes teleradiology using DICOM easy to implement. Access to cable modem service is spotty and dependent on the replacement of the existing coaxial cable infrastructure with fiber optic cable on a neighborhood by neighborhood basis. General cost is about $40/month.

Digital Subscriber Line (DSL)

Stated simply, DSL provides high-speed multimedia services, such as video-on-demand and super-fast Internet access (for teleradiology) to anyone with a standard, copper telephone line. DSL is run over existing copper phone wires, so carriers do not have to run new cable to and within your location. However, users will need to install a DSL modem that communicates with a DSL access multiplexer (DSLAM) at the telco central office. The DSL modem connects to the 10BaseT Ethernet card on your PC.

DSL service operates in frequencies outside those used for voice. Voice or analog transmissions typically fall in the 0 to 3400 Hz range and transmit at speeds from 9.6 to 56 kbps. By extending the top frequency boundary, DSL can operate on the same line without interfering with the analog signal. However, to support DSL, the copper wiring from the central office must meet certain criteria. For example, the line must be free of load coils, which are often added to long local loops to improve voice quality. Thus for DSL, one typically has to be less than 18,000 feet from the central office and the longer the local loop, the slower the DSL rate. DSL deployment to date has not gone as smoothly as carriers originally hoped due to the poor quality of many local loops and oversubscription of current limited deployment, and is gaining heavy competition from cable modem service.

Two of the most common flavors of DSL are Rate Adaptive DSL (RADSL) and asymmetrical DSL (ADSL). Rates in multiples of 256 kbps to over 10 Mbps are available. For 256 kbps DSL service through a local carrier, the rate is around $40/month. Again, typically a hard IP address is given for use by the NIC, which makes teleradiology using DICOM easy to implement.

References

Bellamy, J. *Digital Telephony*. New York, NY: John Wiley; 1991.

Blaine, G.J., Cox, J.R., Jost, R.G. "Networks for electronic radiology." *Radiol Clin North Am* 34:647-65; 1996.

Bidgood, W.D., Horii, S.C. "Introduction to the ACR-NEMA DICOM standard." *RadioGraphics* 12:345-55; 1992.

Day, J.D. "The (un)revised OSI reference model." *Computer Commun. Rev.* 25:1334-40; 1995.

Hinden, R.M. "IP next generation overview." *Commun. ACM* 39:61-71; 1996.

Horii, S.C. "Network and ACR-NEMA protocols." *RadioGraphics* 12:537-48; 1992.

Jain, R. *FDDI Handbook—High-speed Networking Using Fiber and other Media*. Reading, MA: Addison-Wesley; 1994.

Johnson, H.W. *Fast Ethernet—Dawn of a New Network*. Englewood Cliffs, NJ: Prentice Hall; 1996.

Kessler, G.C. *ISDN*, 2nd ed. New York, NY: McGraw-Hill; 1993.

Kim, J.B., Suda, T., Yoshimuri, M. "International standardization of B-ISDN." *Computer Networks and ISDN Systems* 27:5-27; 1994.

Kyas, O. *ATM Networks*. London: International Thompson Publishing; 1995.

Leiner, B.M., Cole, R., Postel, J., Mills, D. "The DARPA internet protocol suite." *IEEE Commun. Magazine* 23:29-34; 1985.

Minoli, D., Alles, A. *LAN, ATM, and LAN Emulation Technologies.* Boston, MA: Artech House; 1996.

Omidyar, C.G., Aldridge, A. "Introduction to SDH/SONET." *IEEE Commun. Magazine* 31:30-3; 1993.

Smith, P. *Frame Relay.* Reading, MA: Addison-Wesley; 1993.

Stallings, W. *Data and Computer Communications,* 5th ed. Upper Saddle River, NJ: Prentice Hall; 1997.

Stallings, W. *Handbook of Computer Communication Standards.* Vol 2, Local Area Network Standards. Carmel, IN: Sams Publishing; 1990a.

Stallings, W. *Handbook of Computer Communication Standards.* Vol 3, The TCP/IP Protocol Suite. Carmel, IN: Sams Publishing; 1990b.

Stewart, B.K. "Local area network topologies, media and routing." In: *Syllabus: A Special Course in Computers for Clinical Practice and Education in Radiology.* Honeyman, J.C., Staab, E.V. (Eds). Oak Brook, IL: RSNA Publications, 79-95; 1992a.

Stewart, B.K. "Local area network topologies, media and routing." *Radiographics* 12: 549-66; 1992b.

Stewart, B.K. "Operational departmentwide picture archiving communication system analysis using discrete event-driven block-oriented network simulation." *Journal of Digital Imaging* 6: 126-39; 1993a.

Stewart, B.K., Dwyer, S.J. "Prediction of teleradiology system throughput by discrete event-driven, block-oriented network simulation." *Investigative Radiology* 1993; 28: 162-168; 1993b.

Tanenbaum, A.S. *Computer Networks,* 3rd ed. Upper Saddle River, NJ:Prentice Hall; 1996.

Ward, S.A., Halstead, R.H. *Computation Structures.* Cambridge , MA: MIT Press, 286-7; 1991.

Introduction to DICOM

Richard L. Kennedy, Mark H. Oskin, J. Anthony Seibert, Stephen T. Hecht
Department of Radiology
University of California-Davis
UC Davis Medical Center
Sacramento, California 95817

What is the Purpose of DICOM?

DICOM (Digital Imaging and Communications in Medicine) is a set of standards-based protocols for exchanging and storing medical imaging data, both as actual images and as text associated with these images. It is an open standard in that the information for developing DICOM-based software applications is public, defined, and regulated by public committees, and that devices or software claiming to support this standard are required to conform to strict and detailed protocol definitions. Also, DICOM requires, as part of the standard, that a specific implementation claiming DICOM conformance must provide documentation of the specific DICOM services and data types supported, and in what manner another implementation could communicate with the proposed system for which the DICOM conformance is claimed.

What this means for Physicists and Information Technology (IT) staff responsible for integrating DICOM conformant devices is that understanding the structure and concepts of the standard itself, as well as being able to understand the documentation that DICOM requires for conformance claims (the Conformance Statement) is critical to success when trying to utilize DICOM to communicate between medical imaging devices. Whether these devices are scanners, archives, workstations, or radiation therapy systems, the DICOM standard provides a high level of structure for defining the possible communications between these systems. Understanding this structure is an important part of attempting DICOM interoperability between imaging systems.

The purpose of this paper is to provide a very basic overview of the DICOM standard, to explain the essential concepts of the standard, and to provide the minimum background required to understand the Conformance Statement documentation that is required for every DICOM implementation. As the DICOM Standard now consists of thousands of pages of documents, covering an increasingly large area of applications, this will be an extremely brief overview to the overall text. What we will provide here is a description of the structure of the Standard specific to medical physics, and a means to approach DICOM in the context of solving actual problems in DICOM interoperability. A companion paper in this syllabus will continue from this introduction to further describe basic analysis and troubleshooting for actual DICOM implementations.

History and Evolution of the Standard

Early in the development of digital imaging systems, the need for a standard method of interchange between different imaging devices was recognized. Work began in the early 1980's to develop such a standard, under the joint auspices of the American College of Radiology (ACR) and the National Electrical Manufacturers Association (NEMA). This culminated with the establishment in 1984 of the predecessor to the DICOM standard, called ACR/NEMA. This was initially envisioned and developed as a hardware-based point-to-point standard, as few of the early generation of imaging systems supported standards-based computer networking, and what networks did exist at that time were not considered fast enough to service the bandwidth requirements of medical imaging.

To put this into the perspective of the history of network development, Bolt, Beranek, and Newman (BBN) installed the first Internet node at UCLA and the first host computer was connected to that network in September 1969. The FDDI standard (the first network protocol as fast as ACR/NEMA II, at 100 megabits per second) for fiber networking was defined formally for Internet Protocol (IP) networks in 1989, (RFC 1103) and IP packets over ATM (at 155 mbs) were defined in 1993 (RFC 1577). Thus the original NEMA 100 mbs-hardware solution, while appearing somewhat quaint in retrospect, was a logical development within the historical context.

With the rapid parallel development of network technology, however, it became apparent that the ACR/NEMA standard needed to be adapted to operate over the emerging network standards, rather than relying on specialized interface hardware for speed. Changes were needed in the standard to facilitate imaging systems operating as parts of larger enterprise-based networks, utilizing standard protocols such as the Transmission Control Protocol/Internet Protocol (TCP/IP). Such systems could then make use of advances in computer networking independent of medical technology. With the growth of the Internet and the advent of technologies such as Fast (100BaseT) and Gigabit Ethernet, the advantages of DICOM as a software standard rather than as a specialized hardware standard are now quite evident. Fortunately, DICOM today runs over general-purpose computer networks, and while it is still common practice to isolate clinical imaging networks on dedicated Local Area Networks (LANs) and Wide Area Networks (WANs) to help manage their bandwidth requirements, many hospitals interoperate their DICOM-based imaging systems with general networks, including desktop systems.

The subsequent development of the DICOM standard—changed in name from ACR/NEMA to reflect the more general scope of medical imaging rather than being specific to Radiology—was formalized in 1993, but the standard was by no means completed at that point. The first 14 parts (described in detail below) have led to the current (189) separate working documents (see appendix 1), representing a tremendous expansion of scope and depth for the standard itself. As a result of this expansion, DICOM now encompasses the imaging aspects of Cardiology, Gastroenterology, Ophthalmology, Pathology, and Radiation Therapy through the addition of new data objects and types.

Essential Concepts of DICOM

In order to describe the structure of DICOM, we must first introduce some, perhaps unfamiliar, terms used in the Standard documentation. These terms come from the OSI *(Open Systems Interconnection)* model, and are used quite formally in the actual Standard, but we will here attempt to present these in a more informal and applied manner. We will present first the formal definition (in Italics) from the Standard text, followed by the less formal definition for the purposes of this paper, with a specific focus of interconnectivity problems that are likely to be faced by medical physicists.

ISO 7-layer network model

7	APPLICATION	Application services
6	PRESENTATION	Code conversion and data reformatting
5	SESSION	Coordinates interaction between end and application process
4	TRANSPORT	End-to-end data integrity and quality of service
3	NETWORK	Switches and routes information
2	DATA LINK	Transfers unit of information to other end of physical link
1	PHYSICAL	Transmits bit streams

DICOM/ISO Model

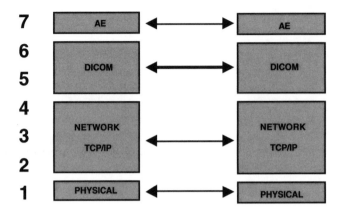

Information Object: *An abstraction of a real information entity (e.g., CT Image, Study, etc.) which is acted upon by DICOM Commands.* A DICOM Object, as described by a DICOM Information Object Descriptor (IOD), is generally a modality-specific software module with certain attributes (gantry position, radionuclide, pulse sequence, etc.) appropriate for a particular modality or function. Thus, as new IODs are added to the DICOM standard, the scope of the standard can be expanded to encompass new areas and new technologies as needed. (Radiotherapy, Positron Emission Tomography (PET), etc.). Although it is inappropriate to think of DICOM as a "file format," a reasonable way of thinking about the IOD is—it is the structure of a DICOM image.

An Information Object is, more generally, a set of related information, grouped into what DICOM calls *Information Entities* (IEs). Each Entity relates to a single real-world item, such as patient name, or a single CT image. An object can be either Composite (consisting of multiple Information Entities) or Normalized (consisting of a single Information Entity). Typically, management services utilize normalized objects, while image services utilize more complicated composite objects.

Application Entities (AE): This refers, in the concrete sense, to the applications (programs and devices) that are to communicate via DICOM. These are named (AE Titles), have certain attributes, and can perform certain services (a CT scanner, for example, might only be able to send CT studies, or it might also be able to print to a DICOM print device.) In the more abstract model, it refers to the functional entities of the OSI model (ISO 7495-1) that participate in this model. Although a particular hardware device may have several AE titles, a reasonable way to think about the AE title in today's market place is—a device has a name, and that name is the AE title.

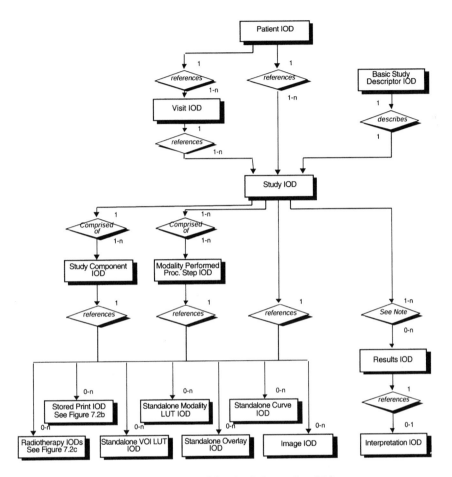

DICOM Information Model—Information Objects
Source: DICOM PS 3.3

<u>Service</u>: In the DICOM context, an action to perform on an Object. Storing (Store), retrieving (Get), locating (Find), responding to diagnostics (Echo), and printing (Print) are examples of Services. Although services are further specialized, it is helpful to catalog devices along these basic functionality lines (Echo, Store, Query/Retrieve, Print, and HIS/RIS), and whether or not the device is a Service Class Provider (SCP) or Service Class User (SCU) of each.

<u>Service-Object-Pair (SOP)</u>: *A Service-Object Pair class is defined by the union of an IOD and a DIMSE (DICOM Message Service Element; for definition, see page 295) Service Group. The SOP Class definition contains the rules and semantics, which may restrict*

the use of the services in the DIMSE Service Group or the Attributes of the IOD. The combination of a DICOM action (Store, Find, etc.) and a DICOM object (CT study, MR study, etc.) is referred to as a SOP ("Store a CT Study," "Find an MR study," etc.). An important point to note here is that a specific implementation is allowed to modify— within very strict bounds—DICOM actions and objects. The Conformance Statement must list these alterations, and looking for the differences and alterations is one of the critical parts of comparing Conformance Statements.

Service-Object-Pair (SOP) instance: *A concrete occurrence of an Information Object and communication context.* In the above example, a specific combination of an action and an object: "Store **this** CT study." This is not particularly relevant for the medical physicist.

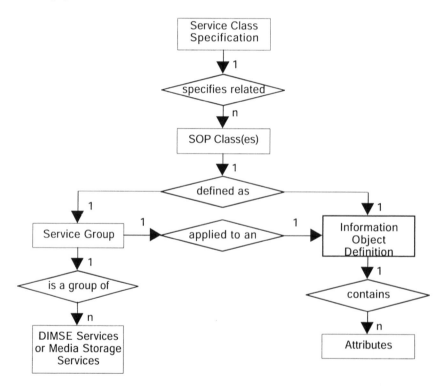

Major Structures of the DICOM Information Model—Service/Object Relationship
Source: DICOM PS 3.3

Service Class: *A collection of SOP classes and/or Meta SOP Classes which are related in that they are described together to accomplish a single application.* A Service Class is specific definition of a service, which will be supported by cooperating devices to perform an action on a specific class of Information Object. The Service Class is extremely relevant for the medical physicist. When comparing two conformance statements to ensure interoperability, the first step is to look at the service classes, and roles supported.

Service Class User (SCU): *The role played by a DICOM Application Entity (DIMSE-Service-User)* **which invokes operations** *and performs notifications on a specific Association.* In the client-server terminology, this is whichever system is performing an operation as a client[1]. In the example of a CT scanner, when sending a study to a PACS, the scanner is performing as a SCU for storage, i.e., it is **using** the storage of the PACS.

Service Class Provider (SCP): *The role played by a DICOM Application Entity (DIMSE-Service-User)* **which performs operations** *and invokes notifications on a specific Association.* In the client-server terminology, this is whichever system is performing an operation as a server[2]. In the example of a PACS, when receiving a study from a CT scanner, the PACS is performing as a SCP for storage, i.e., it is **providing** the storage for the scanner.

SCU/SCP Roles (example):

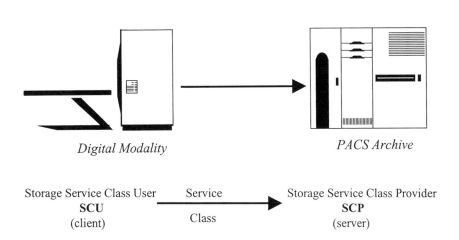

Digital Modality   *PACS Archive*

Storage Service Class User   Service   Storage Service Class Provider
SCU   **SCP**
(client)   Class   (server)

---

[1] Strictly speaking, this is not entirely true. However, it is a useful enough method of thinking about the relationship of SCU and SCP that for almost all practical purposes it holds. The exceptions to this are largely irrelevant to practical DICOM inter-networking.

[2] Similar to SCU, this again is not strictly true, but is generally applicable.

Conformance Statement: *A formal statement associated with a specific implementation of the DICOM standard. It specifies the Service Classes, Information Objects, and Communication Protocols supported by the implementation.* Practically speaking, the Conformance Statement is the document that a vendor must provide to describe what their DICOM implementation can, or by omission, cannot do. For example, a specific CT scanner might be able to send DICOM studies to an archive, but not be able to receive studies from a MR scanner from the same vendor. Or a workstation might be able to receive CT, MR, and CR, but not US. Reading, and comparing, the Conformance Statements of the respective devices is an essential step in attempting DICOM interoperability between those devices. It should be pointed out that, if a vendor claims conformance to the DICOM standard, then the DICOM standard mandates that the vendor make public a conformance statement. The language to this effect is located in Part 2 of the standard, and often comes in handy in leveraging conformance statements out of sly vendors, without signing non-disclosure agreements.

Association: *Association establishment is the first phase of communication between peer DICOM compliant Application Entities. The Application Entities shall use Association establishment to negotiate which SOP Classes can be exchanged and how this data will be encoded.* Negotiating a connection between two devices in order to perform a service or services is called establishing a DICOM Association. It is point that many of the most common interconnectivity problems appear, since several critical aspects of DICOM are negotiated between the devices at this point. The respective roles of the SCP and SCU, the specific service classes that are to be performed, as well the particulars of the communication protocol that are to be used, are all part of this negotiation phase. If the two proposed AEs cannot negotiate a set of services, contexts, and objects, the association will be refused. One of the most common reasons for DICOM devices to refuse an association, for example, is that most (but not all) implementations require that each AE have *a priori* knowledge of each other—such as IP address, port, and AE calling and called title (name). For this reason, it is generally required that both devices attempting to communicate via DICOM be configured to be aware of each other before attempting to communicate. In most cases, this will involve modifying a table of "known" AEs on both devices (scanner, workstation, PACS, etc.) before attempting DICOM communication.

Parts of the Base Standard

The following is a brief description of the first 14 parts of the base standard using the definitions provided above. Our intent here is to provide a "roadmap" of the Standard Parts, describing the purpose and role of each Part in the context of medical physics. Additionally, the concept of HIS/RIS interfacing is presented, as we feel that this is a function that rests equally in the domains of Information Technology (IT) and Medical Physics.

Part 1: "Introduction and Overview"
Defines the structure and scope of the standard itself, introduces basic concepts, and describes the roles and interrelationships of the other 13 Parts. This is essential, and quite approachable, reading.

Part 2: "Conformance"
Defines the structure for the required documentation that must—as per the standard— be provided for every DICOM conformant system. In order to claim DICOM conformance, an implementer **must** provide this documentation, and the document **must** be structured as defined by Part 2. The reason for this rigid structure is that the Conformance Statement is—in effect—the blueprint for a specific DICOM implementation, providing an overview of what the system claims as functionality. A conformance statement specifies the service classes, information objects, and communications protocols used by a specific implementation.

Understanding the DICOM Conformance Statement for an imaging device prior to purchasing it is, we feel, as important as studying the device's physical imaging characteristics, if DICOM interoperability is essential for the device's clinical function. This is probably the single area where the partnership of the IT and Physics groups are most essential to the success of DICOM-based interoperability.

Part 3: "Information Object Definitions"
Defines the structure and kind of data objects that DICOM can manage—some examples of this would be CT or MRI studies, and patient demographic tables. Additionally, Part 3 defines the attributes for these objects (CT gantry position, radiographic technique, patient date of birth, etc.) The particulars of these attributes are defined in Parts 5 and 6, the encoding rules, and data dictionary.

Part 4: "Service Class Specifications"
Defines the services—the operations, such as moving, storing, finding, or printing— that can be performed on the data objects of Part 3. A specific combination of a Service and an Object is termed a "Service Object Pair" or SOP. The SOP is a particularly important concept of DICOM, and constitutes the basic unit of DICOM operability. Another concept that is developed in Part 4 is that of "primitive" vs. higher-level (DICOM Message Service Element, DIMSE) services. The DIMSE services comprise the user-recognizable services for DICOM. One analogy that has been made is that Messages (Part 7) are the verbs acting on the Object (Part 3) nouns: together they can be used to construct a command (SOP), describing what DICOM is being requested to perform ("Store a CT Study"). The structure of the sentence itself is the service (Part 4).

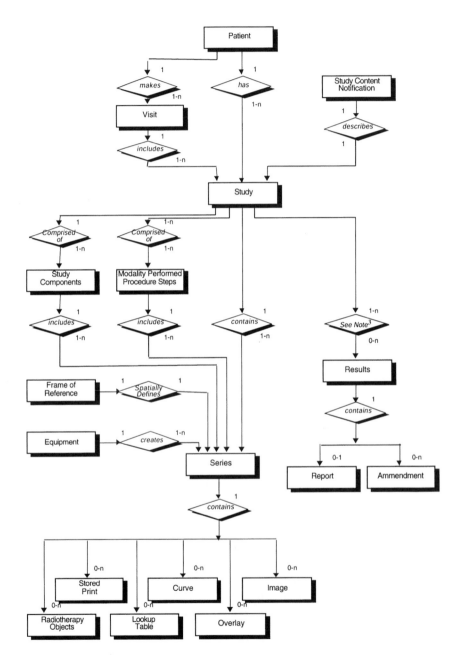

DICOM Model of the Real World
Source: DICOM PS 3.3

---

[3] The relationship between study and result is complex, involving other portions of the standard, and other standards, such as HL7.

Table 1. DIMSE (DICOM Message Service Element) Services

Name	Group	Type
C-Store	DIMSE Composite	Operation
C-Get	DIMSE Composite	Operation
C-Move	DIMSE Composite	Operation
C-Find	DIMSE Composite	Operation
C-Echo	DIMSE Composite	Operation
N-Event-Report	DIMSE Composite	Notification
N-Get	DIMSE Normalized	Operation
N-Set	DIMSE Normalized	Operation
N-Action	DIMSE Normalized	Operation
N-Create	DIMSE Normalized	Operation
N-Delete	DIMSE Normalized	Operation

Part 5: "Data Structures and Encoding"
Defines the actual coding of specific DICOM elements, and the system-dependent technical details of their data. Examples are how the value is stored (little endian (*DEC/Intel ordering*) or big endian (*SUN/Motorola ordering*), etc.), and the possible value representations (VRs: Decimal String, Date, Time, etc.) that are supported within DICOM. Additionally, the mechanism for compressed syntax(es) are defined here as well. JPEG is defined as a specific compression syntax, however the standard is expected to include newer mechanisms as they are completed and accepted (wavelet, JPEG 2000, etc.).

Part 6: "Data Dictionary"
Defines and enumerates the actual data elements that can be used to construct DICOM messages or files. Part 6 is, in effect, a registry of DICOM data elements and identifiers. For each data element (example: "Accession Number") there is a numeric tag (example: (008,0052)); a value representation (example: SH, "Short String"); and a value multiplicity, or the number of instances that a value can have (example: "1"—a study instance can have only one accession number).

Part 7: "Message Exchange"
Defines the structure for DICOM services and messaging. This is a particularly complex portion of the standard, as it relies heavily on the formal OSI Reference Model for its nomenclature. In basic, however, Part 7 defines the services that DICOM can perform (Store, Get, Move, Find, Echo, etc.) (see table 1) in terms of the protocols with

which two DICOM devices (Application Entities, or AEs) can communicate. The process of starting and establishing a basis for a DICOM communication (Association Negotiation), as well as the formal structure for all subsequent DICOM messaging, including error notification and recovery, are covered in this Part. (But take heart—this is the most difficult part of DICOM—from here, it's easier!). Further note, that in order to have a working basic knowledge of how to understand a conformance statement, you do not have to read and understand Part 7. However, it is helpful, when diagnosing complicated DICOM communication errors, to understand Part 7.

Part 8: "Network Communication Support for Message Exchange"
Defines the technical details of DICOM messaging over a host network (typically, and almost always TCP/IP), including the lower-level handshaking for establishing a DICOM message stream. This includes a description of the state machine to understand DICOM's event and error notification process. It is most helpful to refer to this part when, in effect, your "DICOM won't start." Note the concepts of "calling AE" and "called AE," and that of AE titles, as these underlie many basic, and easily resolved, DICOM problems.

Part 9: "Point to Point Communication for Message Exchange"
Defines the older ACR/NEMA point-to-point interface protocol. This is the one Part of the DICOM standard that a physicist can most safely ignore. DICOM supports, as backward compatibility, the older ACR/NEMA 50-pin interface, despite the fact that is now considered a legacy protocol. Unless you are faced with the prospect of interfacing a very old scanner, that just happened to have the ACR/NEMA interface, and cannot, for whatever reason, utilize one of the several vendors now manufacturing DICOM retrofit systems (Merge, DeJarnette, Dicomit, etc.), this part of the standard will probably be of limited relevance. (A common joke among DICOM implementers is that if you took Part 9 of DICOM and *moved* it over to the HL7 standard, it would be a win/win for all involved).

Part 10: "Media Storage and File Format for Data Exchange"
Defines the structure for "portable" DICOM volumes. This is particularly important in mobile applications such as Ultrasound, and in applications such as Cardiac Cath where removable media such as CD-R are especially valuable. With Parts 10, 11, and 12, DICOM defines, in addition to the network messaging protocols described above, a complete means for storing information on disk and tape, and the means by which these volumes can be interchanged between various systems. Some vendors (GE for instance) now utilize DICOM volumes as their "native" disk archive format, thus allowing free interchange of disks between systems supporting this standard. Part 10 defines the file and volume format required for DICOM conformance.

Part 11: "Media Storage Application Profiles"
Defines the specific elements from the other parts of the DICOM standard that are required to support removable media. This is required for these volumes to provide a

complete and "standalone" patient context, once removed from the original host system. A DICOM conformant removable volume will be readable between systems with different native filesystems—this is critical for imaging systems given the number and variation of operating systems in use today, as well as providing a means for reading these volumes in the future.

Part 12: "Media Formats and Physical Media for Data Interchange"
Defines both the allowable physical media (1.44mb floppy, 128mb, 230mb, 540mb, 650mb, 1.2gb, and 2.6gb MO disks, as well as 650mb CD-R, currently) for DICOM removable media. Also, the structure for a "portable" file system for those media (floppy and MO) that do not include this as part of their normative standard, as well as a standard directory structure "DICOMDir" for allowing interoperability between dissimilar operating systems.

Part 13: "Print Management Point to Point Communication Support"
Defines the extensions to DICOM required to support the specialized and more complex application of printer control and image data. Unlike workstations, printers used for radiology typically employ two communications channels—one for control and the other for image pixel transmission. In order to support the specialized requirements of these devices within the scope of the DICOM standard, the standard incorporates a point-to-point physical interface option. As with Part 9, however, the physical interface has been superceded by software control with many current generation print devices. The medical physicist can safely ignore this section.

Part 14: "Greyscale Standard Display Function"
Defines the quantitative relationship between the pixel data of the preceding parts and display values, either as hardcopy (film, paper) or softcopy (workstations). This relationship is defined in terms of human perception of luminance (visual psychophysical values), and given as specific characteristic curves for each display system and type. This section is new and is not implemented by many vendors. However, given the severe lack of quality control by vendors and their software display products, this section should become increasingly relevant as PACS is more widely adopted.

Supplement 10: Basic Worklist Management (Modality Worklist Management SOP Class)
While not part of the initial Parts of the Standard, we have included this here since it represents an area of specific relevance to medical physicists, and one we feel is critical to the practical issues of patient workflow and quality assurance. This section of the Standard includes the definition for Modality Worklist, the ability to exchange patient and study demographic information with imaging modalities, which represents by far the most effective way to ensure that patient and study information is consistent across the modalities, RIS, HIS, and ultimately PACS. This service is described more thoroughly below in the "HIS/RIS interfacing" section.

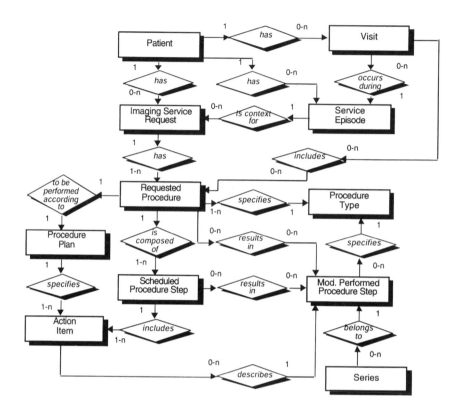

DICOM Information Model—HIS/RIS Interfacing

HIS/RIS Interfacing

While a general model for DICOM image storage involves a modality serving as an SCU, and storing to an external SCP device, the modality worklist model is somewhat different. In modality worklist, the modality device acquires requisite patient/study information from a worklist server (be it a PACS, RIS, or a device dedicated to this service that is interfaced to a HIS or RIS). This can be accomplished via two basic models: A) by having patient data sent to the modality based on an external trigger (patient arrival, study scheduled, etc.) or B) on demand (query) from the modality, based on information available at the point of study initiation (accession number, medical record number, etc.). One example of such a service would be for a scanner to barcode the accession number and initiate a request for the associated HIS/RIS information (patient name, gender, date of birth, medical record number, etc.) from the worklist server.

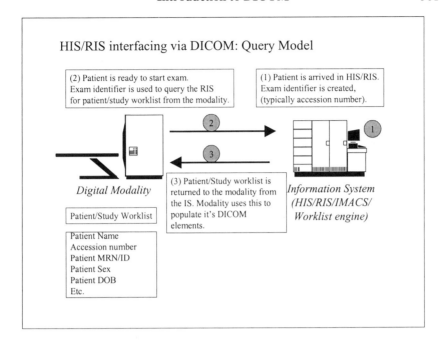

HIS/RIS interfacing via DICOM: Query Model

(2) Patient is ready to start exam. Exam identifier is used to query the RIS for patient/study worklist from the modality.

(1) Patient is arrived in HIS/RIS. Exam identifier is created, (typically accession number).

Digital Modality

Patient/Study Worklist

Patient Name
Accession number
Patient MRN/ID
Patient Sex
Patient DOB
Etc.

(3) Patient/Study worklist is returned to the modality from the IS. Modality uses this to populate it's DICOM elements.

Information System (HIS/RIS/IMACS/ Worklist engine)

The advantages of such a model are tremendous—assuring that PACS data are consistent with HIS/RIS information is critical to PACS, as well as providing essential tools for medical physicists responsible for quality assurance.

The critical importance of HIS/RIS integration is not necessarily obvious from the perspective of image communication, but follows from the realities of how radiology workflow is generally performed in the real world. The non-imaging systems (HIS/RIS) are almost always considered the "authoritative" source for patient demographic information, rather than the PACS or the modalities themselves. While the technologist generally does have the current information from the HIS or RIS at hand when initiating the study, these data are generally manually entered at the modality, and can be subject to many opportunities for incorrect or incomplete data entry. Further, the complete patient information may not be available—even to the HIS or RIS—at the point in time that the exam is performed. The IS systems typically continue, however, to be updated with additional patient information long after the exam is completed, and the images are transmitted. Integration of the PACS and RIS, then, must also be accomplished to facilitate corrections to the PACS archived information.

Another aspect of HIS/RIS integration is worthy of note: that of results management from the modality **to** the PACS. While this service seems to many people counterintuitive—"doesn't the RIS manage the text results?"—the purpose of this service is quite significant. During the course of the study being performed, additional text information is acquired by the modality at the same time as the image data: X-ray dose, contrast specifics, US quantitative values, etc. These data should, properly, be recorded in the

RIS, and ideally be available for the generation of radiology reports. In some areas, such as US Obstetrics, for example, it could be possible to generate much, if not all, of the radiology report itself from the text data available from the modality itself.

It would be accurate to state that complete HIS/RIS integration—including modality worklist, reading worklist, as well as results management—is the greatest current barrier to effective PACS remaining with the current generation of systems. Further, this is an arena demanding the highest level of cooperation between Physicists and IT, as it is rarely the case that IT groups have sufficient expertise in the modalities to succeed in this endeavor.

Some vendors, in fact, have recognized this fundamental barrier to PACS implementation to the extent that they have "bundled" RIS technology into their PACS products in an effort to apply Occam's Razor to the problem of HIS/RIS integration. It is our opinion, however, that such "embedded" RIS solutions have been generally inadequate to serve the other needs of a modern RIS—billing and report management among these. While coming generations of PACS/RIS combination systems may prove themselves, it is not clear at the present that there is an alternative to the complexities of establishing HIS/RIS interfaces with PACS. Fortunately, several vendors are now offering "middleware" (external systems to both the HIS, RIS, and PACS) solutions to facilitate this integration, and this technology is the basis for most current HIS/RIS integration. (Few current RIS speak DICOM, few current PACS speak HL7[4], but the "middleware" systems speak and understand both protocols.)

It is the author's opinion that *no* DICOM device (except printers) should be purchased that does not support HIS/RIS integration. Not only does HIS/RIS integration prove invaluable to functionality, it also demonstrated that a vendor actually is committed to using the DICOM standard. It, along with DICOM printing functionality, is a useful threshold test that measures whether a vendor is really interested in using DICOM, or only interested in having DICOM on their marketing literature.

Acquiring Copies of the Standard

The official source for the Standard documents is the National Electrical Manufactors Association:

       (703) 841-3200 (US)
       (703) 841-3300 (FAX)
or write:
       NEMA
       1300 North 17th Street
       Suite 1847
       Rosslyn, Virginia 22209

---

[4] HL7, Health Level 7, is a protocol for communication of patient text information used widely in RIS and HIS environments. http://www.hl7.org.

The official DICOM documentation itself is sold and distributed through Global Engineering Documents (Global) and Information Handling Services (HIS), in hardcopy, CD-ROM, and Internet access. For more information concerning documentation availability and pricing, please contact Global:

> (800) 854-7179 (within US)
> (303) 397-7956 (International)
> (303) 397-2740 (fax)

or write:

> Global Engineering Documents
> 15 Inverness Way East
> Englewood, Colorado 80112-5776

For individuals that do not require the formal Standard (typically those developing commercial software do so), but are simply interested in understanding it, the final drafts of the Standard are also available online at the NEMA site at no cost:

http://www.nema.org/nema/medical/dicom/

ftp://ftp.nema.org/MEDICAL/Dicom/

While these are not guaranteed to be identical to the information available from the official documents, these serve quite well for the purpose of understanding the Standard itself further.

Merge Technologies (a leading provider of DICOM software and professional services) maintains web site of valuable DICOM resources at:

http://www.merge.com

Learning More about DICOM

An excellent way to learn more about DICOM is by installing a test system and by experimenting with various DICOM configurations using public-domain DICOM and PACS tools. There are currently three principal implementations of DICOM in public domain; that of the Mallinckrodt Institute of Radiology (MIR) at Washington University, that of the University of California Davis Medical Center (UCDMC), and that of the University of Oldenburg. While these implementations differ in their basic software architectures, all serve equally as a means of establishing a DICOM workbench for experimenting with DICOM services and operability. Further, having a DICOM test system available is generally useful, and often required, when attempting to validate DICOM interoperability between commercial devices as it provides an "objective" reference model to define vendor-specific variances in DICOM implementation. As all of the reference implementation packages discussed here can be implemented on low-cost hardware platforms (Intel-based PCs and Sun Microsystems workstations, for example), maintaining a DICOM workbench can often serve as an essential, and affordable, tool for resolving interoperability problems. At present, the Mallinckrodt implementation is by far the best supported of these three toolkits. These packages can be obtained via anonymous ftp at:

http://www.erl.wustl.edu/ftpserve.html
(Mallinckrodt Institute of Radiology (MIR) CTN)

This is the premier DICOM workbench, funded by the Radiological Society of North America and Washington University. This system serves as the Central Test Node (CTN) for the annual Radiological Society of North America (RSNA) DICOM test environment, which now involves dozens of commercial vendors inter-operating at the RSNA. The MIR CTN is considered the "gold standard" for testing DICOM interoperability. As this system is in public domain, many commercial vendors have used this as the basis for their own PACS implementations. It is not uncommon to see CTN-derived PACS components as part of commercial systems.

http://www.erl.wustl.edu/ftpserve.html
(Univ. of Oldenburg)

This is a variation of the MIR toolkit, which has evolved as the basis for European variations from the CTN. One aspect that this package supports particularly well is Modality Worklist—it was the basis for the CAR demonstration of Worklist in 1996.) The CAR'96 DICOM demonstration featured Modality Worklist Management and Image Storage/Query/Retrieval. The available software includes source code and documentation for the worklist management and image storage/query/retrieve server applications, a number of test applications, and all the necessary libraries.

http://imrad.ucdmc.ucdavis.edu/pub
(Univ. of California)

The UCDMC contributions are more a collection of separate projects than a single comprehensive toolkit, and represent the efforts of the UCDMC PACS Laboratory supported by funding from Siemens Medical Systems. Components of the UCDMC toolkit are a DICOM class library written in C++, a small PACS (microPACS) running under Windows NT, a DICOM query-based viewer for Windows '95/'98 and NT (NewView), and a DICOM diagnostic tool (Sleuth). As with the CTN, a number of commercial systems use the UCDMC libraries for their DICOM messaging and printing services, as well as some academic implementations. (Michigan State University).

http://www.efilm.net
(Toronto Hospital)

While not a complete DICOM workbench implementation, the E-Film package from the Toronto Hospital is an exceptionally promising package that—we feel—should be on every physicist's computer. E-Film provides a basic Storage SCP and Query SCU, as well as a fairly robust DICOM viewer. While still in early development—version 1.0 was distributed at RSNA 1998—this will likely be a very effective tool for helping physicists acquire and view DICOM objects from modalities. E-film uses the UCDMC DICOM libraries for its DIMSE services, which has been validated against many of the major DICOM implementations.

Summary

The DICOM Standard is daunting and complex, yet it is the **only** feasible means that we have for building large-scale PACS. The simplicity of "homogeneous" (single-vendor, PACS, and modality) solutions neither scales to large enterprises, nor reflects the current reality of the competitive marketplace for imaging systems. Therefore, we—collectively—must master the DICOM standard as a means to integrate imaging systems with the larger scope of healthcare automation, as well as an essential enabling technology for PACS itself.

Developing expertise in this arena is perhaps intimidating, particularly for individuals not familiar with the object-oriented abstractions that DICOM is based upon. However, tools exist—increasingly—to assist with this process. Experimenting with these tools is an effective (and low-cost) means to develop familiarity with DICOM. Further, reading and analyzing vendor conformance statements for **all** potential purchases is critical—as medical physicists are generally the leaders in developing specifications for new medical imaging systems, as well as those responsible for acceptance testing such systems, it is important that you evaluate DICOM conformance for all such systems. Simply including DICOM testing as part of the acceptance testing process is not sufficient—evaluation of DICOM vendor conformance prior to purchase is essential to the success of a PACS implementation. Even if you are not currently considering a PACS, it most likely that you will be within the lifecycle of any imaging modality you may be purchasing now, therefore it is prudent for us to consider this as a component of all new modality purchases.

Supplements—By Number

Source: David Clunie: http://idt.net/~dclunie/dicom_status/status.html

Supplement	Affected	Title	Status
Supp 1	Part 10	Media Storage and File Format For Media Interchange	Standard
Supp 2	Part 11	Media Storage Application Profiles	Standard
Supp 3	Part 12	Media Format and Physical Media Media Interchange	Standard
Supp 4	Parts 3,4,6	X-Ray Angiographic Image Objects and Media Storage	Standard
Supp 5	Parts 3,4,5,6,11	Ultrasound Application Profile, IOD and Transfer Syntax Extension	Standard
Supp 6	Parts 3,4,6	X-Ray Flouroscopic Image Object	Standard
Supp 7	Parts 3,4,6	Nuclear Medicine Image Object	Standard
Supp 8	Parts 3,4,6	Storage Commitment Service Class	Standard
Supp 9	Parts 2,3,4,5,6	Multi-byte Character Set Support	Standard
Supp 10	Parts 3,4,6	Basic Worklist Management— Modality	Standard
Supp 11	Parts 3,4,6	Radiotherapy Information Objects	Standard
Supp 12	Parts 3,4,6	PET Information Object	Standard
Supp 13	Parts 3,4,6	Queue Management Service Class	Standard
Supp 14	Parts 2,5	Standard Extended SOP Classes and Unknown Value Representation	Standard
Supp 15	Parts 3,4,6	Visible Light Image Object	Work
Supp 16	Parts 3,4,6	Postscript Print Management	Cancelled
Supp 17	Parts 3,4,6	Modality Performed Procedure Step	Standard

Supp 18	Part 11	Media Storage Application Profile for CT and MR Images	Standard
Supp 19	Part 11	General Purpose CD-R Image Interchange Profile	Standard
Supp 20	Part 11	X-Ray Cardiac (1024) Media Application Profile	Standard
Supp 21	Part 11	Nuclear Medicine Media Application Profile	Cancelled
Supp 22	Parts 3,4,6	Presentation LUT	Standard
Supp 23	Parts 3,4,6	Structured Reporting Object	Frozen
Supp 24	Parts 3,4,6	Stored Print	Standard
Supp 25	Part 11	New Ultrasound MOD	Standard
Supp 26	Parts 3,4,6	Ultrasound Structured Interpretation	Draft
Supp 27	Part 12	New 90mm and 130mm MOD Formats	Standard
Supp 28	Part 14	Grayscale Standard Display Function	Standard
Supp 29	Parts 3,4,6	Radiotherapy Treatment Record and Media Extensions	Ballot
Supp 30	Parts 3,6,7,11	Waveform Interchange	Comment
Supp 31	Parts 3,6,7,8	Security Enhancements	Draft
Supp 32	Parts 3,4,6	Digital X-Ray	Standard
Supp 33	Parts 3,4,6	Softcopy Presentation State	Frozen Draft
Supp 34	Parts 3,4,6	Stored Print of Non-Preformatted Images	Cancelled
Supp 35	Parts 3,4,6	Retirement of Referenced Print	Ballot
Supp 36	Parts 3,4,6	Codes and Controlled Terminology	Standard
Supp 37	Parts 3,4,6	Printer Configuration Retrieval	Standard
Supp 38	Parts 3,4,6	New Print Image Overlay Box	Ballot
Supp 39	Parts 3,4,10	Stored Print Media Storage	Standard
Supp 40	Parts 11,12	UDF Media	Comment

Supp 41	Parts 2,5,6,15	Security Enhancements 2 – Digital Signatures	Work
Supp 42	Parts 5,6	MPEG Transfer Syntaxes and Encoding	Work
Supp 43	Parts 3,4,6,10	3D Ultraound objects	Work
Supp 44	Parts 1,9,13	Retirement of Part 9,13 and OSI	Work
Supp 45	Parts 3,6	Ultrasound Protocol Support	Work
Supp 46	Parts 3,4,6	Basic Structured Reporting SOP Classes	Work
Supp ?	Part 11	Dynamic Cardio Review Media Application Profile	Draft (Clinical Study)

Correction Proposals—By Number

Correction	Affected	Title	Status
CP 1-13	Part ?	Various errata and typos	Cancelled
CP 14	Part 5	Encoding of Uncompressed Pixel Data **** NB. Critical Change	Standard
CP 15	Part 3	LUT Data Encoding and Rescale Type	Standard
CP 16	Part 3	Sorter Bin Attribute for Basic Film Session	Standard
CP 17	Part 4	Conformance Statement SOP Class Attributes and Values	Standard
CP 18	Part 3	Open issues for CR IOD	Cancelled
CP 19	Part 4	Image Deletion in Film Session	Standard
CP 20	Part 3	Clarification of Pixel Aspect Ratio	Standard
CP 21	Part 3	Same Attribute in Multiple Modules	Standard
CP 22	Part 3	Units for Frame Time and Vector	Standard
CP 23	Part 3	Numbering of Pixel Origin	Standard

CP 24	Part 5	Correct Definition in Table for VR=SQ	Standard
CP 25	Part 3	Frame of Reference— CT/MR Localizer	Standard
CP 26	Part 2	Standard Extended SOP Classes Adding Required Attributes	Standard
CP 27	Part 3	Patient Orientation "will" to "shall"	Standard
CP 28	Part 7	C-ECHO Message Protocol Description	Standard
CP 29	Part 5	JPEG Transfer Syntax UID Wrong	Standard
CP 30	Part 7	Behaviour of Synchronous/ Asynchronous Operation	Standard
CP 31	Part 5	Explicit VR in Compressed Pixel Data Examples	Standard
CP 32	Part 5	Definition of Enumerated Values	Standard
CP 33	Parts 3,4,7	UID Typo—No Trailing Periods	Standard
CP 34	Part 3	SC and General Equipment/ Image Modules	Standard
CP 35	Part 7	N-CREATE and Empty Data Sets	Standard
CP 36	Part 4	Type 3 Attributes for Patient Events	Standard
CP 37	Part 4	N-CREATE of VOI LUT Box SOP Instance	Standard
CP 38	Part 5	Byte Order of Attribute Tag VR	Standard
CP 39	Part ?	Clarification of Optical Density Units for LUTs	Cancelled
CP 40	Part ?	Correct Scheduled Study Location for multiple locations	Inactive
CP 41	Part ?	Correct the relationship between Results and Studies	Inactive
CP 42	Part ?	Correct the relationship between Results and Studies	Inactive

CP 43	Part 3	Double Occurrence of LUT Number in Module	Standard
CP 44	Part 3	Multiplicity of Sequence Items, Part A (see also CP 83)	Standard
CP 45	Part 5	Clarification on encoding of Type 2 sequence elements	Cancelled
CP 46	Part 3	Wrong Tag for Study Component Sequence	Standard
CP 47	Part 5	Private Creator Required Within Sequences	Standard
CP 48	Part 8	Correct Misnamed Table and Reference	Standard
CP 49	Parts 4,7	Attribute Out of Range Warning Status	Standard
CP 50	Part ?	Correct encoding of designation of character sets	Cancelled
CP 51	Part 3	Include Curves in CR IODs	Standard
CP 52	Part 3	Wrong Attribute Placement in Visit Admission Module	Standard
CP 53	Parts 3,6	Double Entry of Referenced Image Box Sequence Tag	Standard
CP 54	Part 5	Unclear example for AT encoding	Standard
CP 55	Part 3	Pixel Aspect Ratio Example	Standard
CP 56	Part 4	Pixel Aspect Ratio Use Conditional	Standard
CP 57	Part 3	Units of Image Position Co-ordinates are mm.	Standard
CP 58	Part 3	Incorrect Module Names	Standard
CP 59	Parts 3,6	Attribute Names Used Twice (by Overlay Plane Module)	Standard
CP 60	Part 6	Audio Comments Type Specification	Standard
CP 61	Part 4	C-DIMSE Status Codes Clarified	Standard

CP 62	Part ?	Value Representation for Interpretation Text is too short	Cancelled
CP 63	Part 3	Rescale Attributes for MR IOD	Assigned
CP 64	Part 3	Application of Modality LUTs	Assigned
CP 65	Part 3	Add Attribute Pixel Transformation	Cancelled
CP 66	Part 3	Imager Pixel Spacing Attribute added to CR Image Module as Type 3	Standard
CP 67	Part 4	Exceptions to the character repertoire for matching	Standard
CP 68	Supp 9	Forbid Backslash in Person Names	Standard
CP 69	Part 5	Planar Configuration in US Supplement	Standard
CP 70	Part 3	Axis Units CMS2 listed twice with different definitions	Standard
CP 71	Parts 4,6	Modality at the study level	Standard
CP 72	Parts 3,4,6	Optional Worklist Matching Key	Standard
CP 73	Part 3	Need to identify head of patient for RF IOD	Cancelled
CP 74	Parts 4,6	Add number of series related images in Series level keys	Standard
CP 75			Not Used
CP 76	Parts 3,4	Make link from study to study component optional	Standard
CP 77	Part 6	Wrong VR for exposure parameters	Standard
CP 78	Parts 3,6	Attribute for Pixel Transformation (duplicates CP 65 ?)	Cancelled
CP 79	Part 5	JPEG Multiframe Encoding	Standard
CP 80	Part 4	Print Management Clarifications	Standard

CP 81	Part 4	Print Management Clarifications—Negotiate Print Job/Printer SOP Class alone	Standard
CP 82	Part 2	Relax requirement for documenting private attributes	Cancelled
CP 83	Part 3	Multiplicity of Sequence Items, Part B (see also CP 44)	Inactive
CP 84	Part 7	Asynchronous Operations Clarification	Cancelled
CP 85	Parts 3,4,6	Basic Print and Overlays	Cancelled
CP 86	Part 3	Documentation of Repeating Sequences, Attribute Macros	Standard
CP 87	Part 3	Overlay Bits Allocated	Standard
CP 88	Part 3	Overlay Pixel Aspect Ratio	Work
CP 89	Part 3	Overlay Origin Clarification	Standard
CP 90	Part 3	Retire Overlay LUTs	Standard
CP 91	Part 3	Printing Overlays with Different Magnification than the Image	Cancelled
CP 92	Part 4	Storing Overlay Data for Printing	Cancelled
CP 93	Part 4	Storing N-SET of Overlay Sequence in Image Boxes	Cancelled
CP 94	Part 4	Attribute usage when N-SET Attributes same as N-CREATE	Standard
CP 95	Part 3	Define SOP Instance UID same/different criteria	Cancelled
CP 96	Part 3	duplicate of CP 66	Cancelled
CP 97	Part 3	LUT Value Ranges	Work
CP 98	Part 4	Make link from Study to Visit Optional	Cancelled
CP 99	Parts 3,4,6	Extended Query Retrieve Model	Standard
CP 100	Part 4	Printable Matrix Sizes	Assigned
CP 101	Parts 3,5,6	Standard Text VR too short for Information Systems	Cancelled

CP 102	Part 3	Correct condition on Pixel Component Organization	Standard
CP 103	Part 6	Administration Route Code Sequence	Standard
CP 104	Part 3	Typo in File-set Consistency Flag	Standard
CP 105	Part 5	Odd String Attribute Padding	Standard
CP 106	Part 2	Clarify Media Conformance Requirements	Standard
CP 107	Parts 3,5	Add Support for UNICODE Character Set	Inactive
CP 108	Parts 3,4	Requested Image Size Description	Standard
CP 109	Part 4	Fix Film Box N-ACTION	Standard
CP 110	Part 4	Update Conformance Statement to improve annotation description	Work
CP 111	Part 5	Sequence example has wrong table heading	Standard
CP 112	Part 3	Display Shutter for non-1:1 aspect ratio images is unclear	Standard
CP 113	Part 4	Correct example for Scheduled procedure Step Start Time (range matching)	Standard
CP 114	Part 10	Modify Title for Annex A (Normative to Informative)	Standard
CP 115	Part 5	Clarify the Date Time (DT) VR for Years	Standard
CP 116	Part 4	Correct Tag Value for Scheduled Procedure Step Description	Standard
CP 117	Part 8	Correct Field Name for Table 9-23	Cancelled
CP 118	Parts 3,11	Need Frame in Referenced Image Sequence	Standard
CP 119	Part 5	Clarify limit on private Repeating Groups	Standard

CP 120	Part 5	Clarify Padding for Multiframe Encapsulated Pixel Data	Standard Standard
CP 121	Parts 3,4,6	Retire Biplane XA SOP Class	Standard
CP 122	Part 5	Unlimited Text VR	Standard
CP 123	Part 5	Clarification of Unknown VR Byte Order Issues	Work
CP 124	Part 5	Misleading wording regarding data element tags	Work
CP 125	Part 3	Value for Frame Time for Single frame Multi-frame images	Work
CP 126	Parts 4,6	Consistency of Error Codes	Work
CP 127	Part 4	Flexible Print Formatting, Annotation and Layout	Standard
CP 128	Part 7	Status Code Conventions	Work
CP 129	Part 5	Clarification by Correction of Tables	Work
CP 130	Part 4	Specify Date/Time Matching for Query/Retrieve	Work
CP 131	Part 3	Timezone Specification in SOP Common	Work
CP 132	Part 3	Type Definition of Duplicate Attributes	Work
CP 133	Parts 3,6	Add support for associating contours in Bifurcated RT Structures	Work
CP 134	Part 3	Add Instance Number to DICOm RT Objects	Work
CP 135	Parts 3,6	Add Compensator Type to RT Plan Object	Work
CP 136	Part 5	Creation of OL Value Representation	Comment
CP 137	Part 3	Clarification of Image Position Definition	Ballot

CP 138	Part 3	Add Procedure Code Sequence and Action Item Code Sequence to Image IODs	Ballot
CP 139	Part 3	Specify Photometric Interpretation for CR IOD	Ballot
CP 140	Part 3	Remove redundant sequence item encoding descriptions	Ballot
CP 141	Part 4	Additional types to exclude from wildcard matching	Ballot
CP 142	Part 3	Incorrect value range for IS, SL and SS	Ballot
CP 143	Parts 3,5,6	Palette Color LUT Clarifications	Work
CP 144	Part 5	Audio Sample Data VR Clarification	Ballot
CP 145	Parts 5,6	Curve Data VR Clarification	Work
CP 146	Part 4	Clarification of Query Retrieve	Mar 99 VP
CP 147	Parts 3,5	Multi-byte Character Set Clarification	Ballot
CP 148	Part 3	Interpretation Status ID Clarification	Ballot
CP 150	Part 3	16 Bit Palette Color Encoding Clarification	Cancelled—See CP 143
CP 151	Part 3	Anatomic Region Sequence Modifier nesting in Intra-oral Image	Ballot
CP 152	Parts 3,5	Clarification of Type 2 Intention	Work
CP 153	Part 4	N-Event-report and association management in Storage Commitment	Mar 99 VP
CP 155	Parts 3,5	Add support for ISO IR 149 Korean Character Sets	Mar 99 VP
CP 156	Part 5	Clarify Image Pixel Attributes for Compressed Transfer Syntaxes	Work

CP 157	Part 3	Correct Typos in US Image Module	Mar 99 VP
CP 158	Part 4	Print Image Collision Status Clarification	Mar 99 VP
CP 159	Part 4	New Therapy Description Text Attribute	Work
CP 160	Part 6	Correct VR of Performed Procedure Step ID to SH	Mar 99 VP
CP 161	Part 3	Miscellaneous Corrections on Models	Mar 99 VP
CP 162	Part 5	Scope of UID Uniqueness	Mar 99 VP
CP 163	Parts 3,4,6	Support of HL7 Placer/Filler Order Numbers	Mar 99 VP
CP 164	Parts 3,4,6	Correct Tag for Maximum Memory Allocation	Mar 99 VP
CP 165	Part 5	Icon Image Sequence for Composite Image IODs	Work

Diagnostics and Acceptance Testing for DICOM Networks

Experiences at the University of California, Davis Medical Center

Mark Oskin, J. Anthony Seibert, Richard L. Kennedy
Department of Radiology
University of California Davis
UC Davis Medical Center
Sacramento, California 95817

Abstract

The University of California Davis Medical Center (UCDMC) is in the process of implementing a Picture Archiving and Communication System (PACS) for archival storage and primary diagnostic reading within the Radiology department. This is being implemented as a first step toward an enterprise-wide PACS designed for all primary and specialty care departments and affiliates. In the process of implementing clinical imaging networks and acceptance testing vendor "DICOM compatible" equipment, several tools and methods where developed. These tools were developed due to the multi-vendor environment that exists on the UCDMC campus. This multi-vendor environment created an often contentious and charged environment in which a vendor's "DICOM compatible" device was forced to interoperate. Along the way, it became apparent that the *norm* is for "DICOM compatible" devices from different vendors to *not* communicate. Thus, UCDMC developed tools to analyze supposedly "DICOM compatible" transmissions and often played the role of prosecutor, defense, judge, and jury in multi-vendor inter-networking disputes. This paper presents a summary of the incompatibility issues involved, the reason for their existence, how they where discovered, and ultimately resolved. Furthermore, we present a tool for DICOM diagnostic work and, finally, discuss acceptance testing of DICOM image networking equipment.

Introduction

The Digital Imaging and Communications in Medicine (DICOM) standard traces its history back to the early 1980's as a joint effort between the American College of Radiology (ACR) and the National Electronic Manufacturers Association (NEMA). The preceding document to the DICOM standard was termed the ACR-NEMA v2 transmission protocol. The prior ACR-NEMA v2 standard described a point-to-point transmission protocol operating over a dedicated 50-pin hardware interface bus. Furthermore, a tagged data format was described with a standard set of tags for commonly used image attributes. Finally, a simple set of semantics was introduced that allowed

317

for the storage and retrieval of images across the dedicated point-to-point transmission bus.

The DICOM standard is a direct evolution from this original transmission protocol. In many respects the DICOM standard, sometimes referred to as DICOM v3 to indicate it as being derived from the old ACR-NEMA v2 standard resembles the old point-to-point transmission protocol. However, the new standard benefits from both hindsight and technological advancement.

Perhaps the single most important technical change is the addition of underlying protocol semantics for communication over generalized TCP/IP networks. However, broadly significant was the general expansion of the scope of the standard. The standard extended the scope of medical imaging that it attempted to cover. First, Hospital Information System and Radiology Information System (HIS/RIS) interfacing was introduced. Hard-copy film output device semantics were constructed. A new object-based approach to attribute structure was created and this in turn enabled the extension of the standard into all forms of medical imaging modalities. Finally, the standard took on a more formal and accepted form of presentation by following ANSI/IEEE Standard 830-1984 guidelines.

Above all of these enhancements, however, perhaps the single most important addition was the formalizing of what it meant to be "DICOM conformant." The concept of DICOM Conformance was formally introduced, and any vendor claiming DICOM conformance was *required* to provide a document (the Conformance Statement), that described the particular subsections of the standard to which the vendor's device was claiming DICOM conformance. However, the standard did not formalize a testing body, or a method to *prove* a device claiming DICOM conformance actually is conformant.

Therein lies the rub. It is impossible to measure this directly, but perhaps less than a quarter of the medical imaging devices sold today as being "DICOM conformant" actually are. The remainder exist in some hazy world somewhere between "DICOM compatible" and flat out vaporware.

DICOM Conformant vs. "DICOM Compatible"

In this paper we introduce a distinction between being DICOM conformant and DICOM compatible. It is *very* important that these two terms not be confused. In this section we introduce a definition for these two terms and how they interrelate.

> **DICOM conformant**: any device is DICOM conforming if it conforms exactly, to those sections of the DICOM standard the device claims it conforms to within its conformance statement.

DICOM compatible: any device is DICOM compatible if it claims conformance within its conformance statement to various sections of the DICOM standard but despite such claims exhibits behavior in direct contradiction to any subsection of the DICOM standard it claims conformance to.

Some observations about these definitions: First, they are mutually exclusive: a device claiming DICOM conformance is either conformant or compatible. Second, they are inclusive of the entire "DICOM conformance claiming" space, i.e., any device claiming DICOM conformance is either conformant or compatible, no third possibility exists. Finally, the following observations are made:

1. Two DICOM conformant devices that should communicate will communicate.

2. A DICOM compatible device that should communicate with a DICOM conformant device may or may not communicate.

3. Two DICOM compatible devices that should communicate may or may not communicate.

This situation is illustrated in Figure 1. Each sphere represents a device and the space of other devices with which it successfully communicates. Globally, the entire illustration depicts the situation of devices that should communicate, i.e., a device that provides storage of one type of DICOM object as a Service Class User (SCU) and a device that only provides storage for a different type of DICOM object such as a Service Class Provider (SCP) are not illustrated. Hence, all devices depicted in Figure 1 are expected to communicate with each other.

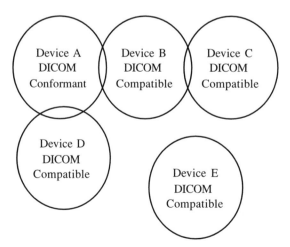

Figure 1

As illustrated, there exists only a single DICOM conformant device. This is an abstract notion since clearly two devices can be DICOM conformant, but not communicate. This situation arises if the two devices where not *meant* to communicate since they do not implement complementary service classes. However, the situation depicted in Figure 1 is supposed to depict devices that *should* communicate; hence, only a single DICOM conformant device is drawn. We denote this device as device A.

However, several DICOM compatible devices are illustrated. As noted, some of these devices, such as device B, successfully communicate with the DICOM conformant A device; however, other devices such as device E are wholly incompatible and fail to communicate with a DICOM conforming device. Furthermore, some DICOM compatible devices, such as device C, can communicate with other DICOM compatible devices such as device B, but not directly with the DICOM conformant device A.

Purchasing of DICOM Devices

Clearly, to ensure communication between two devices, the surest route is to make certain they are both DICOM conformant. However, empirically, UCDMC has found this is rarely the case. It is far more common to find DICOM compatible devices than DICOM conformant ones. Successfully navigating the sea of DICOM compatible devices out there is a challenging process, and we have observed two purchasing methods.

1. **Closed-set model:** The closed set-model of purchasing is this: To have *n* devices that successfully communicate with each other, purchase the first device. Next, purchase the second device requiring that whether or not the first device is DICOM conformant, the second device must communicate with it. Next, purchase the third device requiring that whether or not the first and second device are DICOM conformant, the third device must communicate with the first and second devices. Carry this method out to *n* devices and inductively all *n* devices will successfully communicate with each other.

2. **DICOM conformant-limit model:** The DICOM conformant-limit model is this: To have *n* devices successfully communicate with each other, for each device: do not permit the device to pass acceptance testing until it has been demonstrated with reasonable confidence that the device is DICOM conformant. Then, assuming all *n* devices are DICOM conformant, they should communicate.

Most reasonable buying strategies can be related to one or a mixture of both of these two purchasing models. For instance, the single-vendor buying model most closely resembles the closed-set purchasing model. The multi-vendor open-standards approach to purchasing most closely resembles the DICOM conformant-limit model.

The closed-set purchasing model may seem unattractive at first glance from an open-systems perspective; however, it has an attractive property that the DICOM conformant-limit model lacks. That is, the closed-set purchasing model can be proved to create a set of devices that will successfully communicate. Hence, if success is measured in actually being able to communicate, and not in matching an open-standard of communication, then the closed-set purchasing model is assured to create success.

The DICOM conformant-limit model on the other hand is not. If we assume that it is impossible to prove a device is DICOM conformant beyond *any* doubt, then it is impossible to prove that the DICOM conformant-limit purchasing model will create a set of communicating devices. In fact, the DICOM conformant-limit model cannot even create a set of two communicating devices. This is why it is called the conformant-limit model, because one trys to prove a device is conformant, but doing so is a limiting process where one can only approach the limit of being completely conformant.

On the other hand, the closed-set model has serious down-sides which are not evident from the theory alone. The closed-set model of purchasing assures that equipment will eventually become obsolete, and no vendor, at least at a reasonable cost, will provide equipment that will successfully communicate with your closed-set of communicating devices. A real-world example of this is the number of radiotherapy treatment planning systems that interfaced to the reel-to-reel archive tape generated by the GE Highspeed advantage CT scanner. When GE switched over to the newer product line that archived to magneto-optical media, no backward compatibility with the reel-to-reel tape was provided. Radiology departments that upgraded to the newer CT scanner found themselves unable to provide connectivity to legacy treatment planning systems. Thus departments were faced with a costly choice: stick to the older CT technology, upgrade the legacy treatment planning system, or purchase a costly custom software interface solution.

One might think that the two models can always be mixed to assure success, but this too does not work. Suppose you mix the two models, requiring that devices be both DICOM conformant and will communicate with your existing set of devices. To use a real-world example, a certain workstation installed at UCDMC would issue C-Find requests that were invalid. The device is installed under the assumption that it was DICOM conformant, but then later found to be compatible after acceptance testing is complete. The C-Find request that it issues was largely conformant, with only a slight error in the encoding of the search parameters (in this instance, the search was using a '*' character for a wild-card search on a Unique IDentifier (UID) type attribute, which is illegal). Most DICOM devices were fairly forgiving of this error, but a true DICOM-conformant device should refuse to process the query, and just such a device was later installed at UCDMC (in this case it was a CT scanner). In this instance, the customer is left in a difficult position. The second device is correct in refusing to accept the query. On the other hand, you have already acceptance tested and paid for the workstation device which is found to be in error. The vendor who wrote the workstation does not care to fix the problem since you have paid for everything, and it is an uphill battle with the vendor of the CT scanner to convince him to make its software intentionally non-conformant in order to communicate with your nonconformant workstation.

Thus, it would appear that no solution exists, that it is impossible to purchase a set of n devices that will communicate and will follow an open-standard. Unfortunately, this is true in theory and in practice. But, in general, despite the mixture of these two purchasing models being unable to assure success, it has been UCDMC's practice to pursue the mixed approach to purchasing. Therefore, when implementing a real-world PACS we are left with an unfortunate choice:

1. Purchase a DICOM compatible device, and do not permit the device to pass acceptance testing until it is proved DICOM conformant.

or

2. Purchase a DICOM compatible device, and do permit the device to pass acceptance testing once successful, reliable communication is achieved with all existing devices at the institution.

It has been a practice of UCDMC to formulate as part of acceptance testing both the successful installation of the device, and successful proof that a device is DICOM conformant. Our practice has been to make the finding of DICOM conformance a component of the acceptance testing phase of the equipment. Hence, a partial payment is usually made to the vendor upon delivery of the equipment, without respect to DICOM conformance. Full payment should be withheld until conformance is demonstrated.

The first step in ensuring DICOM conformance is to have in writing as part of any purchasing contract that a device shall be DICOM conformant as a mandatory condition for payment. In general, at our institution the full payment for a device is split into two or more components. The first installment of this payment is usually sent to the vendor upon delivery of the equipment. The second installment, comprising the remainder of the payment, is sent upon successful completion of acceptance testing of the device.

I do not recommend this practice. In general, vendors recover the true cost or more of the goods upon payment of the delivery component. After payment of this first component they have been less than forthcoming in fixing any DICOM nonconformance issues found. Unfortunately a substantial amount of leverage is lost by the customer as soon as that first payment is sent to the vendor, and here at UCDMC venders have demonstrated an unusual amount of laxness in trying to fix incompatibilities in order to receive the balance of payment.

To save you a substantial amount of time going "toe to toe" with a vendor over particular DICOM incompatibilities, I suggest not sending any payment until a device is demonstrated to be effectively communicating with all existing DICOM devices at the site. Then, reserve the balance of payment for when a device can be demonstrated to be fully DICOM conformant. To do this I suggest that all purchasing contracts contain specific language mandating that all devices be not only fully DICOM conformant, but also must communicate with all existing DICOM conformant and compatible devices at the institution. List, in writing, all existing devices with which the new device must successfully communicate. Put this list in the contract.

Acceptance Testing DICOM Devices

Although the most desirable choice for purchasing DICOM devices is (1) above, the purchase of DICOM conformant devices, acceptance testing devices to demonstrate they are DICOM conformant is a complicated issue. A number of practical challenges exist in doing so, namely:

a. How do you go about proving a device is DICOM conformant, when the device may claim conformance to several hundred pages of the DICOM standard?

b. How do you bring together the required resources in terms of acceptance testing equipment and individuals knowledgeable enough to perform the acceptance testing in a timely and cost-effective manner?

c. If a device is found to not be DICOM conformant, how do you convince the vendor to implement any required changes to bring the device into conformance in a timely fashion?

d. What if DICOM compatible devices are already existing on-site, and although they were previously acceptance tested, during subsequent testing of a new DICOM device you find nonconformant behavior from an existing device?

To purchase only DICOM conformant devices, a method must exist to demonstrate that a device is in fact conformant. This is no trivial task. Fortunately, three software tools are available to make this task tractable.

- **ADVT (Agfa DICOM Validation Tool)**: This tool, written by the Agfa Corporation is invaluable in discovering minute DICOM incompatibilities. There are only two major drawbacks to this tool:

  –The first is that the tool originates from a commercial vendor. This would not be an issue, except it makes it more difficult to use the results to convince any commercial vendor except Agfa that they should change their products based upon what the ADVT indicates. However, in my experience the ADVT has been correct, every time, and I strongly recommend you use it for your own acceptance testing. To overcome the commercial vendor issue, you must become familiar with the DICOM standard and before approaching a vendor about a potential DICOM nonconformance issue, fully research what information the ADVT tells you and then approach the vendor with specific sections from the DICOM standard they are not following, not just the results of the ADVT.

–The second problem with the ADVT is that to use it you must be very familiar with the internal workings of the DICOM standard. The ADVT was constructed for use by programmers, not individuals performing acceptance testing. Despite the primitive interface, it is well worth your time to investigate this tool and *use it* in your acceptance testing procedures. A healthy understanding of the DICOM standards inner workings is helpful anyway in order to deal with day-to-day DICOM communication issues. (http://medical.agfa.com/dicom.html)

• **DICOM-check**: This tool, developed by WDS Technologies is invaluable in acceptance testing. Free copies were distributed at the annual meeting of the Radiological Society of North America (RSNA) under the name "Pap-check," in 1996. The tool will load a "DICOM file" from a number of different, widely accepted formats, and will verify the attributes within the file match the requirements of the particular Information Object Definition (IOD) specified in Parts 3, 5, and 6 of the DICOM standard. This tool is most useful in verifying that a modality is generating acceptable images for an enterprise PACS. (http://www.wds.ch)

• **DICOM Sleuth**: Developed at UCDMC, the Sleuth was developed primarily as a diagnostic tool for DICOM network transmissions. The Sleuth is a passive network device that "listens" to the local-area network and reconstructs successful or failed DICOM transmissions. The Sleuth was designed to trouble-shoot installation of DICOM devices. Most PACS workstation, archive, and modality devices provide virtually useless feedback if a DICOM transmission fails. The Sleuth provides a detailed transmission dump that can be used to trace DICOM failures back to particular device failures. Another benefit the Sleuth provides is that DICOM transmissions can be observed, and the image components of a storage request can be saved to disk. This is useful for providing data for the DICOM-check tool mentioned above. The next section of this paper demonstrates various DICOM communication errors that were isolated using the Sleuth.
(http://imrad.ucdmc.ucdavis.edu/pub/sleuth)

These three software packages provide a reasonable collection of tools that should be in every hospitals toolkit. Acceptance testing of DICOM devices can then proceed as follows:

First, install the device for clinical functioning. This is not a trivial matter. Successfully getting two DICOM compatible devices to communicate can be a nerve-racking ordeal. If the vendor's on-site support cannot resolve any particular DICOM connection issue, you should first install and run the Sleuth on the transmission. The Sleuth, once installed, tends to quickly pinpoint configuration errors.

Unfortunately, this phase of the installation and acceptance testing process can be quite long. Here at UCDMC, particularly troublesome installations have taken well over a year and counting, between delivery of a PACS device and successful acceptance of the networking components.

Assuming the device is successfully installed, it is tempting to sign-off on the device as being installed; however, it is important to not do so. At this point the ADVT tool should be executed against the new device.

After a thorough investigation by the ADVT, if the device is a modality such as a CT or MR scanner, then a raw DICOM image should be acquired from the device. This can be done with the Sleuth, or with any number of free DICOM storage SCPs available. This captured DICOM image should be read into the DICOM-check tool. DICOM-check is quite thorough, and you should investigate any errors it reports. If they are valid concerns, you should force the vendor to fix them *before* final payment is made.

Diagnosing Installation Problems for DICOM Devices

Most device installations (including those at UCMDC) perform the installation and configuration of DICOM devices before acceptance testing. Although this is perhaps not the best choice technically, pressures are usually placed on the technical staff to obtain successful communication right away, and then worry about acceptance testing only if it fails. This is not the correct way to install a complicated software component, but it the most often used approach.

If the device is installed, configured, and it worked perfectly on the first try, then count yourself among the very lucky few. When an installation goes astray, we have generally found that vendors are usually helpless to explain why and generally look for someone to blame rather than for a solution. There are really two reasons for this. The first is that diagnostic error codes and messages from devices are usually useless. Reporting a message similar to "Error in transmission" on a failed transmission is just about useless, but messages like it are the most common form of feedback we see from DICOM devices when they fail. For this reason, we highly recommend the use of DICOMSleuth when installing DICOM devices. It is to be hoped that as vendors gain more experience with installing DICOM devices, their programmers will provide more intelligent feedback to their installation support staff, in the form of more meaningful diagnostic messages.

DICOMSleuth is a major time-saver during DICOM device installations, and for this reason we will spend the next few pages discussing some actual DICOM installation problems, and how DICOMSleuth was used to resolve them. Each of these problems came up during real installations of vendor devices at UCDMC.

Successful Association

In this paper we will introduce how to diagnose DICOM network issues by first look-ing at a successful connection. This allows us to point out important things to look at, as well what the normal-case should look like. Here is a transcript from DICOMSleuth of a successful association creation, and activity using the DICOM Validation Service-Object Pair (SOP) class:

```
DICOMwhif  - A Network Analyzer for DICOM Image Transmissions
(C) 1999 U.C. Davis Medical Center    Dev. By: Mark Oskin
                       mhoskin@ucdavis.edu
 New TCP: x.x.x.x (4926) -> y.y.y.y (104)       (1)
Close TCP: x.x.x.x (4926) -> y.y.y.y (104)
------------>
[byte - 1] PDU Type      : 0x01 - AAssociate-RQ
[byte - 1] Reserved      : 0x00
[u32 - 4] PDU Length     : 199
[u16 - 2] ProtocolVersion : 0x0001 (0x0001=DICOM)
[byte - 2] Reserved      : 0x0000
[s  - 16] CalledApTitle  : 'MHO1       '        (2)
[s  - 16] CallingApTitle : 'test_node  '        (3)
[byte - 33] Reserved3     : (00, 00, 00, 00, 00, 00, ...)
 [byte - 1] Item Type     : 0x10 - Application Context
 [byte - 1] Reserved      : 0x00
 [u16 - 2] Length     : 21
 [byte - 21] AppContext    : '1.2.840.10008.3.1.1.1'
 [byte - 1] Item Type     : 0x20 - Presentation Context
 [byte - 1] Reserved      : 0x00
 [u16 - 2] Length     : 46
 [byte - 1] PCID         : 3 - 0x03        (4)
 [byte - 3] Reserved     : (00, 00, 00)
  [byte - 1] Item Type     : 0x30 - Abstract Syntax
  [byte - 1] Reserved      : 0x00
  [u16 - 2] Length     : 17
  [byte - 17] AbsSyntax    : '1.2.840.10008.1.1'     (5)
  [byte - 1] Item Type     : 0x40 - Transfer Syntax
  [byte - 1] Reserved      : 0x00
  [u16 - 2] Length     : 17
  [byte - 17] TrnSyntax    : '1.2.840.10008.1.2'     (6)
 [byte - 1] Item Type     : 0x50 - User Information
 [byte - 1] Reserved      : 0x00
 [u16 - 2] Length     : 52
  [byte - 1] Item Type     : 0x51 - Maximum Sub-Item
  [byte - 1] Reserved      : 0x00
  [u16 - 2] Length     : 4
  [byte - 1] MaxSub-item Lng : 16384 - 0x00004000
  [byte - 1] Item Type     : 0x52 - Implementation Class
```

```
  [byte - 1] Reserved      : 0x00
  [u16 - 2] Length         : 26
  [byte - 26] ImpClass     : 'UCDMC/gcc2.5.8/DECMIPS/MHO'
  [byte - 1] Item Type     : 0x55 - Implementation Version
  [byte - 1] Reserved      : 0x00
  [u16 - 2] Length         : 10
  [byte - 10] ImpVersion   : '0.1B/OTHER'
<------------
[byte - 1] PDU Type        : 0x02 - AAssociate-AC
[byte - 1] Reserved        : 0x00
[u32 - 4] PDU Length       : 178
[u16 - 2] ProtocolVersion  : 0x0001 (0x0001=DICOM)
[byte - 2] Reserved        : 0x0000
[s  - 16] CalledApTitle    : 'MHO1            '
[s  - 16] CallingApTitle   : 'test_node       '
[byte - 33] Reserved3      : (00, 00, 00, 00, 00, 00, ...)
 [byte - 1] Item Type      : 0x10 - Application Context
 [byte - 1] Reserved       : 0x00
 [u16 - 2] Length          : 21
 [byte - 21] AppContext    : '1.2.840.10008.3.1.1.1'
 [byte - 1] Item Type      : 0x21 - Presentation Context - In Accept
 [byte - 1] Reserved       : 0x00
 [u16 - 2] Length          : 25
 [byte - 1] PCID           : 3 - 0x03       (7)
 [byte - 3] Reserved       : 00
 [byte - 3] Result         : 00 - Acceptance
 [byte - 3] Reserved       : 00
  [byte - 1] Item Type     : 0x40 - Transfer Syntax
  [byte - 1] Reserved      : 0x00
  [u16 - 2] Length         : 17
  [byte - 17] TrnSyntax    : '1.2.840.10008.1.2'
 [byte - 1] Item Type      : 0x50 - User Information
 [byte - 1] Reserved       : 0x00
 [u16 - 2] Length          : 52
  [byte - 1] Item Type     : 0x51 - Maximum Sub-Item
  [byte - 1] Reserved      : 0x00
  [u16 - 2] Length         : 4
  [byte - 1] MaxSub-item Lng : 16384 - 0x00004000
  [byte - 1] Item Type     : 0x52 - Implementation Class
  [byte - 1] Reserved      : 0x00
  [u16 - 2] Length         : 26
  [byte - 26] ImpClass     : 'UCDMC/gcc2.5.8/DECMIPS/MHO'
  [byte - 1] Item Type     : 0x55 - Implementation Version
  [byte - 1] Reserved      : 0x00
  [u16 - 2] Length         : 10
  [byte - 10] ImpVersion   : '0.1B/WIN32'
------------>
[byte - 1] PDU Type        : 0x04 - P-DATA-TF
[byte - 1] Reserved        : 0x00
[u32 - 4] PDU Length       : 74
 [u32 - 4] PDV Length      : 70
 [byte - 1] PresContext ID : 3
```

```
    [byte - 1] Message Header : 03 - Command Set / Last
VR:(0000, 0000, 00000004h): 38 00 00 00
VR:(0000, 0002, 00000012h): 31 2e 32 2e 38 34 30 2e 31 30 30 30 38 2e
31 2e ...
VR:(0000, 0100, 00000002h): 30 00                    (8)
VR:(0000, 0110, 00000002h): 01 00
VR:(0000, 0800, 00000002h): 01 01
<------------
[byte - 1] PDU Type       : 0x04 - P-DATA-TF
[byte - 1] Reserved       : 0x00
[u32 - 4] PDU Length      : 84
 [u32 - 4] PDV Length     : 80
 [byte - 1] PresContext ID : 3
 [byte - 1] Message Header : 03 - Command Set / Last
VR:(0000, 0000, 00000004h): 42 00 00 00
VR:(0000, 0002, 00000012h): 31 2e 32 2e 38 34 30 2e 31 30 30 30 38 2e
31 2e ...
VR:(0000, 0100, 00000002h): 30 80                    (9)
VR:(0000, 0120, 00000002h): 01 00
VR:(0000, 0800, 00000002h): 01 01
VR:(0000, 0900, 00000002h): 00 00
------------>
[byte - 1] PDU Type       : 0x05 - ARelease-RQ
[byte - 1] Reserved       : 0x00
[u32 - 4] PDU Length      : 4
[byte - 4] Reserved       : 0x00000000
<------------
[byte - 1] PDU Type       : 0x06 - ARelease-RP
[byte - 1] Reserved       : 0x00
[u32 - 4] PDU Length      : 4
[byte - 4] Reserved       : 0x00000000
<------------
```

This transmission appeared to work. If it did not, then investigate the object logs for further information. From a network stand point here are the things known: a TCP/IP connection was successfully established. A DICOM connection was successfully established. There was some upper-layer message traffic that occurred. The DICOM connection was properly torn down using the normal Part 8 mechanisms which do not indicate an error occurred. If this transmission did not work, then it was because of an SOP/DIMSE class service level problem.

There are nine separate things we wish to point out about this log-file. The log-file itself is displayed with these nine items highlighted in bold so that they can be easily identified. They are:

1. The first item we wish to bring to your attention is the notion of the TCP/IP connection creation and closure. Here, we have slightly altered the log-file for security reasons, but this log was captured by DICOMSleuth, and shows a connection from

host x.x.x.x to host y.y.y.y. The significant thing about this line is the number *after* y.y.y.y. This number (104) is the port the client x.x.x.x attempted to connect to. Vendors use several different numbers. Common ones in use are 104, 3002, 4006, and 4008. It is important that the client (in this case the host at x.x.x.x) be configured to connect to the correct port.

2. Item two is the "called application title." This field must be the application title (AE title) of the "server," in this case, the machine at y.y.y.y.

3. Item three is the "calling application title." This field must be the application title (AE title) of the "client," in this case the machine at x.x.x.x. These first three items (port and AE title setups) comprise the bulk of DICOM connection problems. Make sure they are set-up correctly on both sides of the connection before proceeding further in diagnosing a failing DICOM link.

4. The PCID, or Presentation Context Identifier, is the first of the really ugly details about DICOM with which you need to become familiar. If you look at item 4 and item 7, you will notice that the PCID is the same number (in this case 3). This is not an accident. The "client" in this case (x.x.x.x) *proposes* a presentation context. The "server" in this case (y.y.y.y) *accepts* or *rejects* a presentation context. Within an association a presentation context is given a unique identifier. This identifier should always be an odd number, between 1 and 255. What is a presentation context? A presentation context is a way for the client to say to the server that it wishes to potentially communicate during the association, certain messages pertaining to a particular SOP class. In English, let us say the client is a CT scanner wishing to store an object to a PACS archive. Then it would propose the CT Storage service class. This service class has a unique identity in DICOM (see item 5). When it proposes the CT storage class, it also proposes one or more potential encoding methods (called transfer-syntaxes in DICOM, see item 6) to be used for communication.

5. Item 5 is the UID of the class being proposed for the presentation context. In this example, the UID means the Verification Service Class. See Part 6 of the DICOM standard for a listing of service classes.

6. Item 6 is the UID of the transfer-syntax being proposed for this service class to be communicated with. There may be multiple transfer-syntaxes proposed for a single service class. In this example, only one, the DICOM default transfer-syntax, is proposed.

7. Item 7. Here we wish to point out the similarity with Item 4.

8. Item 8 is a dump of an upper-layer transaction. In this case, the transaction is a C-Echo-request message. You can tell this because of two things. First, the group-

codes for the attributes in the message are all 0x0000. Second, item 0x0000, 0x0100 is 3000. DICOM upper-layer messages are encoded in the byte-ordering specified for the transfer syntax. In the DICOM default transfer syntax (see item 6), the byte-ordering is little-endian, hence you need to read 3000 *byte-swapped*, as 0030.

9. Item 9 is the dump of an upper-layer transaction from the server back to the client. Here you can see that is a response to the C-Echo message (in this case a C-Echo-Response message). The command is 3080, which again needs to be flipped to be 8030.

Association Rejection

Now that we have seen a successful connection between two DICOM entities, we will start to look at unsuccessful ones. First, let us look at an unsuccessful connection which is correctly rejected by a server. In this situation the server is a GE Advantage Windows workstation, and the client is a diagnostic program developed by UCDMC.

```
DICOMwhif  - A Network Analyzer for DICOM Image Transmissions
(C) 1999 U.C. Davis Medical Center    Dev. By: Mark Oskin
                        mhoskin@ucdavis.edu
 New TCP: x.x.x.x (4958) -> y.y.y.y (4006)
Close TCP: x.x.x.x (4958) -> y.y.y.y (4006)
------------>
[byte - 1] PDU Type      : 0x01 - AAssociate-RQ
[byte - 1] Reserved      : 0x00
[u32 - 4] PDU Length     : 199
[u16 - 2] ProtocolVersion : 0x0001 (0x0001=DICOM)
[byte - 2] Reserved      : 0x0000
[s  - 16] CalledApTitle  : 'wrong          '     (1)
[s  - 16] CallingApTitle : 'test_node      '
[byte - 33] Reserved3    : (00, 00, 00, 00, 00, 00, ...)
 [byte - 1] Item Type    : 0x10 - Application Context
 [byte - 1] Reserved     : 0x00
 [u16 - 2] Length     : 21
 [byte - 21] AppContext   : '1.2.840.10008.3.1.1.1'
 [byte - 1] Item Type    : 0x20 - Presentation Context
 [byte - 1] Reserved     : 0x00
 [u16 - 2] Length     : 46
 [byte - 1] PCID       : 3 - 0x03
 [byte - 3] Reserved    : (00, 00, 00)
  [byte - 1] Item Type    : 0x30 - Abstract Syntax
  [byte - 1] Reserved     : 0x00
  [u16 - 2] Length     : 17
  [byte - 17] AbsSyntax    : '1.2.840.10008.1.1'
  [byte - 1] Item Type    : 0x40 - Transfer Syntax
  [byte - 1] Reserved     : 0x00
```

```
[u16 - 2] Length       : 17
[byte - 17] TrnSyntax    : '1.2.840.10008.1.2'
[byte - 1] Item Type     : 0x50 - User Information
[byte - 1] Reserved      : 0x00
[u16 - 2] Length       : 52
  [byte - 1] Item Type     : 0x51 - Maximum Sub-Item
  [byte - 1] Reserved      : 0x00
  [u16 - 2] Length       : 4
  [byte - 1] MaxSub-item Lng : 16384 - 0x00004000
  [byte - 1] Item Type     : 0x52 - Implementation Class
  [byte - 1] Reserved      : 0x00
  [u16 - 2] Length       : 26
  [byte - 26] ImpClass      : 'UCDMC/gcc2.5.8/DECMIPS/MHO'
  [byte - 1] Item Type     : 0x55 - Implementation Version
  [byte - 1] Reserved      : 0x00
  [u16 - 2] Length       : 10
  [byte - 10] ImpVersion    : '0.1B/OTHER'
<------------
[byte - 1] PDU Type     : 0x03 - AAssociate-RJ
[byte - 1] Reserved     : 0x00
[u32 - 4] PDU Length    : 4
[byte - 1] Reserved     : 0x00
[byte - 1] Result       : 0x01 - Rejected-Perament
[byte - 1] Source       : 0x01 - DICOM UL Service User
[byte - 1] Reason       : 0x07 - Called AP Title Not Recognized (2)
<------------
```
The association was rejected by the remote side. The initiator attempted
to open a connection from (ip=x.x.x.x port=4958) to (ip=y.y.y.y
port=4006) The remote side (y.y.y.y/4006) rejected the association with
a Result=1 Source=1 Reason=7. Symbolically this means: Result=1 -
Rejected-Permanent (Reason=7 Source=1) - Called AP Title Not Recognized
The remote side has rejected the title the initiator tried to use for
the other side. Another words, the initiator (x.x.x.x - 4958) tried to
connect to the receiver (y.y.y.y - 4006) and the initiator thinks the
receiver has an application name of "wrong   " The receiver disagrees,
or at least, is not accepting connections from the initiator as this
name. The most likely cause of the problem is the initiator of the connection is miss-configured it's entry for what the remote host is
configured as.

Here we want to draw your attention to two items. The first item is labeled one. Here we note the called AE title of "wrong," which was intentionally set to the incorrect AE title for the host/port combination of y.y.y.y/4006. In this case the GE Advantage Windows workstation correctly rejected the association, and indicated the reason for the rejection as 0x07 (item 2), which corresponds to the called AE title being incorrectly specified.

When a connection problem occurs, the following steps are advised:

1. Go to a third computer and ping both hosts. This ensures they are available on your network.

2. Use a "telnet" tool to telnet into the "server" host's DICOM port. If it connects, but then nothing else happens, then some type of server is running on the port, so you probably have the right IP/port setup. If you get a "connection refused," then most likely the problem is the port or the IP is incorrect.

3. Run DICOMSleuth and see what the summary error report says. Most common DICOM configuration errors will be detected by DICOMSleuth and an informative message provided.

Association Rejection with a Nonconformant Device

From here on we are going to look at more challenging problems to pinpoint. These problems arise because of DICOM nonconformant devices. The first problem we are going to look at it is association rejection due to incorrect called AE title (just like the problem presented above), but the association is rejected incorrectly, providing a challenging diagnostic problem to resolve. In this situation the server is a Cemax Archive Manager v3.5 device, and the client is a diagnostic program developed by UCDMC. This problem first appeared at UCDMC when attempting to connect a GE "CTi" scanner to the Cemax Archive Manager product. The association would be created and then drop for unexplained reasons.

```
DICOMwhif  - A Network Analyzer for DICOM Image Transmissions
(C) 1999 U.C. Davis Medical Center    Dev. By: Mark Oskin
                      mhoskin@ucdavis.edu
 New TCP: x.x.x.x (4962) -> y.y.y.y (3002)
Close TCP: x.x.x.x (4962) -> y.y.y.y (3002)
------------>
[byte - 1] PDU Type      : 0x01 - AAssociate-RQ
[byte - 1] Reserved      : 0x00
[u32 - 4] PDU Length     : 199
[u16 - 2] ProtocolVersion : 0x0001 (0x0001=DICOM)
[byte - 2] Reserved      : 0x0000
[s  - 16] CalledApTitle  : 'wrong         '     (1)
[s  - 16] CallingApTitle : 'test_node     '
[byte - 33] Reserved3    : (00, 00, 00, 00, 00, 00, ...)
 [byte - 1] Item Type    : 0x10 - Application Context
 [byte - 1] Reserved     : 0x00
 [u16 - 2] Length    : 21
 [byte - 21] AppContext   : '1.2.840.10008.3.1.1.1'
 [byte - 1] Item Type    : 0x20 - Presentation Context
 [byte - 1] Reserved     : 0x00
 [u16 - 2] Length    : 46
 [byte - 1] PCID     : 3 - 0x03
 [byte - 3] Reserved     : (00, 00, 00)
```

```
 [byte - 1] Item Type    : 0x30 - Abstract Syntax
 [byte - 1] Reserved     : 0x00
 [u16 - 2] Length        : 17
 [byte - 17] AbsSyntax    : '1.2.840.10008.1.1'
 [byte - 1] Item Type    : 0x40 - Transfer Syntax
 [byte - 1] Reserved     : 0x00
 [u16 - 2] Length        : 17
 [byte - 17] TrnSyntax    : '1.2.840.10008.1.2'
[byte - 1] Item Type     : 0x50 - User Information
[byte - 1] Reserved     : 0x00
[u16 - 2] Length         : 52
 [byte - 1] Item Type     : 0x51 - Maximum Sub-Item
 [byte - 1] Reserved     : 0x00
 [u16 - 2] Length         : 4
 [byte - 1] MaxSub-item Lng : 16384 - 0x00004000
 [byte - 1] Item Type     : 0x52 - Implementation Class
 [byte - 1] Reserved     : 0x00
 [u16 - 2] Length         : 26
 [byte - 26] ImpClass     : 'UCDMC/gcc2.5.8/DECMIPS/MHO'
 [byte - 1] Item Type     : 0x55 - Implementation Version
 [byte - 1] Reserved     : 0x00
 [u16 - 2] Length         : 10
 [byte - 10] ImpVersion   : '0.1B/OTHER'
<------------
[byte - 1] PDU Type     : 0x02 - AAssociate-AC
[byte - 1] Reserved     : 0x00
[u32 - 4] PDU Length    : 180
[u16 - 2] ProtocolVersion : 0x0001 (0x0001=DICOM)
[byte - 2] Reserved     : 0x0000
[s  - 16] CalledApTitle  : 'wrong        '
[s  - 16] CallingApTitle : 'test_node    '
[byte - 33] Reserved3    : (00, 00, 00, 00, 00, 00, ...)
 [byte - 1] Item Type    : 0x10 - Application Context
 [byte - 1] Reserved     : 0x00
 [u16 - 2] Length        : 21
 [byte - 21] AppContext   : '1.2.840.10008.3.1.1.1'
 [byte - 1] Item Type    : 0x21 - Presentation Context - In Accept
 [byte - 1] Reserved     : 0x00
 [u16 - 2] Length        : 25
 [byte - 1] PCID         : 3 - 0x03
 [byte - 3] Reserved     : 00
 [byte - 3] Result       : 00 - Acceptance
 [byte - 3] Reserved     : 00
  [byte - 1] Item Type    : 0x40 - Transfer Syntax
  [byte - 1] Reserved     : 0x00
  [u16 - 2] Length        : 17
  [byte - 17] TrnSyntax    : '1.2.840.10008.1.2'
 [byte - 1] Item Type    : 0x50 - User Information
 [byte - 1] Reserved     : 0x00
 [u16 - 2] Length        : 54
  [byte - 1] Item Type    : 0x51 - Maximum Sub-Item
  [byte - 1] Reserved     : 0x00
```

```
[u16 - 2] Length      : 4
[byte - 1] MaxSub-item Lng : 16384 - 0x00004000
[byte - 1] Item Type    : 0x52 - Implementation Class
[byte - 1] Reserved     : 0x00
[u16 - 2] Length      : 22
[byte - 22] ImpClass    : '1.2.840.113674.6.15.95'
[byte - 1] Item Type    : 0x55 - Implementation Version
[byte - 1] Reserved     : 0x00
[u16 - 2] Length      : 16
[byte - 16] ImpVersion   : 'CEMAX-DOL-V3.5.0'
------------>
[byte - 1] PDU Type     : 0x04 - P-DATA-TF
[byte - 1] Reserved     : 0x00
[u32 - 4] PDU Length    : 74
 [u32 - 4] PDV Length   : 70
 [byte - 1] PresContext ID : 3
 [byte - 1] Message Header : 03 - Command Set / Last
VR:(0000, 0000, 00000004h): 38 00 00 00
VR:(0000, 0002, 00000012h): 31 2e 32 2e 38 34 30 2e 31 30 30 30 38 2e
31 2e ...
VR:(0000, 0100, 00000002h): 30 00
VR:(0000, 0110, 00000002h): 01 00
VR:(0000, 0800, 00000002h): 01 01
------------>
```

No A-ASSOCIATE-RELEASE message has been sent (and no A-ASSOCIATE-ABORT)
but, the connection has been dropped. This may be because of a poorly
written software on the part of the initiator or receiver in this transmission. It may also be because of a network failure. The only source
of further information is the object-dump logs (if the switch is enabled
on the command line. In which case you can investigate the upper layer
protocols to see if there is more in site to be gained there.

This log-file demonstrates a more challenging error to debug. We clearly know the connection did not work, but when we investigate the network traffic, it appears as though
the remote host (y.y.y.y) accepted the connection. The true source of error in this transmission was really the misconfigured called AE title on the Archive Manager side, but
there are no obvious signs that this is the reason. Discovering this bug required a lot
of patience, and a bit of luck. Unfortunately, much time was wasted by the authors con-
figuring remote devices to communicate with the DICOM server device (Archive
Manager) because the device did not correctly report association failure reasons.

Association Failures Due to Message Encoding Errors

The third type of DICOM connection problem we are going to look at is even more
difficult to spot than the previous AE title setup issue. This problem manifested itself
because a workstation (a Siemens MagicView MV1000) was not able to query an
archive (a GE HiSpeed Advantage MRI scanner). Images could be stored to the

archive, and the archive could store back to the workstation, but the query/retrieve facilities did not work. Here is the log file:

```
New TCP: x.x.x.x (33201) -> y.y.y.y (104)
Close TCP: x.x.x.x (33201) -> y.y.y.y (104)
------------>
[byte - 1] PDU Type      : 0x01 - AAssociate-RQ
[byte - 1] Reserved      : 0x00
[u32 - 4] PDU Length     : 780
[u16 - 2] ProtocolVersion : 0x0001 (0x0001=DICOM)
[byte - 2] Reserved      : 0x0000
[s  - 16] CalledApTitle  : 'UCD_MRS1_IC0  '
[s  - 16] CallingApTitle : '001S01DC77DQRY '
[byte - 33] Reserved3    : (00, 00, 00, 00, 00, 00, ...)
 [byte - 1] Item Type    : 0x10 - Application Context
 [byte - 1] Reserved     : 0x00
 [u16 - 2] Length        : 21
 [byte - 21] AppContext  : '1.2.840.10008.3.1.1.1'
 [byte - 1] Item Type    : 0x20 - Presentation Context
 [byte - 1] Reserved     : 0x00
 [u16 - 2] Length        : 102
 [byte - 1] PCID         : 1 - 0x01
 [byte - 3] Reserved     : (00, 00, 00)
  [byte - 1] Item Type    : 0x30 - Abstract Syntax
  [byte - 1] Reserved     : 0x00
  [u16 - 2] Length        : 27
  [byte - 27] AbsSyntax    : '1.2.840.10008.5.1.4.1.2.1.1'
  [byte - 1] Item Type    : 0x40 - Transfer Syntax
  [byte - 1] Reserved     : 0x00
  [u16 - 2] Length        : 19
  [byte - 19] TrnSyntax    : '1.2.840.10008.1.2.2'
  [byte - 1] Item Type    : 0x40 - Transfer Syntax
  [byte - 1] Reserved     : 0x00
  [u16 - 2] Length        : 19
  [byte - 19] TrnSyntax    : '1.2.840.10008.1.2.1'
  [byte - 1] Item Type    : 0x40 - Transfer Syntax
  [byte - 1] Reserved     : 0x00
  [u16 - 2] Length        : 17
  [byte - 17] TrnSyntax    : '1.2.840.10008.1.2'
 [byte - 1] Item Type    : 0x20 - Presentation Context
 [byte - 1] Reserved     : 0x00
 [u16 - 2] Length        : 102
 [byte - 1] PCID         : 3 - 0x03
 [byte - 3] Reserved     : (00, 00, 00)
  [byte - 1] Item Type    : 0x30 - Abstract Syntax
  [byte - 1] Reserved     : 0x00
  [u16 - 2] Length        : 27
  [byte - 27] AbsSyntax    : '1.2.840.10008.5.1.4.1.2.2.1'
  [byte - 1] Item Type    : 0x40 - Transfer Syntax
  [byte - 1] Reserved     : 0x00
  [u16 - 2] Length        : 19
  [byte - 19] TrnSyntax    : '1.2.840.10008.1.2.2'
```

```
[byte - 1] Item Type    : 0x40 - Transfer Syntax
[byte - 1] Reserved     : 0x00
[u16 - 2] Length        : 19
[byte - 19] TrnSyntax    : '1.2.840.10008.1.2.1'
[byte - 1] Item Type    : 0x40 - Transfer Syntax
[byte - 1] Reserved     : 0x00
[u16 - 2] Length        : 17
[byte - 17] TrnSyntax    : '1.2.840.10008.1.2'
[byte - 1] Item Type    : 0x20 - Presentation Context
[byte - 1] Reserved     : 0x00
[u16 - 2] Length        : 102
[byte - 1] PCID         : 5 - 0x05
[byte - 3] Reserved     : (00, 00, 00)
 [byte - 1] Item Type    : 0x30 - Abstract Syntax
 [byte - 1] Reserved     : 0x00
 [u16 - 2] Length        : 27
 [byte - 27] AbsSyntax    : '1.2.840.10008.5.1.4.1.2.3.1'
 [byte - 1] Item Type    : 0x40 - Transfer Syntax
 [byte - 1] Reserved     : 0x00
 [u16 - 2] Length        : 19
 [byte - 19] TrnSyntax    : '1.2.840.10008.1.2.2'
 [byte - 1] Item Type    : 0x40 - Transfer Syntax
 [byte - 1] Reserved     : 0x00
 [u16 - 2] Length        : 19
 [byte - 19] TrnSyntax    : '1.2.840.10008.1.2.1'
 [byte - 1] Item Type    : 0x40 - Transfer Syntax
 [byte - 1] Reserved     : 0x00
 [u16 - 2] Length        : 17
 [byte - 17] TrnSyntax    : '1.2.840.10008.1.2'
[byte - 1] Item Type    : 0x20 - Presentation Context
[byte - 1] Reserved     : 0x00
[u16 - 2] Length        : 102
[byte - 1] PCID         : 7 - 0x07
[byte - 3] Reserved     : (00, 00, 00)
 [byte - 1] Item Type    : 0x30 - Abstract Syntax
 [byte - 1] Reserved     : 0x00
 [u16 - 2] Length        : 27
 [byte - 27] AbsSyntax    : '1.2.840.10008.5.1.4.1.2.1.2'
 [byte - 1] Item Type    : 0x40 - Transfer Syntax
 [byte - 1] Reserved     : 0x00
 [u16 - 2] Length        : 19
 [byte - 19] TrnSyntax    : '1.2.840.10008.1.2.2'
 [byte - 1] Item Type    : 0x40 - Transfer Syntax
 [byte - 1] Reserved     : 0x00
 [u16 - 2] Length        : 19
 [byte - 19] TrnSyntax    : '1.2.840.10008.1.2.1'
 [byte - 1] Item Type    : 0x40 - Transfer Syntax
 [byte - 1] Reserved     : 0x00
 [u16 - 2] Length        : 17
 [byte - 17] TrnSyntax    : '1.2.840.10008.1.2'
[byte - 1] Item Type    : 0x20 - Presentation Context
[byte - 1] Reserved     : 0x00
```

```
[u16 - 2] Length       : 102
[byte - 1] PCID        : 9 - 0x09
[byte - 3] Reserved    : (00, 00, 00)
 [byte - 1] Item Type    : 0x30 - Abstract Syntax
 [byte - 1] Reserved     : 0x00
 [u16 - 2] Length      : 27
 [byte - 27] AbsSyntax    : '1.2.840.10008.5.1.4.1.2.2.2'
 [byte - 1] Item Type    : 0x40 - Transfer Syntax
 [byte - 1] Reserved     : 0x00
 [u16 - 2] Length      : 19
 [byte - 19] TrnSyntax    : '1.2.840.10008.1.2.2'
 [byte - 1] Item Type    : 0x40 - Transfer Syntax
 [byte - 1] Reserved     : 0x00
 [u16 - 2] Length      : 19
 [byte - 19] TrnSyntax    : '1.2.840.10008.1.2.1'
 [byte - 1] Item Type    : 0x40 - Transfer Syntax
 [byte - 1] Reserved     : 0x00
 [u16 - 2] Length      : 17
 [byte - 17] TrnSyntax    : '1.2.840.10008.1.2'
[byte - 1] Item Type    : 0x20 - Presentation Context
[byte - 1] Reserved    : 0x00
[u16 - 2] Length       : 102
[byte - 1] PCID        : 11 - 0x0b
[byte - 3] Reserved    : (00, 00, 00)
 [byte - 1] Item Type    : 0x30 - Abstract Syntax
 [byte - 1] Reserved     : 0x00
 [u16 - 2] Length      : 27
 [byte - 27] AbsSyntax    : '1.2.840.10008.5.1.4.1.2.3.2'
 [byte - 1] Item Type    : 0x40 - Transfer Syntax
 [byte - 1] Reserved     : 0x00
 [u16 - 2] Length      : 19
 [byte - 19] TrnSyntax    : '1.2.840.10008.1.2.2'
 [byte - 1] Item Type    : 0x40 - Transfer Syntax
 [byte - 1] Reserved     : 0x00
 [u16 - 2] Length      : 19
 [byte - 19] TrnSyntax    : '1.2.840.10008.1.2.1'
 [byte - 1] Item Type    : 0x40 - Transfer Syntax
 [byte - 1] Reserved     : 0x00
 [u16 - 2] Length      : 17
 [byte - 17] TrnSyntax    : '1.2.840.10008.1.2'
[byte - 1] Item Type    : 0x50 - User Information
[byte - 1] Reserved    : 0x00
[u16 - 2] Length       : 47
 [byte - 1] Item Type    : 0x51 - Maximum Sub-Item
 [byte - 1] Reserved     : 0x00
 [u16 - 2] Length      : 4
 [byte - 1] MaxSub-item Lng : 16384 - 0x00004000
 [byte - 1] Item Type    : 0x52 - Implementation Class
 [byte - 1] Reserved     : 0x00
 [u16 - 2] Length      : 15
 [byte - 15] ImpClass    : '1.3.12.2.1107.9'
 [byte - 1] Item Type    : 0x55 - Implementation Version
```

```
    [byte - 1] Reserved    : 0x00
    [u16 - 2] Length       : 16
    [byte - 16] ImpVersion   : 'Siemens_DICOM_10'
<------------
[byte - 1] PDU Type      : 0x02 - AAssociate-AC
[byte - 1] Reserved      : 0x00
[u32 - 4] PDU Length     : 211
[u16 - 2] ProtocolVersion : 0x0001 (0x0001=DICOM)
[byte - 2] Reserved      : 0x0000
[s  - 16] CalledApTitle  : 'UCD_MRS1_IC0  '
[s  - 16] CallingApTitle : '001S01DC77DQRY '
[byte - 33] Reserved3    : (00, 00, 00, 00, 00, 00, ...)
 [byte - 1] Item Type    : 0x10 - Application Context
 [byte - 1] Reserved     : 0x00
 [u16 - 2] Length     : 21
 [byte - 21] AppContext    : '1.2.840.10008.3.1.1.1'
 [byte - 1] Item Type     : 0x21 - Presentation Context - In Accept
 [byte - 1] Reserved      : 0x00
 [u16 - 2] Length       : 8
 [byte - 1] PCID        : 1 - 0x01
 [byte - 3] Reserved     : 00
 [byte - 3] Result       : 03 - Abstract Syntax Not Supported
 [byte - 3] Reserved     : 00
  [byte - 1] Item Type    : 0x40 - Transfer Syntax
  [byte - 1] Reserved     : 0x00
  [u16 - 2] Length      : 0
  [byte - 0] TrnSyntax    : ''
 [byte - 1] Item Type     : 0x21 - Presentation Context - In Accept
 [byte - 1] Reserved      : 0x00
 [u16 - 2] Length       : 25
 [byte - 1] PCID        : 3 - 0x03
 [byte - 3] Reserved     : 00
 [byte - 3] Result       : 00 - Acceptance
 [byte - 3] Reserved     : 00
  [byte - 1] Item Type    : 0x40 - Transfer Syntax
  [byte - 1] Reserved     : 0x00
  [u16 - 2] Length      : 17
  [byte - 17] TrnSyntax    : '1.2.840.10008.1.2'
 [byte - 1] Item Type     : 0x21 - Presentation Context - In Accept
 [byte - 1] Reserved      : 0x00
 [u16 - 2] Length       : 8
 [byte - 1] PCID        : 5 - 0x05
 [byte - 3] Reserved     : 00
 [byte - 3] Result       : 03 - Abstract Syntax Not Supported
 [byte - 3] Reserved     : 00
  [byte - 1] Item Type    : 0x40 - Transfer Syntax
  [byte - 1] Reserved     : 0x00
  [u16 - 2] Length      : 0
  [byte - 0] TrnSyntax    : ''
 [byte - 1] Item Type     : 0x21 - Presentation Context - In Accept
 [byte - 1] Reserved      : 0x00
 [u16 - 2] Length       : 8
```

```
[byte - 1] PCID       : 7 - 0x07
[byte - 3] Reserved   : 00
[byte - 3] Result     : 03 - Abstract Syntax Not Supported
[byte - 3] Reserved   : 00
 [byte - 1] Item Type     : 0x40 - Transfer Syntax
 [byte - 1] Reserved      : 0x00
 [u16 - 2] Length      : 0
 [byte - 0] TrnSyntax     : ''
[byte - 1] Item Type      : 0x21 - Presentation Context - In Accept
[byte - 1] Reserved       : 0x00
[u16 - 2] Length       : 25
[byte - 1] PCID        : 9 - 0x09
[byte - 3] Reserved    : 00
[byte - 3] Result      : 00 - Acceptance
[byte - 3] Reserved    : 00
 [byte - 1] Item Type      : 0x40 - Transfer Syntax
 [byte - 1] Reserved       : 0x00
 [u16 - 2] Length       : 17
 [byte - 17] TrnSyntax     : '1.2.840.10008.1.2'
[byte - 1] Item Type       : 0x21 - Presentation Context - In Accept
[byte - 1] Reserved        : 0x00
[u16 - 2] Length        : 8
[byte - 1] PCID         : 11 - 0x0b
[byte - 3] Reserved     : 00
[byte - 3] Result       : 03 - Abstract Syntax Not Supported
[byte - 3] Reserved     : 00
 [byte - 1] Item Type      : 0x40 - Transfer Syntax
 [byte - 1] Reserved       : 0x00
 [u16 - 2] Length       : 0
 [byte - 0] TrnSyntax      : ''
[byte - 1] Item Type       : 0x50 - User Information
[byte - 1] Reserved        : 0x31
[u16 - 2] Length        : 8
 [byte - 1] Item Type       : 0x51 - Maximum Sub-Item
 [byte - 1] Reserved        : 0x38
 [u16 - 2] Length        : 4
 [byte - 1] MaxSub-item Lng : 30000 - 0x00007530
------------>
[byte - 1] PDU Type     : 0x04 - P-DATA-TF
[byte - 1] Reserved     : 0x00
[u32 - 4] PDU Length    : 94
 [u32 - 4] PDV Length    : 90
 [byte - 1] PresContext ID : 3
 [byte - 1] Message Header : 03 - Command Set / Last
VR:(0000, 0000, 00000004h): 4c 00 00 00
VR:(0000, 0002, 0000001ch): 31 2e 32 2e 38 34 30 2e 31 30 30 30 38 2e
35 2e ...
VR:(0000, 0100, 00000002h): 20 00
VR:(0000, 0110, 00000002h): 0a 00
VR:(0000, 0700, 00000002h): 00 00
VR:(0000, 0800, 00000002h): 00 00
------------>
```

```
[byte - 1] PDU Type     : 0x04 - P-DATA-TF
[byte - 1] Reserved     : 0x00
[u32 - 4] PDU Length     : 104
 [u32 - 4] PDV Length    : 100
 [byte - 1] PresContext ID : 3
 [byte - 1] Message Header : 02 - Data Set / Last
VR:(0008, 0020, 0000000ah): 2d 31 39 39 38 30 32 31 32 20
VR:(0008, 0030, 0000000ch): 2d 32 34 30 30 30 30 2e 30 30 30 30 (1)
VR:(0008, 0052, 00000006h): 53 54 55 44 59 20
VR:(0008, 1030, 00000002h): 2a 20
VR:(0010, 0010, 00000002h): 2a 20
VR:(0010, 0020, 00000002h): 2a 20
VR:(0020, 000d, 00000000h):
VR:(0020, 1208, 00000000h):
<------------
[byte - 1] PDU Type     : 0x04 - P-DATA-TF
[byte - 1] Reserved     : 0x00
[u32 - 4] PDU Length     : 168
 [u32 - 4] PDV Length    : 164
 [byte - 1] PresContext ID : 3
 [byte - 1] Message Header : 03 - Command Set / Last
VR:(0000, 0000, 00000004h): 96 00 00 00
VR:(0000, 0001, 00000004h): 8a 00 00 00
VR:(0000, 0002, 0000001ch): 31 2e 32 2e 38 34 30 2e 31 30 30 30 38 2e
35 2e ...
VR:(0000, 0100, 00000002h): 20 80
VR:(0000, 0120, 00000002h): 0a 00
VR:(0000, 0800, 00000002h): 01 01
VR:(0000, 0900, 00000002h): 04 c0
VR:(0000, 0902, 00000036h): 20 28 20 36 35 35 33 35 2c 20 36 35 35 33
35 20 ...
------------>
[byte - 1] PDU Type     : 0x07 - AAbort-RQ
[byte - 1] Reserved     : 0x00
[u32 - 4] PDU Length     : 4
[byte - 1] Reserved     : 0x00
[byte - 1] Reserved     : 0x00
[byte - 1] Source       : 0x00 - *Unknown*
[byte - 1] Reason       : 0x00 - Reason Not Specified
------------>
```

An A-ASSOCIATE-ABORT message was sent. However, some P-DATA-TF traffic occurred. This may be an upper-layer problem (i.e. with the actual encoding of the data. I suggest using the Object-Capture feature to, and to re-run this connection. Then post-analyze the objects sent using the "test" utility ("test -v filename"). The answer is beyond this applications scope. Another possibility, which needs to be mentioned, is that the client sent an A-ASSOCIATE-ABORT instead of an A-ASSOCIATE-RELEASE. Some do this. In such a case, this may not be an error at all, just a minor tweak of the DICOM standard on the part of the client. a case, this may not be an error at all, just a minor tweak of the DICOM standard on the part of the client.

Finding the bug in this transmission was quite difficult. The workstation would associate with the archive, but the archive would not respond to the C-Find request. As it turns out, the problem was when the workstation sent the C-Find request, it included a set of query parameters. One of these query parameters, attribute (0x0008, 0x0030), contained the time query string of "-240000.0000." What the workstation intended by this query string was that all studies with times between "000000" (midnight, in the morning), and "-240000.0000" were to be included. However, Part 5 of the DICOM standard indicates that time "240000" is invalid since it is ambiguous. Hence, the archive was correctly refusing to service the query.

Transfer-syntax Decoding Errors

This next problem appeared when trying to send data from a GE QA workstation attached to a Fuji FCR9000 Computed Radiography device. The GE QA workstation was attemping to send to a Cemax v3.5 Archive Manager device. The GE QA would successfully "test" against the archive device, but it was unable to send an image. Here is the log-file of the transmission:

```
New TCP: 152.79.18.11 (41644) -> 152.79.49.104 (3002)
Close TCP: 152.79.18.11 (41644) -> 152.79.49.104 (3002)
------------>
[byte - 1] PDU Type      : 0x01 - AAssociate-RQ
[byte - 1] Reserved      : 0x00
[u32 - 4] PDU Length     : 332
[u16 - 2] ProtocolVersion : 0x0001 (0x0001=DICOM)
[byte - 2] Reserved      : 0x0000
[s  - 16] CalledApTitle  : 'DS02_UCDMC      '
[s  - 16] CallingApTitle : 'gecrrad2        '
[byte - 33] Reserved3    : (00, 00, 00, 00, 00, 00, ...)
 [byte - 1] Item Type     : 0x10 - Application Context
 [byte - 1] Reserved      : 0x00
 [u16 - 2] Length         : 21
 [byte - 21] AppContext   : '1.2.840.10008.3.1.1.1'
 [byte - 1] Item Type     : 0x20 - Presentation Context
 [byte - 1] Reserved      : 0x00
 [u16 - 2] Length         : 54
 [byte - 1] PCID          : 1 - 0x01
 [byte - 3] Reserved      : (00, 00, 00)
  [byte - 1] Item Type     : 0x30 - Abstract Syntax
  [byte - 1] Reserved      : 0x00
  [u16 - 2] Length         : 25
  [byte - 25] AbsSyntax    : '1.2.840.10008.5.1.4.1.1.1'
  [byte - 1] Item Type     : 0x40 - Transfer Syntax
  [byte - 1] Reserved      : 0x00
  [u16 - 2] Length         : 17
  [byte - 17] TrnSyntax    : '1.2.840.10008.1.2'
 [byte - 1] Item Type     : 0x20 - Presentation Context
 [byte - 1] Reserved      : 0x00
```

```
[u16 - 2] Length      : 56
[byte - 1] PCID       : 3 - 0x03
[byte - 3] Reserved   : (00, 00, 00)
 [byte - 1] Item Type    : 0x30 - Abstract Syntax
 [byte - 1] Reserved     : 0x00
 [u16 - 2] Length     : 25
 [byte - 25] AbsSyntax    : '1.2.840.10008.5.1.4.1.1.1'
 [byte - 1] Item Type     : 0x40 - Transfer Syntax
 [byte - 1] Reserved     : 0x00
 [u16 - 2] Length     : 19
 [byte - 19] TrnSyntax    : '1.2.840.10008.1.2.2'
[byte - 1] Item Type    : 0x20 - Presentation Context
[byte - 1] Reserved     : 0x00
[u16 - 2] Length      : 54
[byte - 1] PCID       : 5 - 0x05
[byte - 3] Reserved   : (00, 00, 00)
 [byte - 1] Item Type    : 0x30 - Abstract Syntax
 [byte - 1] Reserved     : 0x00
 [u16 - 2] Length     : 25
 [byte - 25] AbsSyntax    : '1.2.840.10008.5.1.4.1.1.7'
 [byte - 1] Item Type     : 0x40 - Transfer Syntax
 [byte - 1] Reserved     : 0x00
 [u16 - 2] Length     : 17
 [byte - 17] TrnSyntax    : '1.2.840.10008.1.2'
[byte - 1] Item Type    : 0x50 - User Information
[byte - 1] Reserved     : 0x00
[u16 - 2] Length      : 59
 [byte - 1] Item Type    : 0x51 - Maximum Sub-Item
 [byte - 1] Reserved     : 0x00
 [u16 - 2] Length     : 4
 [byte - 1] MaxSub-item Lng : 100000 - 0x000186a0
 [byte - 1] Item Type    : 0x52 - Implementation Class
 [byte - 1] Reserved     : 0x00
 [u16 - 2] Length     : 20
 [byte - 20] ImpClass    : '1.2.840.113619.6.62'
 [byte - 1] Item Type    : 0x53 - Not sure
 [byte - 1] Reserved     : 0x00
 [u16 - 2] Length     : 4
 [byte - 1] Item Type    : 0x55 - Implementation Version
 [byte - 1] Reserved     : 0x00
 [u16 - 2] Length     : 15
 [byte - 15] ImpVersion   : 'GE-ACRQADCM1197'
<------------
[byte - 1] PDU Type      : 0x02 - AAssociate-AC
[byte - 1] Reserved      : 0x00
[u32 - 4] PDU Length     : 239
[u16 - 2] ProtocolVersion : 0x0001 (0x0001=DICOM)
[byte - 2] Reserved      : 0x0000
[s  - 16] CalledApTitle  : 'DS02_UCDMC    '
[s  - 16] CallingApTitle : 'gecrrad2      '
[byte - 33] Reserved3    : (00, 00, 00, 00, 00, 00, ...)
 [byte - 1] Item Type    : 0x10 - Application Context
```

```
[byte - 1] Reserved     : 0x00
[u16 - 2] Length      : 21
[byte - 21] AppContext   : '1.2.840.10008.3.1.1.1'
[byte - 1] Item Type   : 0x21 - Presentation Context - In Accept
[byte - 1] Reserved    : 0x00
[u16 - 2] Length      : 25
[byte - 1] PCID       : 1 - 0x01
[byte - 3] Reserved     : 00
[byte - 3] Result     : 00 - Acceptance
[byte - 3] Reserved     : 00
 [byte - 1] Item Type    : 0x40 - Transfer Syntax
 [byte - 1] Reserved     : 0x00
 [u16 - 2] Length     : 17
 [byte - 17] TrnSyntax    : '1.2.840.10008.1.2'
[byte - 1] Item Type   : 0x21 - Presentation Context - In Accept
[byte - 1] Reserved    : 0x00
[u16 - 2] Length      : 27
[byte - 1] PCID       : 3 - 0x03
[byte - 3] Reserved     : 00
[byte - 3] Result     : 00 - Acceptance
[byte - 3] Reserved     : 00
 [byte - 1] Item Type    : 0x40 - Transfer Syntax
 [byte - 1] Reserved     : 0x00
 [u16 - 2] Length     : 19
 [byte - 19] TrnSyntax   : '1.2.840.10008.1.2.2'
[byte - 1] Item Type   : 0x21 - Presentation Context - In Accept
[byte - 1] Reserved    : 0x00
[u16 - 2] Length      : 25
[byte - 1] PCID       : 5 - 0x05
[byte - 3] Reserved     : 00
[byte - 3] Result     : 00 - Acceptance
[byte - 3] Reserved     : 00
 [byte - 1] Item Type    : 0x40 - Transfer Syntax
 [byte - 1] Reserved     : 0x00
 [u16 - 2] Length     : 17
 [byte - 17] TrnSyntax    : '1.2.840.10008.1.2'
[byte - 1] Item Type   : 0x50 - User Information
[byte - 1] Reserved    : 0x00
[u16 - 2] Length      : 53
 [byte - 1] Item Type    : 0x51 - Maximum Sub-Item
 [byte - 1] Reserved     : 0x00
 [u16 - 2] Length     : 4
 [byte - 1] MaxSub-item Lng : 16384 - 0x00004000
 [byte - 1] Item Type    : 0x52 - Implementation Class
 [byte - 1] Reserved     : 0x00
 [u16 - 2] Length     : 22
 [byte - 22] ImpClass    : '1.2.840.113674.6.15.95'
 [byte - 1] Item Type    : 0x55 - Implementation Version
 [byte - 1] Reserved     : 0x00
 [u16 - 2] Length     : 15
 [byte - 15] ImpVersion   : 'CEMAX-DOL-PROTO'
------------>
```

```
[byte - 1] PDU Type     : 0x04 - P-DATA-TF
[byte - 1] Reserved     : 0x00
[u32 - 4] PDU Length     : 160
 [u32 - 4] PDV Length    : 156
 [byte - 1] PresContext ID : 1
 [byte - 1] Message Header : 03 - Command Set / Last
VR:(0000, 0000, 00000004h): 8e 00 00 00
VR:(0000, 0002, 0000001ah): 31 2e 32 2e 38 34 30 2e 31 30 30 30 38 2e
35 2e ...
VR:(0000, 0100, 00000002h): 01 00
VR:(0000, 0110, 00000002h): 00 00
VR:(0000, 0700, 00000002h): 02 00
VR:(0000, 0800, 00000002h): 00 00
VR:(0000, 1000, 0000003ch): 31 2e 32 2e 38 34 30 2e 31 31 33 36 31 39
2e 32 ...
------------>
[byte - 1] PDU Type      : 0x04 - P-DATA-TF
[byte - 1] Reserved      : 0x00
[u32 - 4] PDU Length     : 16384
 [u32 - 4] PDV Length    : 16380
 [byte - 1] PresContext ID : 1
 [byte - 1] Message Header : 00 - Data Set / Continues
VR:(0008, 0005, 0000000ah): 49 53 4f 5f 49 52 20 31 30 30
VR:(0008, 0008, 00000010h): 44 45 52 49 56 45 44 5c 50 52 49 4d 41 52
59 20
VR:(0008, 0016, 0000001ah): 31 2e 32 2e 38 34 30 2e 31 30 30 30 38 2e
35 2e ...
VR:(0008, 0018, 0000003ch): 31 2e 32 2e 38 34 30 2e 31 31 33 36 31 39
2e 32 ...
VR:(0008, 0020, 00000008h): 31 39 39 38 30 37 31 38
VR:(0008, 0021, 00000008h): 31 39 39 38 30 37 31 38
VR:(0008, 0022, 00000008h): 31 39 39 38 30 37 31 38
VR:(0008, 0023, 00000008h): 31 39 39 38 30 37 31 38
VR:(0008, 0030, 00000006h): 30 39 34 33 30 30
VR:(0008, 0031, 00000006h): 30 39 34 33 30 30
VR:(0008, 0032, 00000006h): 30 39 34 33 30 30
VR:(0008, 0033, 0000000ah): 30 39 34 32 33 31 2e 30 30 20
VR:(0008, 0050, 0000000eh): 31 39 39 38 30 37 31 38 30 39 34 32 33 31
VR:(0008, 0060, 00000002h): 43 52
VR:(0008, 0070, 00000030h): 46 75 6a 69 20 50 68 6f 74 6f 20 46 69 6c
6d 20 ...
VR:(0008, 0080, 00000014h): 55 2e 43 2e 20 44 41 56 49 53 20 4d 45 44
20 43 ...
VR:(0008, 0090, 00000000h):
VR:(0008, 1010, 0000000ah): 67 65 63 72 72 61 64 32 2d 41
VR:(0008, 1030, 0000000eh): 43 2d 53 50 49 4e 45 20 41 50 5f 4f 42 4c
VR:(0010, 0010, 0000000eh): 48 49 44 59 5e 4c 49 4e 44 41 5e 5e 5e 5e
VR:(0010, 0020, 00000008h): 31 33 33 33 33 36 30 20
VR:(0010, 0030, 00000008h): 31 39 36 34 31 30 30 33
VR:(0010, 0040, 00000002h): 46 20
VR:(0018, 0010, 00000000h):
VR:(0018, 0015, 0000000eh): 43 2d 53 50 49 4e 45 20 41 50 5f 4f 42 4c
```

```
VR:(0018, 1020, 0000000eh): 47 45 4d 53 20 41 43 52 51 41 20 32 2e 30
VR:(0018, 1164, 0000000eh): 30 2e 31 35 30 30 5c 30 2e 31 35 30 30 20
VR:(0018, 1400, 0000000eh): 43 2d 53 50 49 4e 45 20 41 50 5f 4f 42 4c
VR:(0018, 1401, 00000004h): 30 31 30 31
VR:(0018, 5101, 00000000h):
VR:(0018, 6000, 00000004h): 20 31 38 33
VR:(0020, 000d, 00000032h): 31 2e 32 2e 38 34 30 2e 31 31 33 36 31 39
2e 32 ...
VR:(0020, 000e, 00000032h): 31 2e 32 2e 38 34 30 2e 31 31 33 36 31 39
2e 32 ...
VR:(0020, 0010, 0000000eh): 31 39 39 38 30 37 31 38 30 39 34 32 33 31
VR:(0020, 0011, 00000004h): 32 35 37 20
VR:(0020, 0013, 00000006h): 33 31 33 33 38 20
VR:(0020, 0020, 00000000h):
VR:(0020, 0060, 00000000h):
VR:(0020, 4000, 0000000eh): 43 2d 53 50 49 4e 45 20 41 50 5f 4f 42 4c
VR:(0023, 0010, 00000016h): 47 45 4d 53 5f 41 43 52 51 41 5f 32 2e 30
20 42 ...
VR:(0023, 0020, 00000016h): 47 45 4d 53 5f 41 43 52 51 41 5f 32 2e 30
20 42 ...
VR:(0023, 0030, 00000016h): 47 45 4d 53 5f 41 43 52 51 41 5f 32 2e 30
20 42 ...
VR:(0023, 0040, 00000016h): 47 45 4d 53 5f 41 43 52 51 41 5f 32 2e 30
20 42 ...
VR:(0023, 1000, 00000004h): 30 31 30 31
VR:(0023, 1010, 0000000eh): 43 2d 53 50 49 4e 45 20 41 50 5f 4f 42 4c
VR:(0023, 1020, 00000002h): 30 20
VR:(0023, 1030, 00000004h): 32 2e 31 20
VR:(0023, 1040, 00000002h): 30 31
VR:(0023, 1050, 00000002h): 63 00
VR:(0023, 1060, 0000000ah): 61 30 36 34 31 36 36 30 37 63
VR:(0023, 1070, 0000000ah): 20 20 20 20 20 20 20 20 20 20
VR:(0023, 1080, 00000002h): 31 20
VR:(0023, 1090, 00000004h): 2a 31 2e 30
VR:(0023, 2000, 00000002h): 00 00
VR:(0023, 2010, 00000004h): 2a 31 2e 30
VR:(0023, 2020, 00000002h): 46 20
VR:(0023, 2030, 00000004h): 31 2e 31 20
VR:(0023, 2040, 00000004h): 30 2e 36 30
VR:(0023, 2050, 00000004h): 30 2e 35 30
VR:(0023, 2060, 00000002h): 50 20
VR:(0023, 2070, 00000004h): 30 2e 35 20
VR:(0023, 2080, 00000002h): 05 00
VR:(0023, 2090, 00000000h):
VR:(0023, 3000, 00000004h): 30 2e 30 20
VR:(0023, 3010, 00000002h): 00 00
VR:(0023, 3020, 00000004h): 30 2e 30 20
VR:(0023, 3030, 00000002h): 00 00
VR:(0023, 3040, 00000002h): 00 00
VR:(0023, 3050, 00000002h): 42 20
VR:(0023, 3060, 00000002h): 41 20
VR:(0023, 3070, 00000006h): 41 43 33 49 44 54
```

```
VR:(0023, 3080, 00000002h): 20 20
VR:(0023, 3090, 00000014h): 54 61 3d 20 2c 54 62 3d 20 2c 54 63 3d 20
2c 54 ...
VR:(0023, 30f0, 00000008h): 41 2d 30 37 31 38 39 38
VR:(0028, 0002, 00000002h): 01 00
VR:(0028, 0004, 0000000ch): 4d 4f 4e 4f 43 48 52 4f 4d 45 31 20
VR:(0028, 0010, 00000002h): b8 07
VR:(0028, 0011, 00000002h): 28 06
VR:(0028, 0030, 0000000eh): 30 2e 31 35 30 30 5c 30 2e 31 35 30 30 20
VR:(0028, 0100, 00000002h): 10 00
VR:(0028, 0101, 00000002h): 0a 00
VR:(0028, 0102, 00000002h): 09 00
VR:(0028, 0103, 00000002h): 00 00
VR:(0028, 1050, 00000004h): 35 31 31 20
VR:(0028, 1051, 00000004h): 31 30 32 34
VR:(7fe0, 0010, 005f0980h): 8c 00 8c 00 8c 00 8c 00 8c 00 8c 00 8c 00
8c 00 ...------------>
[byte - 1] PDU Type     : 0x04 - P-DATA-TF
[byte - 1] Reserved     : 0x00
[u32 - 4] PDU Length    : 16384
 [u32 - 4] PDV Length    : 16380
 [byte - 1] PresContext ID : 1
 [byte - 1] Message Header : 00 - Data Set / Continues
------------>
[byte - 1] PDU Type     : 0x04 - P-DATA-TF
[byte - 1] Reserved     : 0x00
[u32 - 4] PDU Length    : 16384
 [u32 - 4] PDV Length    : 16380
 [byte - 1] PresContext ID : 1
 [byte - 1] Message Header : 00 - Data Set / Continues
------------>
```

No A-ASSOCIATE-RELEASE message has been sent (and no A-ASSOCIATE-ABORT) but, the connection has been dropped. This may be because of a poorly written software on the part of the initiator or receiver in this transmission. It may also be because of a network failure. The only source of further information is the object-dump logs (if the switch is enabled on the command line. In which case you can investigate the upper layer protocols to see if there is more in site to be gained there.

What caused this transmission to fail? First, the symptoms. Although the workstation would "test" fine against the archive, it would not store an image. The "test" was actually doing a C-Echo on the Validation service class. The C-Echo is a command only message (there is no data section). When an image was sent, it would tend to appear as though a large quantity of network traffic would occur before failure, since the failure was not instantaneous, but rather took time. Furthermore, stranger still, we could send the image to another DICOM device successfully, and from that device, send it over to the archive. Hence, there was nothing inherently wrong with the attribute encoding.

The problem turns out to not be what you can see from the log file, but what you *don't* see. What you don't see are group-length codes within the data-section of the C-Store message. Although DICOM clearly specifies group-length codes as optional, it turns out the archive device was buggy and would not accept images without group-length codes. A small test program was written that verified this to be true.

Invalid Encoding of Attributes

We conclude our look at DICOM communication problems by looking at a subtle problem that although does not currently disrupt transmission does throw an archive's database into chaos. In this instance, a new GE Lightspeed CT scanner sends objects to a PACS archive. The transmission works, and the images are stored in the archive, but they are not reconciled into the correct patient folders. If we examine a DICOM object created with this scanner, it becomes obvious why this occurs:

```
[-------DICOM Object: 4_9_921955079.v2--------]
Object: (0008, 0000, 4, UL, IdentifyingGroupLength) 492
Object: (0008, 0005, 10, CS, SpecificCharacterSet) "ISO_IR 100"
Object: (0008, 0008, 22, CS, ImageType) "ORIGINAL\PRIMARY\AXIAL"
Object: (0008, 0012, 8, DA, InstanceCreationDate) "19990319"
Object: (0008, 0013, 6, TM, InstanceCreationTime) "130527"
Object: (0008, 0016, 26, UI, SOPClassUID) "1.2.840.10008.5.1.4.1.1.2"
Object: (0008, 0018, 52, UI, SOPInstanceUID)
"1.2.840.113619.2.55.1.1762525482.1730.921862866.917"
Object: (0008, 0020, 8, DA, StudyDate) "19990319"
Object: (0008, 0021, 8, DA, SeriesDate) "19990319"
Object: (0008, 0022, 8, DA, AcquisitionDate) "19990319"
Object: (0008, 0023, 8, DA, ImageDate) "19990319"
Object: (0008, 0030, 6, TM, StudyTime) "124931"
Object: (0008, 0031, 6, TM, SeriesTime) "130105"
Object: (0008, 0032, 6, TM, AcquisitionTime) "130459"
Object: (0008, 0033, 6, TM, ImageTime) "130527"
Object: (0008, 0050, 0, SH, AccessionNumber) (null)
Object: (0008, 0060, 2, CS, Modality) "CT"
Object: (0008, 0070, 18, LO, Manufacturer) "GE MEDICAL SYSTEMS"
Object: (0008, 0080, 32, LO, InstitutionName) "UC Davis Health Sys
Ellison ACC "
Object: (0008, 0090, 6, PN, ReferringPhysicianName) "MURIN "
Object: (0008, 1010, 8, SH, StationName) "CTI3_OC0"
Object: (0008, 1030, 18, LO, StudyDescription) "COMBO 4 NECK/CHEST"
Object: (0008, 103e, 4, LO, SeriesDescription) "NECK"
Object: (0008, 1060, 6, PN, PhysicianReadingStudy) "STAFF "
Object: (0008, 1070, 2, PN, OperatorName) "KB"
Object: (0008, 1090, 16, LO, ManufacturerModelName) "LightSpeed QX/i "
Object: (0009, 0000, 4, LT, ?) "b"
Object: (0009, 0010, 12, LT, ?) "GEMS_IDEN_01"
Object: (0009, 1001, 14, Type Unknown) "CT_LIGHTSPEED "
Object: (0009, 1002, 4, Type Unknown) [860443715|33495443]
Object: (0009, 1004, 16, Type Unknown) "LightSpeed QX/i "
```

```
Object: (0009, 1027, 4, Type Unknown) [921848465|36f24a91]
Object: (0009, 10e3, 0, Type Unknown) (null)
Object: (0010, 0000, 4, UL, PatientGroupLength) 100
Object: (0010, 0010, 14, PN, PatientName) "LAST, FIRST"        (1)
Object: (0010, 0020, 8, LO, PatientID) "1467949 "
Object: (0010, 0030, 8, DA, PatientBirthDate) "19580308"
Object: (0010, 0040, 2, CS, PatientSex) "M "
Object: (0010, 1010, 4, AS, PatientAge) "041Y"
Object: (0010, 21b0, 16, LT, AdditionalPatientHistory) "TOXIC EXPOSURE
"
Object: (0018, 0000, 4, UL, AcquisitionGroupLength) 290
Object: (0018, 0010, 14, LO, ContrastBolusAgent) "150ML OMNI 300"
Object: (0018, 0022, 12, CS, ScanOptions) "HELICAL MODE"
Object: (0018, 0050, 8, DS, SliceThickness) "5.000000"
Object: (0018, 0060, 4, DS, KVP) "120 "
Object: (0018, 0090, 10, DS, DataCollectionDiameter) "250.000000"
Object: (0018, 1040, 2, LO, ContrastBolusRoute) "IV"
Object: (0018, 1100, 10, DS, ReconstructionDiameter) "146.000000"
Object: (0018, 1110, 10, DS, DistanceSourceToDetector) "949.075012"
Object: (0018, 1111, 10, DS, DistanceSourceToPatient) "541.000000"
Object: (0018, 1120, 8, DS, GantryDetectorTilt) "0.000000"
Object: (0018, 1130, 10, DS, TableHeight) "137.800003"
Object: (0018, 1140, 2, CS, RotationDirection) "CW"
Object: (0018, 1150, 4, IS, ExposureTime) "600 "
Object: (0018, 1151, 4, IS, XrayTubeCurrent) "250 "
Object: (0018, 1152, 4, IS, Exposure) "1500"
Object: (0018, 1170, 6, IS, GeneratorPower) "30000 "
Object: (0018, 1190, 8, DS, FocalSpot) "1.200000"
Object: (0018, 1210, 8, SH, ConvolutionKernel) "STANDARD"
Object: (0018, 5100, 4, CS, PatientPosition) "HFS "
Object: (0019, 0000, 4, US, ?) 286 0
Object: (0019, 0010, 12, IS, DistanceSourceToSourceSideCollimator)
"GEMS_ACQU_01"
Object: (0019, 1002, 4, Type Unknown) [912|390]
Object: (0019, 1003, 10, Type Unknown) "389.750000"
Object: (0019, 1004, 8, Type Unknown) "1.023900"
Object: (0019, 100f, 12, Type Unknown) "-163.300003 "
Object: (0019, 1011, 2, Type Unknown) (1|1)
Object: (0019, 1018, 2, Type Unknown) (8265|2049)
Object: (0019, 101a, 2, Type Unknown) (8275|2053)
Object: (0019, 1023, 10, Type Unknown) "11.250000 "
Object: (0019, 1024, 10, Type Unknown) "518.451233"
Object: (0019, 1025, 2, Type Unknown) (1|1)
Object: (0019, 1026, 4, Type Unknown) [357|165]
Object: (0019, 1027, 8, Type Unknown) "1.000000"
Object: (0019, 102c, 4, Type Unknown) [6146|1802]
Object: (0019, 102e, 8, Type Unknown) "0.000000"
Object: (0019, 102f, 10, Type Unknown) "984.000000"
Object: (0019, 1039, 2, Type Unknown) (4|4)
Object: (0019, 1042, 2, Type Unknown) (0|0)
Object: (0019, 1043, 2, Type Unknown) (0|0)
Object: (0019, 1047, 2, Type Unknown) (1|1)
```

```
Object: (0019, 1052, 2, Type Unknown) (1|1)
Object: (0020, 0000, 4, UL, ImageGroupLength) 362
Object: (0020, 000d, 52, UI, StudyInstanceUID)
"1.2.840.113619.2.55.1.1762525482.1730.921862866.736"
Object: (0020, 000e, 52, UI, SeriesInstanceUID)
"1.2.840.113619.2.55.1.1762525482.1730.921862866.877"
Object: (0020, 0010, 4, SH, StudyID) "403 "
Object: (0020, 0011, 2, IS, SeriesNumber) "4 "
Object: (0020, 0012, 2, IS, AcquisitionNumber) "1 "
Object: (0020, 0013, 2, IS, ImageNumber) "9 "
Object: (0020, 0032, 32, DS, ImagePositionPatient) "-69.099998\-
73.000000\-20.000000"
Object: (0020, 0037, 54, DS, ImageOrientationPatient)
"0.998047\0.000000\0.000000\0.000000\0.998047\0.000000 "
Object: (0020, 0052, 62, UI, FrameOfReferenceUID)
"1.2.840.113619.2.55.1.1762525482.1730.921862866.736.1633.0.11"
Object: (0020, 1040, 2, LO, PositionReferenceIndicator) "SN"
Object: (0020, 1041, 10, DS, SliceLocation) "-20.000000"
Object: (0021, 0000, 4, IS, ReconstructionNumber) "J"
Object: (0021, 0010, 12, DS, Zoom) "GEMS_RELA_01"
Object: (0021, 1003, 2, Type Unknown) (4|4)
Object: (0021, 1035, 2, Type Unknown) (0|0)
Object: (0021, 1091, 2, Type Unknown) (0|0)
Object: (0021, 1092, 4, Type Unknown) [0|0]
Object: (0021, 1093, 4, Type Unknown) [0|0]
Object: (0023, 0000, 4, Type Unknown) [36|24]
Object: (0023, 0010, 12, Type Unknown) "GEMS_STDY_01"
Object: (0023, 1070, 8, Type Unknown) 00(e Unknown)
[1158449302|450c8896]
Object: (0043, 1042, 4, Type Unknown) [0|0]
Object: (0043, 1043, 4, Type Unknown) [0|0]
Object: (0043, 1044, 4, Type Unknown) [1|1]
Object: (0043, 1045, 4, Type Unknown) [1|1]
Object: (0043, 1046, 4, Type Unknown) [3|3]
Object: (0043, 104d, 4, Type Unknown) [0|0]
Object: (0043, 104e, 4, Type Unknown) [1086836948|40c7d0d4]
Object: (0045, 0000, 4, Type Unknown) [296|128]
Object: (0045, 0010, 14, Type Unknown) "GEMS_HELIOS_01"
Object: (0045, 1001, 2, Type Unknown) (4|4)
Object: (0045, 1002, 4, Type Unknown) [3|3]
Object: (0045, 1003, 2, Type Unknown) (5|5)
Object: (0045, 1004, 2, Type Unknown) (29|1d)
Object: (0045, 1006, 14, Type Unknown) "OUT OF GANTRY "
Object: (0045, 1007, 4, Type Unknown) [0|0]
Object: (0045, 1008, 2, Type Unknown) (0|0)
Object: (0045, 1009, 2, Type Unknown) (230|e6)
Object: (0045, 100a, 4, Type Unknown) [0|0]
Object: (0045, 100b, 4, Type Unknown) [0|0]
Object: (0045, 100c, 2, Type Unknown) (0|0)
Object: (0045, 100d, 2, Type Unknown) (0|0)
Object: (0045, 100e, 4, Type Unknown) [0|0]
Object: (0045, 100f, 4, Type Unknown) [0|0]
```

```
Object: (0045, 1010, 2, Type Unknown) (0|0)
Object: (0045, 1011, 2, Type Unknown) (0|0)
Object: (0045, 1012, 2, Type Unknown) (0|0)
Object: (0045, 1013, 2, Type Unknown) (0|0)
Object: (0045, 1014, 2, Type Unknown) (0|0)
Object: (0045, 1015, 2, Type Unknown) (0|0)
Object: (0045, 1016, 2, Type Unknown) (0|0)
Object: (0045, 1017, 2, Type Unknown) (0|0)
Object: (0045, 1018, 2, Type Unknown) (0|0)
Object: (0045, 1021, 2, Type Unknown) (0|0)
Object: (0045, 1022, 2, Type Unknown) (0|0)
Object: (7fe0, 0000, 4, UL, PixelDataGroupLength) 524296
Object: (7fe0, 0010, 524288, OW, PixelData) f830  f830  f830  f830  f830
f830  f830  f830  f830  f830  f830
```

If you examine item one highlighted above, you will note that patient name is encoded as "LAST, FIRST." This is clearly a violation of the DICOM standard which indicates that this name should be encoded as "LAST^FIRST" in the ANSI standard format for names. This throws these images into the "to be reconciled" bin on the PACS archive and creates chaos for the database administrator. Furthermore if these images are not properly reconciled, it makes retrieving them at a later date difficult by name searching alone.

Conclusion

This paper introduces the notion of DICOM conformance versus DICOM compatibility. How these notions of DICOM capabilities affect real-world purchases is discussed. Three tools are discussed that can be used for both diagnosing DICOM network problems, as well as acceptance testing. Finally, a summary of several DICOM related transmission problems is demonstrated, which can serve as guidance for resolving your own DICOM-related connection errors.

PACS Brokers: The RIS and HIS

Richard L. Morin, Ph.D.
Dept. of Radiology
Mayo Clinic Jacksonville
4500 San Pablo Road
Jacksonville FL
(904) 953-8752 (V)
(904) 953-2894 (F)
morin@mayo.edu

Introduction

PACS is not an island. An electronic radiology practice can be characterized as demonstrated in Figure 1.

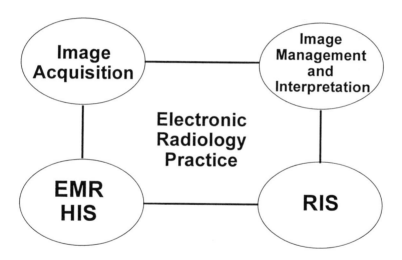

Figure 1. Diagram of the electronic radiology practice and its components.

Image acquisition combined with image management and interpretation are generally considered together as the Picture Archiving and Communication System (PACS). The communication of the PACS with the other electronic systems in the radiology department and institution is essential to fully realize the implementation and benefit afforded by automation. Even though the effect of PACS is far greater outside the radiology department, the function of PACS within the department can be markedly different depending upon the proper design and function of these interfaces. It is not often appreciated that the full realization of efficiency and expense reduction is dependent upon these active communications. In this chapter, we shall examine the nature and design of the interfaces that allow PACS to become a cornerstone of the electronic radiology practice. We shall proceed with this examination, using as a model the electronic radiology practice at Mayo Clinic Jacksonville. We shall begin with a brief description of the practice and motivation for the electronic radiology practice and proceed with the design and function of these interfaces, with particular attention to the clinical experience gained over the last few years.

Practice Description

The medical practice at Mayo Clinic Jacksonville is performed at two primary sites: Mayo Clinic Jacksonville and St. Luke's Hospital. In addition, there are nine additional Family Medicine practices, which refer patients to the primary locations, some of which provide radiology imaging. The staff consists of 215 physicians covering 23 medical and 12 surgical specialties. Approximately 200,000 patient visits occur each year. Approximately 40% of patients come from Jacksonville/North Eastern Florida area, 30% from the rest of Florida, 26% from the rest of the United States, and 4% from international locations. The practice at the hospital, in addition to Mayo physicians, consists of approximately 200 community physicians, who supply services in a facility licensed for 279 beds and provides all medical specialties except for pediatrics. The average length of hospital stay is approximately 5 days. The radiology practice consists of 19 radiologists, 2 fellows, and approximately 117 technologists and support personnel at both sites. The department volume is approximately 180,000 exams per year with approximately 120,000 being performed at the Clinic.

The motivation for the implementation of electronic imaging stemmed from a desire to increase efficiency while decreasing expenses. The previous screen-film based practice was very efficient from the referring physician's perspective. The chest examination (original film plus report) was available to the referring physician within 45 minutes of the completion of the exam within the department. Standard radiography exams were routinely available within 60 minutes and specialty exams [CT/MR/US/NM (computed tomography/magnetic resonance/ultrasound/nuclear medicine)] were available within 120 minutes. Upon special request, certain examinations such as orthopedic studies were available to the referring physician within 15 minutes following the completion of radiography. The major difficulty was that this efficiency was not without a cost. The largest component of that cost was the personnel expenses; on average eight different persons handled the film from the radiologic technologist to the referring physician. Hence, the motivating factor to implement this style of practice was to reduce cost and simultaneously to improve an already very efficient process.

Automated Radiology Practice

Prior to the electronic imaging practice design and implementation, the clinic had embarked upon a project to eliminate the paper medical record and its transportation throughout the facility and institutional system. This project was termed the Automated Clinical Practice (ACP). This identification was chosen to reflect the fact that the implementation of the electronic medical record was not meant to be simply an electronic facsimile of the paper medical record, but rather a change in practice involving physicians and nursing and desk staff, as well as all other support services. In order to parallel this activity and express the same sentiment, the implementation of the electronic imaging in radiology was termed the Automated Radiology Practice (ARP). The project was envisioned as demonstrated in Figure 2.

Electronic Imaging- Mayo Clinic Jacksonville

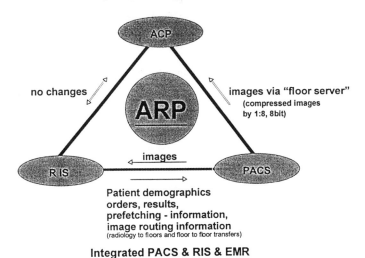

Figure 2. Diagram of the components and data interchange or the automated radiology practice.

The design and implementation of the PACS must be closely and intimately interconnected to the ACP as well as the already established Radiology Information System (RIS). As seen in Figure 2, there was envisioned a great deal of information flow between the RIS and PACS, as well as primary image flow between the ACP and PACS. The high level of interconnection already established between the ACP and RIS would continue without significant change (particularly from the user perspective).

A schematic representation of the PACS at Mayo Clinic Jacksonville is given in Figures 3 and 4.

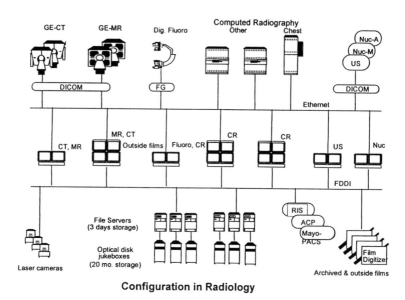

Figure 3. Configuration of the ARP within Radiology.

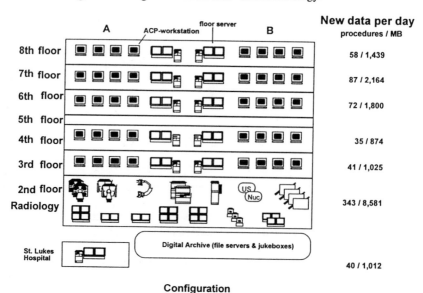

Figure 4. Configuration of the ARP at Mayo Clinic Jacksonville.

Figure 3 is a depiction of the devices and layout within the radiology department and Figure 4 demonstrates the activity and devices within the clinic building within the department (Figure 3). Conversion of radiography to Computed Radiography (CR) with interfacing to the institutional backbone was an essential first step. In addition, current existing systems for CT, MR, US, and NM were to be interfaced via the Digital Imaging and Communication in Medicine (DICOM) standard. The data would then be interpreted via workstations (rather than light boxes) with subsequent transmission to electronic archives on magnetic disk, optical disk, and tape. In addition, image distribution throughout the facility (Figure 4) was to be accomplished by transmission, upon completion, to servers on each clinical floor, which would then provide images to the ACP workstation in each physician examination room or office (approximately 500 workstations).

It is most important to point out that the single line connecting the RIS and ACP in Figures 3 and 4 actually became over 25 separate interfaces. A subset of these interfaces is presented in Table 1.

Table 1. Sample of ARP-RIS-ACP interfaces

Device/Systems	Function	Method
Fuji 9000 ↔ RIS	Demographics to CR Reader	HL7
Siemens Digiscan 2T ↔ RIS	Demographics to Chest CR System	HL7
SIENET ↔ RIS	Reports to SIENET for Display	HL7
SIENET ↔ RIS	Radiology Pre-Fetch List	HL7
SIENET ↔ RIS	Floor Server Pre-Fetch List	HL7
CERNER acp ↔ RIS ↔ SIENET	Images to ACP Workstation	HL7
Dejarnette ↔ RIS ↔ SIENET	Demographics to Digitizer	Bar-code
GE ↔ RIS	Demographics to CT	Bar-code
GE ↔ RIS	Demographics to MR	Bar-code
Acuson ↔ ALI ↔ RIS	Demographics to Ultrasound	Bar-code
ADAC ↔ RIS	Demographics to Nuclear Medicine	Bar-code

We shall now examine the information and image flow which necessitates the design and function of these interfaces.

Data and Image Flow

There are two primary types of image flow: (1) the production of new images and their distribution for interpretation and clinical review and (2) the retrieval of prior images to radiologists for interpretation/comparison and to clinicians for patient consultation and review.

To illustrate the data and image flow we shall examine the production and use of radiography images. An examination is ordered either through the ACP ordering software or through the RIS. An Accession Number is generated by the RIS. The order is sent by the RIS to a computer which can communicate with both the RIS and the ACP. This device is commonly called the PACS broker. Other terms for this device are: HIS broker or HIS/SCP (DICOM terminology). This device is capable of speaking a language which is a standard for hospital information systems (HIS) or electronic medical record systems (EMR) which is known as HL-7. This is an acronym for Health Level-7. In addition, the device can also communicate with the RIS either through HL-7 or DICOM. The necessity for such a brokering device is present at this time because the various HIS and RIS systems do not have embedded and inherent communication with one another. Upon patient arrival, the order is updated on the broker to capture any changes in demographics or examination information. The transfer of demographics and examination information occurs in one of two ways depending upon the imaging system. At discrete intervals (every 3 minutes) the digital chest system requests the work list from the HIS broker. The work list is presented at the acquisition console and the technologist selects the appropriate patient from the list. All patient and examination information is encoded in the image header. For radiography using CR plates, a query upon demand approach is used. Prior to performing the examination, the technologist uses the bar code reader on the CR image identification terminal (IDT) to read the Accession Number on the work sheet.

A query to the RIS is performed through the HIS broker and patient demographics are downloaded to the IDT. Following plate identification, the proper demographics are associated with each plate at the CR reader and coded into each image header. This interface is shown schematically in Figure 5.

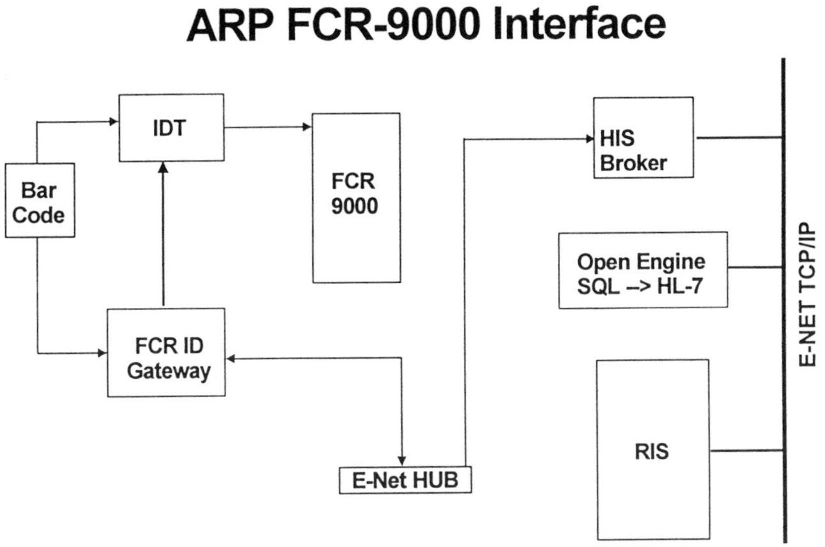

ARP FCR-9000 Interface

Figure 5. Diagram of the on-demand Computed Radiography interface.

Following interpretation, the ordering location within the RIS is utilized to direct image flow to the referring physician.

We shall now discuss the image flow for a radiography examination. As images are produced, they are transmitted via an image gateway to a quality control workstation. After the image folder is properly prepared, the folder is sent for interpretation to an electronic workstation. In addition, the images are sent to the electronic archives which verifies the header information with the available RIS orders. Additional information from the RIS order is then utilized to build the PACS database so that it is consistent with the RIS database. Upon notification that the examination has been interpreted, the archive forwards the image folder to the floor server for distribution to the physician's workstation.

The RIS interface, fundamentally, is the set of communication protocols for exchange of patient information between systems. Such exchange includes the transmittal of patient data to the acquisition device. The transmission of the RIS Accession Number to the acquisition device is crucial so that that number can be built into the DICOM header. This is important, because this provides a unique key to associate a set of images with the proper radiology report. If such a system is not utilized, individual databases must continually inform each other of changes in either the examination folder ID or the RIS examination ID. This feature is essential to the maintenance of both the integrity, as well as security, of both databases. Hence the fundamental reason for electronic interfaces between clinical systems, such as CR and the RIS, center on issues of data integrity and workflow. From an integrity standpoint there are two fundamental areas that are of importance: the PACS database and the accurate recording of patient demographics.

Database integrity has not been identified as a problem with film and human handling. The reason for this is that it is common for personnel to re-label films with the proper demographic information. This however, is a significant problem with electronic imaging systems and PACS. Some of the items which are important to properly record are: the patient's address, date of birth, indications of certain clinical aspects such as allergies. While these are important, perhaps even more important is the proper recording of the name and identification number. For instance, the names specified in Table 2 would all be interpreted by electronic systems as different individuals. Hence this would result in six distinct patient image examination folders which the electronic systems interpret as six individual persons.

Table 2. Configuration of patient names.

- Charles R. Morin
- Morin, Charles
- Charles Morin
- MORIN, CHARLES
- MORIN CHARLES
- MORIN, CHARLES R.

While this certainly is resolved by human intervention, the primary difficulty lies in automated retrieval for either prior exam review by radiologists or distribution to physician offices. In addition and in a similar fashion, the proper formatting of identification numbers as demonstrated in Table 3 is also crucial.

Table 3. Configuration of patient identification numbers.

- 3 965 619 4
- 3-965-619-4
- 03-965-619-4

Once again, these would represent three separate individuals even though the number is the same. Hence, both the format as well as the style is crucial for electronic retrieval of image data. In this case, acquisition is not the problem; retrieval is the problem. In studies conducted at Mayo Clinic Jacksonville, Mayo Clinic Rochester, and other sites, manual entry of these data resulted in 15-20% errors in the setting of CT and MR. For a department with 200 exams a day, this could result in 12-24 hours per week for database corrections in order to assure database integrity. In addition to issues of integrity, manual entry creates potential problems for workflow within the department. Either bottlenecks can occur at identification devices or many different individuals are involved in manual entry, leading to a promulgation of errors as described above. These features vary from practice to practice and are heavily dependent upon the workflow, either within the department in the conventional practice mode or the intended workflow as the practice implements electronic imaging.

Summary

The interface of PACS with other electronic systems in the institution is crucial, not only for the electronic practice of radiology but also the electronic practice of medicine.

Medical and Radiology practices cannot realize the benefits of automation without efficient and standardized interfaces. The presence of PACS brokers to accomplish this interfacing will be necessary until all systems can communicate utilizing standard procedures and techniques. Adherence to standards such as HL-7 and DICOM is essential for these devices to have continued use over their necessary lifetime.

Integrated Medical Imaging: Web Browsers and the Future of Image Distribution

Amit Mehta, M.D., Keith, J. Dreyer, D.O. Ph.D., James Thrall, M.D.
Department of Radiology, Massachusetts General Hospital,
Harvard Medical School, Boston, MA

Corresponding Author
Amit Mehta, M.D.
8 Whittier Place, 19D
Boston, MA
02114
mehta@helix.mgh.harvard.edu

Basic Concepts

Terminology

At the heart of electronic radiology are several systems. The first is the radiology information system or RIS. The RIS encompasses transcription, reporting, ordering, scheduling, and billing. Next is the PACS or Picture Archiving and Communication System. This encompasses acquisition, interpretation, and storage of images. Integration of the RIS and PACS involves synchronization of data, validation, interpretation, and results reporting. The success of these technologies coupled with the need for review of images and reports by referring physicians has brought about the need for electronic distribution of images. The images are transferred along networks using standard communication "languages."

Communication Protocols

The transfer of images to the referring physician along a network pathway involves several communication protocols not only to ensure the information requested is the information that is received but also to ensure security and conformance. The primary method of transfer within web-based enterprise image distribution solutions involves the use of the TCP/IP or transfer communication protocol/Internet protocol. The TCP/IP is a standard communications protocol used by the entire Internet. Specific to the healthcare industry exist further integrated protocols that serve essentially as layers on these existing communication methods and additionally ensure the maintenance of predefined standards. The first of these protocols named HL-7 (Health Level 7) standardizes and allows communication between devices dealing with patient data and/or Hospital Information Systems (HIS). With HL-7 compliance, a RIS is guaranteed to be able to communicate with the HIS and successfully transfer radiology report data to the integrated hospital information solution. Next, specific to the image market has been the development of the DICOM (Digital Imaging Communications in Medicine) v3.0 standard. This standard helps define certain conformance issues between radiology devices. DICOM compliance guarantees that acquisition, communication or display devices will be compliant with all other types of similar devices. Lastly, the use of the web as a solution for distribution of images through a medical enterprise involves the use of the Hyper-Text Transport Protocol or HTTP. HTTP is a protocol or language that dictates the method in which data are transferred over the world wide web (WWW). It defines the transfer and transport protocols that web browsers and pages use to distribute information.

Image Compression

If images are to be distributed throughout the enterprise using internal networks, the Internet or dedicated phone lines, image compression becomes a necessity. Compression allows reduction in large file sizes to more manageable sizes for transfer via networks. One bit is similar to a light switch with possible "ON" or "OFF", (0 or 1 values). One byte is equal to 8 bits with 256 values or '0000'0000' to '1111'1111'. One kilobyte (KB) is equal to 1,000 bytes, one megabyte (MB) is equal to 1,000 KB, one gigabyte (GB) is 1,000 MB, one terabyte (TB) 1,000 GBs, and one Petabyte (PB) 1,000 TB. The average radiology exam is approximately equal to 20 MB. With these large file sizes, compression allows the reduction of memory size of an image by efficiently re-representing redundancies.

Images are ultimately compressed to decrease storage requirements and decrease network transmission times. Compression is accomplished by a lossless (e.g., JPEG - 2 to 1) method where all data are preserved or lossy (e.g., Wavelet - 20 to 1) where all clinically relevant data are preserved. An example of lossless compression is as follows: if the number set 7777 6666 1111 0000 is lossless compressed, it will be stored as 74 64 14 04 which with the appropriate decompression algorithm will expand and display 7777 6666 1111 0000. In this particular example, the compression algorithm without losing any data has been able to reduce 16 bytes to 8 bytes. With a 2:1 compression ratio all data are preserved within half the storage space. An example of lossy compression is as follows: when the same number set, 7777 6666 1111 0000 is compressed using a lossy method, it will be stored as 78 18 and when expanded and displayed again with an appropriate decompression algorithm, the following will be displayed 7777 7777 1111 1111. A reduction from 16 bytes to 4 bytes is achieved representing a 4:1 compression ratio. In this situation, however, there is loss of the original data, which in certain instances are non-consequential. This method ultimately serves to employ only 1/4 of the storage space of the original data. With the average radiology examination using 20 MB of storage space, lossless compression such as JPEG with a 2:1 compression scheme results in each exam using more than 10 MB of storage space.

Utilizing lossy compression such as wavelet algorithms, the same study with a 20:1 compression ratio will use just greater than 1 MB per exam. There are emerging technologies such as JPEG 2000 that, when completed, will combine lossless techniques with lossy wavelets and achieve standards-based wavelet compression algorithms.

Integrated Medical Imaging

Introduction

With the installation of PACS into many institutions around the country, the task of distributing images to referring clinicians becomes apparent. In the legacy system, physicians who wished to view their images relied on obtaining their films from the radiology department's film library. Often, these films were used to communicate with patients, family members, and consultants for patient education and patient management. The advent of PACS has eliminated this classic workflow. Industry and leaders in the field of PACS have proposed solutions to solve this dilemma, but few have been implemented. The use of existing networks such as WWW has gained momentum and acceptance within the enterprise due to its ubiquity, portability, and cost. The Internet and its associated Intranets have increasingly become the technological basis for both image management within the radiology department and distribution to the enterprise. Despite the fact that current PACS installations have not been designed around WWW technology, they are able to add web-based solutions with relative ease. Central to the appeal of web-based distribution includes the ability for any physician, whether at home or within the clinical setting, to use a personal computer (PC) to become a virtual light box and to view radiological studies.

Visionaries in the PACS arena cited early in the process that the problem of image management and distribution should be approached from an enterprise point of view creating a parallel structure in radiology with respect to the development of the electronic medical record. The guiding principle in system design should be that images go wherever alphanumeric medical information goes; a task achieved by the flexible, integrated web-based solution.

Costs

The immediate benefit to utilizing the WWW as the basis for image viewing outside the radiology department stems from two further fundamentals. First, the cost of primary interpretation workstations on the current UNIX platform can reach up to $70,000 and thus are not a viable alternative for each referring physician who requires the review of their ordered examinations. Second, the current ubiquity of the desktop PC is a resource that obviates the need for custom-designed distribution channels. For example, the Partners HealthCare System Inc., Boston, the parent corporation of the

Massachusetts General Hospital (MGH) and the Brigham and Women's Hospital have approximately 30,000 PCs currently on the information systems network; utilizing this resource is at no cost to our radiology department.

There remains a confusion of pricing of web solutions within the industry. The alternatives range for the radiology department from cost per user, cost per view, cost per maximum users, cost per studies stored to one time cost in annual licensing. These pricing structures often create confusion when comparing products using a price performance analysis, but generally these systems result in five digit one-time capital expenses. These capital expenditures do include the hardware and software for the server component as well as the software for the clients.

Massachusetts General Hospital Experiences

Overview

We implemented a WWW-based solution in 1995 as we felt it was a solution that would allow the radiology department to automatically and cost-effectively maneuver radiology images to all clinicians. The growing popularity of the WWW over the past 5 years guaranteed a degree of familiarity with the client software and was, additionally, easy to use and to install with low support costs from the parent Information System (IS) group. The web server solution could layer onto the basic system coded access numbers, encryption, and virtual private network (VPN) technology that enabled the radiology group to appropriately ensure security and patient confidentiality regardless of the referring physician's Internet access provider.

We currently have four Web/Intranet Image Servers as the default DICOM destination of 13 digital modalities [6 CT (Computed Tomography), 4 MR (Magnetic Resonance), 2 CR (Computed Radiography), and 1 Digital Fluoro]. Each of the web servers is set up to include a Java-based interface to the RIS and a DICOM autorouter to storage devices as well as the PACS. Incorporated into the web-based solution is the use of a wavelet image compressor/decompressor that preserves compatibility with DICOM workstations and a server to distribute images throughout the enterprise.

These web servers enable sub-second, on-demand image distribution without any impact on our PACS resources as the servers contain their own archives. A 23 GB RAID solution in each web server caches over two months of studies. The use of wavelet compression preserves the 12-bit data and allows interactive window/level and magnification control within common web browsers such as Netscape Navigator and Microsoft Internet Explorer. An encoded auto-layout capability initially displays CR and digitized film at a reduced resolution to desktops with smaller screens while making full resolution available on demand.

Hardware

The Client

Clients that are able to utilize the HTTP protocol are available on nearly all platforms, not inclusive of Macintosh and PC. Despite the wide availability of the Internet, the implementations of JAVA virtual machines, protocols, and scripting language interpreters often render these platforms as unique as they were before the Internet. This becomes particularly true for radiology enterprise applications which involve medical image display.

The Server

Current web servers solutions predominately utilize the NT or UNIX operating systems. A variety of tools provided by the NT server pack simplify web deployment and are able to run on commonly available Intel-based machines. Our server hardware includes a 200 MHz Pentium Pro Microsoft Windows NT server with 64 MB RAM. The acquisition and compression times for typical studies using this hardware are as follows: CT (512×512×12 bit; 60 slices) 30 MB raw, 4 MB estimated compressed—4 minutes, MR (256×256×12 bit; 120 slices) 15 MB Raw, 3 MB estimated compressed—3 minutes and CR (2500 × 2000 × 12 bit; 3 images) 30 MB raw, 3 MB estimated compressed—4 minutes. Our archive size pending the above hardware assumes a typical 3 MB compressed study with 3 GB free disk space including 1000 studies. The communication and transfer of images is accomplished through an Intranet with 10 Mbps Ethernet TCP/IP and 28.8 kb/s modem lines for remote configuration.

Workflow

Access to the image servers is accessed, as mentioned, over the Web or Intranet using Netscape Navigator or Internet Explorer. The minimal client resides on conventionally available PCs, typically 100 MHz Pentium PCs with 24 MB of RAM, with either Microsoft Windows 95 or Microsoft Windows NT, a TCP/IP stack, and a PPP connection to an Internet/Intranet service provider. The wavelet compression method that our web server solution uses will transmit the full 12-bit data set to the Web browser allowing the user to interactively modify the window and level settings that specify the translation from 4096 to 256 shades of gray. This wavelet plug-in is available for most major platforms with other platforms accessing images using the JPEG format. The JPEG compression format, however, does not allow for interactive manipulation of the grayscale transformation with the system ultimately automatically making a guess for the proper window and level values based on an intelligent algorithm that utilizes the image data, the radiologic modality, and study description information.

Trends

Many institutions still regard the superiority of Sun hardware a necessity for the central components of PACS. Current trends are illustrating a migration of classic PACS client hardware as well as web componentry to cheaper, often faster, and commonly available Intel platforms. Custom monitors and display cards are proving to be too costly and troublesome with significant differences between consumer counterparts transparent.

On the other hand, web hardware remains an area of debate. The hardware surrounding web servers fall into the realm of the mission critical main PACS computers. As these servers best serve images through the institution, they are best likened to devices or computers which currently provide services such as printing, email, storage, and applications services. MGH's choices are commonplace throughout the medical arena and have seen the installation of over 200 NT servers that have been purchased for these purposes last year alone. With the understanding that with redundancy comes stability and with the observation that there has been and will be a rapid maturation of NT server features, the institution has been able to experience decreased costs of ownership with improving functionality.

Future Applications

Despite the ability to distribute images throughout the enterprise using web server technology, certain issues still exist. The necessity of providing copies of radiologic studies performed to the patient remains an issue in every radiology department due to disparate geographical locations and interdisciplinary communication. Conventionally, film libraries have provided original films, pending the recipient confirms their return.

With a fundamental goal of PACS to reduce costs, the costs associated with printing copies of films including film, envelopes, and printers as well as supplies necessitates an alternate format. Enabling the radiology department to provide images to patients in an electronic format obviates the need to print copies of films and ultimately saves in operating budgets. Secondly, an electronic distribution format provides the patient with a permanent copy of the radiologic studies performed in their healthcare management should they desire this information. Globally within the healthcare system, additional savings can be achieved as repeated radiologic studies can be eliminated.

The Personal Medical Record Solution

Utilizing a relatively inexpensive and commonly available storage format such as the compact disc recordable (CDR) format allows the complete elimination of film in the transfer of studies from one institution to another. The use of a browser on this CDR and a transfer engine application performing a DICOM transfer from one compliant PACS to another allows a permanent personal electronic imaging record for each patient. In the far future, alternate forms of media will decrease the cost of producing a copy of the electronic image. Currently, smart cards are becoming a reality in parts of the country as a test medium for other applications. Once a storage medium as such becomes commonly available, it is foreseeable that each patient will be able to download onto a card, copies of all imaging studies performed in their healthcare management. This record will be easily accessible by referring physicians with smart card readers, which may be installed in physician offices for alternate purposes such as obtaining the patient's medical record. In the nearer future, we will see the creation of high capacity, portable storage devices in the capacity ranges of 1.0 to 3.0 GB and should these storage media become commonplace, radiology departments can explore issues of using these as alternate forms of storage for patients requiring large amounts of studies in their record.

Conclusions

The benefits of web server utilization for image distribution stem from the ability to convert DICOM and RIS to Web protocols. The WWW allows the referring physician to receive text as well as images in a similar fashion without the need to learn different viewers to manipulate the data. In addition, this system allows the use of standard queries with familiar search-engine interface hyperlinks from electronic medical records systems and DICOM requests from radiologist workstations or PACS. The addition of web servers to our electronic imaging effort has allowed an added level of convenience and ease of use to our clinicians including those who are unfamiliar with our existing IS network. For the future, our web service will prove to be an essential component of our PACS as it is already accomplishing and will hopefully allow us to completely eliminate film in CT, MRI (Magnetic Resonance Imaging), and ultrasonography.

Image Compression and Encryption

Nicholas J. Hangiandreou, Ph.D.
Department of Diagnostic Radiology
Mayo Clinic
Rochester, Minnesota

Learning Objectives:

To understand the basic concepts of general transform-based image compression algorithms

To understand in greater detail the specific implementation of two common irreversible compression algorithms (JPEG & wavelet)

To understand the general effects of irreversible compression on radiological images, and factors affecting the acceptability of compressed images

To understand basic concepts pertaining to image encryption

Section I: Image Compression

Introduction

The use of image compression in the practice of diagnostic radiology has a long history and is in routine use in virtually every radiology department today. The compression referred to here includes that which occurs in several areas during image acquisition and printing:

1. Sonographer selecting a small subset of still images from the hundreds of dynamic images which are observed during an ultrasound examination; this subset of images will be viewed by the radiologist during primary interpretation

2. Radiologist selecting a small subset of fluoro-spot images from the hundreds observed during a GI fluoroscopy examination; this subset of images is used to document the case and support the radiologist's interpretation

3. Technologist printing CT or MR images using a only a limited number of 8-bit window settings, of the many that might be selected from the 12-bit reconstructed image data set

Other, similar examples undoubtedly exist. All of these situations involve original access to a large amount of image data, and the "compression" of the original data into a more limited data set that is used for primary interpretation of the examination. The compression used in these situations would have to be termed "irreversible" since there

369

are usually no means by which the "original" image data may be recovered. In spite of the irreversible data compression which occurs, the procedures described have been proven to provide a very high standard of radiological practice.

The introduction and growing use of digital imaging devices in radiology has provided another opportunity to implement image compression, by processing and re-coding the digital image data files themselves so that the resulting files are smaller than the originals. The two primary motivations for computational image compression are reduced image storage costs and reduced network transmission times. As the transition towards electronic radiology practice continues, radiology departments will need to grapple with the costs of digital storage of image data. In a large department (say performing 250,000 imaging examinations annually), approximately 7 terabytes (TB) of image data will be generated each year. The common desire to have all image data available on-line in an archive jukebox during the legally-dictated period of medical records retention (typically ~ 7 years) will required that ~50 TB of storage be available on the network. This problem is made even more challenging by recent trends toward acquiring more images per examination (e.g., in MR and CT). Many teleradiology applications require the transmission of image data over very slow wide area networks (WANs). Depending on the location of the sending site, it is possible that the analog telephone system and a modem is the only cost-effective WAN option available. Transmission of a single digital radiograph will require 30 minutes or longer, with current modem speeds and image data sizes. At best, an average case would require approximately 105 minutes. The problems of storage capacity and cost, and network transmission speed are encountered in combination when institutional electronic medical record systems are considered. In this case, there are more departments than radiology providing large volumes of image data which must be stored (e.g., cardiology, pathology, dermatology, and others), the number of potential users desiring access to these data range into the hundreds, and these systems are often deployed on low cost, low bandwidth standard networks (e.g., 10 megabit/second ethernet). Image compression potentially offers solutions to all of these problems.

Image compression algorithms may be broken into two general categories: reversible and irreversible. Reversible algorithms, as the name implies, are those in which the original image and the compressed image are identical on a bit-by-bit basis. No alteration of the original image data is produced. These algorithms are also sometimes referred to as lossless, or bit-preserving. Reduction in image size using reversible algorithms is achieved by removing redundancy that naturally exists in the image data due to spatial, spectral or temporal correlations between pixels. The redundancy present in images can be analyzed using the tools of information theory (e.g., the definition of entropy as a measure of information content) [Rabbani et al. 1991]. Common reversible image compression algorithms include run-length encoding, differential pulse code modulation (DPCM), Huffman encoding, and arithmetic encoding [Rabanni et al. 1991]. In general, reversible techniques result in compression ratios (i.e., the ratio of the original image size to the compressed image size) ranging between 2:1 and 3:1. To effectively solve image data management problems in radiology (see for example the teleradiology problem discussed above) larger compression ratios are often required.

Larger compression ratios are provided by the second category, irreversible compression, which is also known as "lossy" compression. The larger compression ratios come at the price of alterations in the compressed image data as compared to the original image data. These alterations are introduced into the image data by the algorithm to increase the amount of redundancy in the resulting data set, which is then compressed using reversible methods. These alterations may be so subtle that the original and compressed images cannot be distinguished from one another by human observers, in which case the compression is referred to as "visually lossless." In other instances, to achieve higher compression ratios, images may be compressed such that alterations may be detected by the observer, but are not severe enough to degrade the practical diagnostic utility of the image. This situation is referred to as "diagnostically lossless." In certain situations, an irreversibly compressed image may be preferred by observers to the original image. These instances underscore the misleading connotations that accompany the use of the term "lossy," and in this article, the terms "irreversible" and "reversible" will be used.

Because of the lack of data alteration implicit in reversible compression techniques, these should be always employed for data storage and transmission wherever feasible, unless irreversible methods are chosen. The rest of this manuscript will focus primarily on irreversible compression methods as applied to single frame, grayscale, radiological images. General principles regarding irreversible compression will be discussed, and two common irreversible compression algorithms, JPEG and wavelet, will be detailed. From this point on in the article, the term "compression" should be interpreted to mean "irreversible compression" unless otherwise specified.

Basic Concepts

In general, compression algorithms follow three basic steps:

1. Image transformation

2. Quantization

3. Encoding

Image transformation is performed using one of a variety of basis function decompositions. The image data are transformed into a spectral domain defined by the particular basis function set. Transformation is performed in an effort to redistribute the image signal energy into a small number of spectral coefficients, thus making the data set inherently more compressible. Signal energy is defined as the magnitude of the transform coefficients or pixels values of the data in the spectral domain. Two common transformations used in compression algorithms are the discrete cosine transform (DCT; closely related to the Fourier transform), and the wavelet transform. Figure

1 shows an original head MR image, along with Fourier and wavelet transforms. Figure 2 shows histograms for the three representations of the data. It is evident in the transform images and the histograms that the transform step does indeed concentrate the image data into a smaller range of pixel values. The wavelet transform is especially efficient in mapping the original image pixel values into a small number of pixel values at either end of the pixel value range. The transform images illustrate that the image information is primarily focused in the lowest spatial frequency spectral components (in the center of the Fourier transform, and the upper left corner of the wavelet transform). The transformation step does not produce any data compression in and of itself, and is fully reversible.

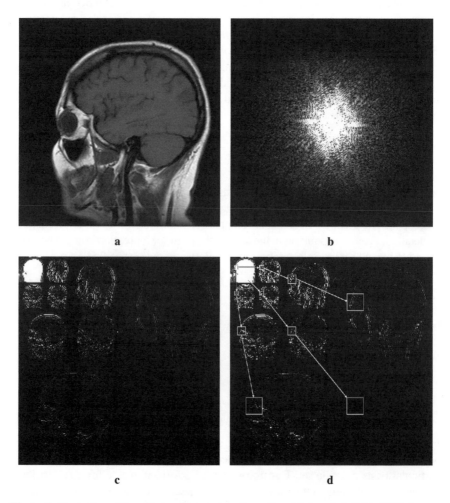

Figure 1. Illustration of the effects of image transformation. (a) An original head MR image. The images in (b) and (c) show the results of discrete Fourier transformation, and a three level wavelet transformation, respectively. The wavelet transform image has been enhanced to better display data in the high-frequency subbands. (d) An illustration of the hierarchical tree or pyramid organization of the wavelet transform data.

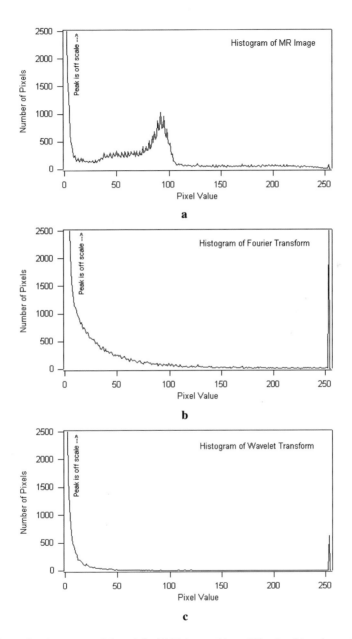

Figure 2. Histograms of the original MR image (a), and Fourier (b) and wavelet (c) transform images shown in Figure 1.

As previously mentioned, the discrete cosine transform is very closely related to the familiar discrete Fourier transform (DFT). The DCT is used in compression work because it does not exhibit the same types of frequency space discontinuities inherent in the DFT which may give rise to problematic high-frequency transform coefficients. Also, the DCT results in real, as opposed to complex, spectral coefficients, which simplifies implementation of the algorithm. Two dimensional (2D) discrete cosine transforms are obtained by serial applications of 1D DCT along orthogonal directions (i.e., the discrete cosine transform is separable).

The term "wavelet transform" is a misleading one, in that it implies that there is a single unique set of wavelet basis functions similar to the role of the sine and cosine functions in Fourier transform theory. This is not the case, as there are numerous "families" of wavelet basis functions that may be used in compression applications [Schomer et al. 1998, Harpen 1998]. Wavelet transformation is perhaps most easily understood as an iterative filtering process, in which a specific pair of complementary filter functions (one high-pass, the other low-pass) are used to split a signal into low- and high-frequency components. The filter outputs are then down-sampled by a factor of 2, resulting in an identical number of total data elements between the two filter outputs as was present in the original input signal. The same filter pair (i.e., with identical relative band-pass characteristics) is then applied to the low-pass result from the previous stage. This process is shown in Figure 3 for a 1D signal. The subscript on the high- and low-frequency components is decremented with successive filtration stages, and correlates qualitatively with spatial frequency (i.e., higher stage indices indicate higher spatial frequency information).

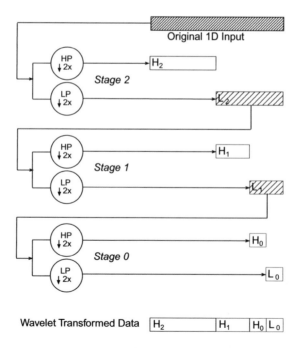

Figure 3. Schematic diagram illustrating the filtration steps corresponding to a one dimensional wavelet transformation. The shaded data elements are fed into the following filter stage, while the open data elements are retained and contribute directly to the final wavelet transformed 1D data set.

Two dimensional wavelet transformation may be obtained as for the 2D DCT, by successively applying 1D transforms in orthogonal directions. Each 2D filter step results in a set of spectral coefficients with four distinct regions representing (1) high-frequency x-direction information & high-frequency y-direction information (HH), (2) high-frequency x-direction information & low-frequency y-direction information (HL), (3) low-frequency x-direction information & high-frequency y-direction information (LH), and (4) low-frequency x-direction information & low-frequency y-direction information (LL). In the next step of the process, the same filter pair is applied to the LL result from the previous stage. An example of a three-stage 2D wavelet transformation process is illustrated in Figure 4.

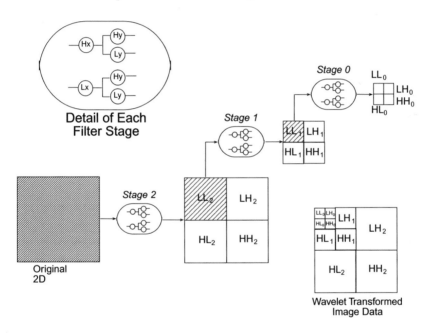

Figure 4. Schematic diagram illustrating the filtration steps corresponding to a two dimensional wavelet transformation. As for the 1D wavelet transform, the shaded data elements are fed into the following filter stage, while the open data elements are retained and contribute directly to the final wavelet transformed 2D data set.

Figure 1(c) shows an example of a wavelet transformed head MR image. Each labeled region in the transform data set (e.g., LH_1) is called a subband. Examination of this transformed image supports the data organization discussed above. The LH components tend to emphasize edges (high-frequency information) perpendicular to the x-direction, while the HL components emphasize edges perpendicular to the y-direction. The level of spatial detail in the image tends to decrease as the stage index gets smaller. It is evident in the transform image that considerable spatial information is preserved by the wavelet transform. This is in stark contrast to the discrete cosine transform shown in Figure 1(b). Whereas the cosine basis functions of the DCT are perfectly localized in frequency and completely unlocalized in spatial position, wavelet basis functions tend to be partially localized in both frequency and space. If a square group of pixels in the LL_0 subband is identified and then correlated with pixels in other subbands that correspond to the same spatial location in the original image, a hierarchical tree or pyramid structure is produced, as shown in Figure 1(d). The hierarchical levels correspond to filter stages, groups of subbands, and qualitative spatial frequency content. The larger number of associated pixels in each successive level of the hierarchy reflects the 2x down-sampling that occurs in each filter stage.

The previous discussion suggests that a particular wavelet transformation can be specified by indicating the choice of filter functions, and the number of iterative filtration steps that are utilized. The wavelet algorithm used in this work is one based on the 9tap/7tap biorthogonal filter functions described in [Antonini et al. 1992], with five filter stages. This algorithm also includes other refinements [Said et al. 1993, Said et al. 1996, Manduca et al. 1996].

Quantization of the spectral coefficients follows the image transformation step. The goal of this step is to reduce the precision of the set of spectral coefficients in order to increase redundancy and make the coefficient set amenable to very efficient encoding using reversible techniques (which occurs in the final step of the irreversible compression process). This reduction in precision is imposed while maintaining the fidelity of the compressed image as much as possible. This is the single step of the compression process that introduces irreversible alteration of the image data. Quantization produces a set of spectral coefficients that is an approximation of the original coefficient set. The accuracy of the approximation is typically best for low spatial frequency components (and will be 100% for many coefficients), since these coefficients contain the majority of the signal energy as seen in Figures 1(b) and 1(c). Accuracy typically decreases for higher spatial frequency components, and may be 0% for many of the highest frequency coefficients. The overall level of quantization during the compression process is generally selectable. Higher levels of quantization produce larger compression ratios and larger discrepancies between the compressed and original images.

One common approach to quantization involves dividing individual spectral coefficients by predetermined quantization factors and rounding the results to integer values. The full set of reduced-precision coefficients are then efficiently encoded and written to the compressed image file. This approach focuses on altering the precision of individual coefficients. A second approach to quantization is one in which the spectral coefficients are ordered according to their role in maintaining the fidelity of the compressed image, regardless of spatial frequency. Quantization is then completed by truncating this list at some point such that the "most important" coefficients are retained with greatest precision and accuracy, while the remaining coefficients are discarded (i.e., are maintained with 0% accuracy). The "importance" of the coefficients is commonly determined by assessing their relative magnitudes. This approach to quantization focuses primarily on altering the precision of the coefficient set as a whole as opposed to individual specific coefficients, although some schemes will initially send only approximations to important coefficients and then progressively refine the accuracy of the approximation as more data are written to the compressed image file.

In some applications, the full coefficient list may be stored, but when the image is requested only the smallest number of coefficients are provided, corresponding to the requested compression ratio, transmission time, or fidelity level of the compressed image. If all of the original coefficients are provided, the original image is perfectly reproduced upon decompression. Compression algorithms providing this type of progressive storage or transmission are often referred to as "embedded." The two approaches to quantization discussed above may be used alone or in combination; although if both approaches are used, decompression of the embedded compressed image will never produce the original image.

Encoding of the quantized spectral coefficients is the final step of the irreversible compression process. This step, like the image transformation step, is also fully reversible and does not introduce any alteration into the image data. Common encoding algorithms used in irreversible image compression applications include run-length encoding, DPCM, Huffman encoding, and arithmetic encoding. These algorithms may also be applied without quantization to provide reversibly compressed data sets. The basic strategies employed in the encoding step are well-illustrated by the common run-length and Huffman encoding schemes [Huang 1996].

Run-length encoding, as the name implies, exploits sequences of neighboring pixels in image lines or columns (or along other paths through image space) that are found to have the same value. These sequences are encoded using three quantities: (1) a code value signaling that the following two data values in the file encode a run; (2) the length of the run; and (3) the value of the pixels in the run. The encoding process proceeds by considering pixels in a predetermined order through the image (e.g., row by row), and either determining and storing the run codes if a run is encountered, or storing the individual pixel values when no runs are present. Run-length encoding may alternatively be applied to difference images in which long runs of "0"s may exist (assuming a high degree of correlation between neighboring pixels in the original image).

Huffman encoding attempts to reduce the size of the encoded data file by replacing the original pixel values with bit sequences of non-uniform length. The pixel values in the original image to be encoded typically are all represented by the same number of bits (e.g., 8 bits per pixel). The Huffman encoding process computes the histogram of the image and determines the frequency of occurrence of each pixel value. The most frequently occurring pixel values will be encoded with the codes having fewest bits, while those occurring least frequently will be encoded using more bits. In an image with 3 bits per pixel, a list of all possible original pixel values is

$$000, 001, 010, 011, 100, 101, 110, 111,$$

and one list of corresponding Huffman codes might be

$$0, 111, 110, 100, 1011, 10101, 101001, 101000.$$

Note that a Huffman code value may be as short as a single bit in length, and that no code value begins with a sequence of bits equivalent to a complete shorter code value. The particular set of optimum Huffman code values for an image will be a function of the particular frequencies of occurrence of the original pixel values. Once the set of Huffman code values are determined, the encoding process proceeds by replacing the original pixel values by the corresponding Huffman code values, and then storing the new pixel values row- and column-wise (or along another predetermined path through the image).

The approach described in the above section on quantization for producing an embedded compressed image requires a more sophisticated encoding method than simple run-length or Huffman encoding. This is because the spectral coefficients are ordered according to their importance in providing a high-fidelity compressed image, independent of their position in the frequency space pixel matrix. These important coefficients may have arbitrary positions in frequency space and so must be encoded along with positional information. (The simple run-length and Huffman encoding schemes described above assume that spectral coefficients are encoded and stored according to a predefined trajectory through frequency space.) Embedded zero tree encoding [Shapiro 1993] is a common approach which exploits the hierarchical structure of the wavelet transform to encode data in an embedded manner. This approach has been modified by Said and Pearlman [Said et al. 1993, Said et al. 1996] and these modifications have been incorporated into the particular implementation of wavelet compression used at Mayo Clinic over the past several years [Manduca et al. 1996, Savcenko et al. 1998, Erickson et al. 1998]. This algorithm is called set partitioning in hierarchical trees (SPIHT) wavelet compression. It was also used to produced all the examples of wavelet compression in this manuscript. Other encoding schemes have been suggested which facilitate progressive decompression to a desired matrix size, and which produce optimum image quality at only a particular region of interest in the decompressed image [Boliek et al. 1997].

Two Common Compression Algorithms

Currently, the most common irreversible compression algorithms in use for medical image compression are JPEG and wavelet-based methods. In this section, details of the operation of these algorithms will be provided (using the Mayo SPIHT algorithm as a particular example of wavelet compression). A more in-depth treatment of the JPEG algorithm can be found in references [Rabanni et al. 1991, Wallace 1991], while references [Said et al. 1993, Said et al. 1996, Manduca et al. 1996] detail the SPIHT wavelet algorithm more completely.

The JPEG compression algorithm was named for the standards committee that established it, the Joint Photographic Experts Group. It can be used with both color and grayscale images. It is not a single unique algorithm, in that there are several supported variations that can be implemented. This discussion will focus on the baseline JPEG implementation. It follows the general steps, outlined above, of image transformation, quantization, and encoding.

Image transformation utilizes the discrete cosine transform, but the DCT is applied to individual 8 × 8 pixel blocks instead of to the whole image, as shown in Figure 5. (Application of the DCT to the whole image is sometimes referred to as full-frame DCT, and there have been compression algorithms reported based on this full-frame DCT transformation.) The use of small blocks allows either more rapid transformation by addressing all blocks simultaneously in parallel, or implementation of the algorithm with minimal computer memory requirements.

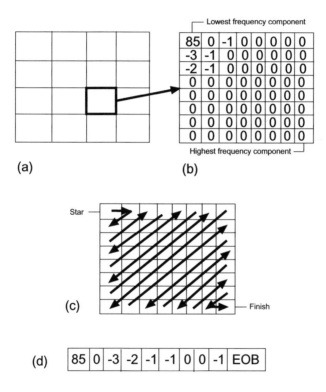

(a) (b)

(c)

(d)

Figure 5. Schematic diagram of the JPEG compression algorithm. (a) Schematic illustration of a 32 × 32 pixel image segmented into 8 × 8 pixel blocks. (b) The results of the DCT and quantization steps for one of the blocks. The order in which the spectral coefficients are encoded is shown in (c). The resulting spectral data sequence for the block following simple run-length encoding is shown in (d). "EOB" stands for "end of block" and indicates that all of the remaining quantized coefficients are equal to zero.

Quantization is performed using an 8 × 8 table of divisors (the quantization table, q_{ij}, where i and j specify the location in the 8 × 8 table), and a quality factor (Q) that is specified by the user for each image to be compressed. Each element in the DCT matrix is quantized in a manner similar to

$$DCT_{ij}' = NINT(Q * DCT_{ij} / q_{ij}),\qquad(1)$$

where DCTij' is the quantized approximation to the original DCT coefficient, DCTij, and NINT indicates the nearest integer operation. The elements of the quantization table are typically small for low frequency positions (near i=j=0) and larger for high-frequency positions (near i=j=8), resulting in more accurate DCT coefficient estimation for low frequency components. The quality factor typically ranges between 1 and 100, with higher values producing more accurate overall DCT coefficient estimation. In the example shown in Figure 5, it is evident that many of the highest frequency DCT coefficients have been quantized to zero.

Encoding is performed by first ordering the quantized DCT coefficients according to a zigzag pattern through frequency space. This pattern is illustrated in Figure 5. This pattern exploits the fact that the lower frequency components are generally larger than the higher frequency components, and many of the higher frequency quantized coefficients are zero. The components are ordered so that they can be efficiently represented by run length methods. The ordered coefficients from all of the 8×8 blocks are then efficiently encoded using a combination of run length and Huffman encoding schemes. The manner in which the JPEG quantization and encoding are performed shows that a user cannot specify a desired compression ratio (R), but can only specify a desired quality factor, Q. The quality factor and resulting compression ratio are inversely related (i.e., as Q decreases, R increases, and vice versa), but a desired compression ratio for any particular image can only be obtained via trial and error.

The wavelet compression technique described here is the Mayo implementation of the SPIHT wavelet algorithm, as described in references [Manduca et al. 1996, Erickson et al. 1998].

Image transformation utilizes the wavelet transform defined by the 9tap/7tap biorthogonal filters described in [Antonini et al. 1992]. An example of a MR image wavelet-transformed using three stages of these filters is shown in Figure 1(c).

Quantization and encoding are both performed by application of the SPIHT (set partitioning in hierarchical trees) algorithm as described in references [Said et al. 1993, Said et al. 1996. Manduca et al. 1996]. Quantization is not performed by simple division and rounding of the wavelet transform coefficients as was done for JPEG. The SPIHT algorithm proceeds by identifying the coefficients that are most important in maintaining the fidelity of the compressed image by comparing their magnitudes to a series of thresholds which start large and decrease in successive steps. The thresholds are all of the form 2^n, so the thresholding operations can be understood as examining successive bit-planes of the wavelet transformed data, starting with the most significant bit plane. At each threshold level, the coefficients with values exceeding the threshold are identified, and the non-zero bits are encoded and written to the compressed data file. In this manner, as the threshold is lowered, data are stored which allow the approximations of all important coefficients to be refined and more and more closely approximate the original wavelet coefficient. Coefficient refinement is essentially accomplished by storing bits from successively lower and lower bit-planes. It is evident in Figure 1(c) that the magnitudes of lower frequency wavelet coefficients tend to be larger than for coefficients corresponding to higher spatial frequencies. This causes the lower frequency information to be preferentially preserved by the SPIHT algorithm at the expense of the lower frequency information. It is also evident in Figure 1(d) that there is a high degree of correlation of important wavelet coefficients along trees between the subbands. This correlation is exploited to allow efficient encoding of the refinement data in a manner allowing determination of the locations in the transform matrix corresponding to the specific bits of refinement information. The sequence of bits produced by the SPIHT algorithm may also be processed by an arithmetic encoder, but this option is not usually enabled as little compression of the SPIHT bit stream is generally realized. The SPIHT algorithm continues writing data to the compressed image file until the requested compression ratio (i.e., size of the compressed image file) is achieved, at which point the algorithm is halted and the file closed. The desired compression ratio can thus be delivered with high accuracy. The resulting decompressed image is very nearly optimized with respect to root-mean-square (RMS) error per compressed file size.

An alternative application of the SPIHT wavelet compression algorithm is to run the algorithm until all bit planes of the transform data set have been stored. In this case the resulting file represents a reversibly compressed image with modest compression ratio, on the order of 23:1. When the image is requested, decompression of this file can be halted at any point resulting in delivery of an irreversibly compressed image to the requester. This mode of operation may be useful in matching the fidelity of the decompressed image to the task, network bandwidth and desired transmission time, or available display quality.

Alterations in Image Quality Caused by Compression

The two main types of image data alteration caused by irreversible compression algorithms are blurring and artifacts. This is generally true for all irreversible compression algorithms. The blurring results from the fact that quantization is preferentially targeted towards the high spatial frequency components in the image. It is these spectral components which are responsible for the depiction of small structures and edges in the image signal. At very low compression ratios (on the order of 5:1), no degradation of the image signal may result if the signal happens to contains no (or little) energy in the highest spatial frequency components. Since image noise generally contains appreciable contributions from all spatial frequency components, the noise will tend to be reduced, even at the lowest compression ratios. An image with little high-frequency content irreversibly compressed to a very small ratio may be judged by observers to be superior to the original image due to this noise reduction effect [Erickson et al. 1997-1]. As the compression ratio is increased, due to the relative weakness of higher spatial frequency components with respect to the overall image signal, subtle signal alterations will occur but will not be readily discernible. The images produced at these (and lower) compression ratios are considered to be visually lossless. Figures 6(b) and 6(c) are examples of MR images compressed with the SPIHT wavelet algorithm to compression ratios of 5:1 and 10:1, respectively. These compressed images are both considered to be visually lossless. The corresponding difference images in Figure 6 (produced in each case by subtracting the compressed image from the original) support this assessment. (The subtle noise difference observed in the image background is caused by differences in the nature of the noise in the background of the uncompressed MR image.) Figure 6(f) shows only noise, and no structured signal, while Figure 6(g) is only beginning to demonstrate subtle correlation.

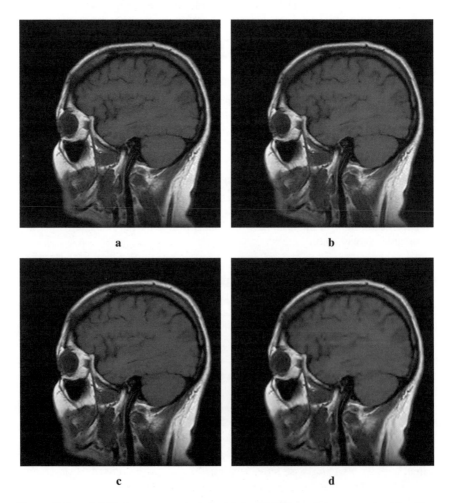

Figure 6. Sample MR images compressed with the SPIHT wavelet compression algorithm with compression ratios of (a) 1:1 = original image, (b) 5:1, (c) 10:1, (d) 20:1, and (e) 40:1. The difference images in (f), (g), (h), and (i) have all been enhanced to the same degree, and correspond to compression ratios of 5:1, 10:1, 20:1, and 40:1 respectively.

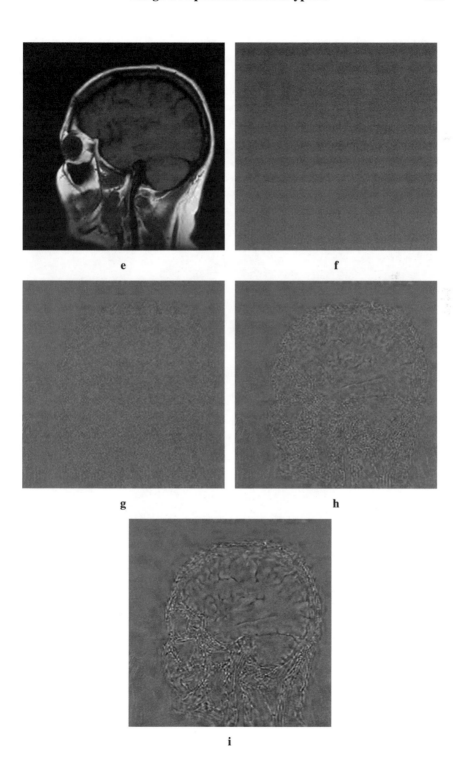

e

f

g

h

i

As the compression ratio is increased, spectral components corresponding to progressively lower spatial frequencies will be altered by the quantization, and blurring of the image will become evident. This is shown in Figures 6(d) and 6(e). Although the blurring effect is common to all irreversible compression algorithms, the compression ratio at which the blurring becomes evident will depend on the details of the specific algorithm as well as the frequency distribution of the signal energy.

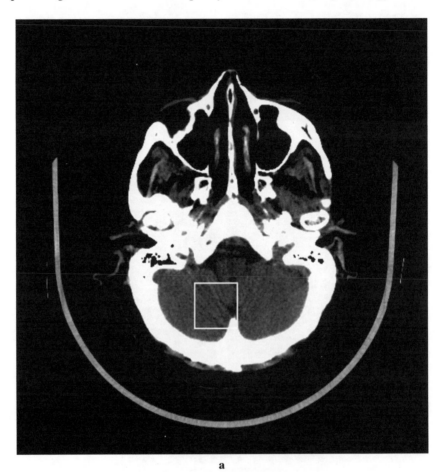

a

Figure 7. Artifacts caused by irreversible compression. An original CT image and a detail from this image are shown in (a) and (b). A detail from the CT image after compression with the SPIHT wavelet algorithm at 20:1 is shown in (c). A schematic diagram of the general shape of a wavelet basis function is shown in (d). A detail of the CT image after compression with the JPEG algorithm to approximately 20:1 (quality factor = 20) is shown in (e).

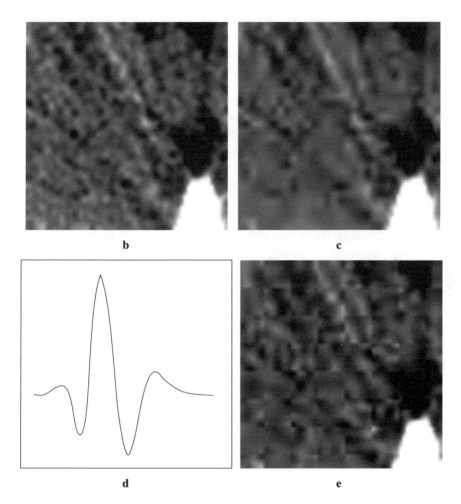

b

c

d

e

As the compression ratio is further increased, blurring becomes more severe and artifacts are introduced into the image. The artifacts are a strong function of the particular compression algorithm being used. Artifacts characteristic of the wavelet algorithm tend to have a grainy appearance with alternating regions of hyper- and hypo-intense signal. These artifacts may be either vertically or horizontally oriented. Examples may be seen in Figure 6(d), and also in Figure 7(c). The artifact pattern correlates with the general shape of the wavelet basis functions shown in Figure 7(d) [Schomer et al. 1998, Harpen 1998]. This observation suggests that these artifacts become appreciable when the quantization process removes all but one or two primary wavelet components from a region, in which case the shapes of these individual basis function components become visible.

Two artifacts characteristic of the JPEG algorithm are shown in Figure 7(e). The most obvious is the so-called "blocking" artifact caused by the division of the image into 8×8 pixel blocks prior to discrete cosine transformation. These blocks are quantized independently of one another and so there is no guarantee of pixel value continuity from block-to-block in the compressed image. At high quantization levels (low quality factors), these discontinuities are observed as artifacts. The second artifact is very similar in nature to the wavelet artifact discussed above. At high quantization levels only one or two primary spectral components in a block of pixels may be retained, causing the shapes of these basis functions to become visible. In the case of JPEG utilizing the DCT, the basis functions are cosines, and these appear in the image as alternating bands of hyper- and hypo-intense signals extending across the full width of the blocks.

Factors Affecting the Acceptability of Compressed Images

There are several key factors which affect the acceptability of irreversibly compressed images.

Compression ratio. As discussed in the previous section and demonstrated in Figure 6, the compression ratio is highly correlated with the quality of the compressed image. This is due to the fact that as the compression ratio increases, so does the level of quantization and data alteration. The end result is increased blurring and incidence of artifacts as the compression ratio is increased.

Compression algorithm. As discussed in the previous section and demonstrated in Figure 7, the particular compression algorithm will strongly influence the general appearance and the specific artifacts present in the compressed image. In general, we have found that wavelet methods are superior to JPEG in that they provide higher quality images at the same compression ratio [Manduca et al. 1996, Manduca 1993]. This is due primarily to the presence of JPEG blocking artifacts at higher compression ratios and the inability of the JPEG algorithm to exploit correlations in the image over ranges exceeding 8×8 pixels. However, in some special circumstances, we have found that JPEG appears to out-perform the SPIHT wavelet algorithm [Persons et al. 1999].

Imaging modality. Another factor that must be considered is the imaging modality used to create the images to be compressed. Because quantization tends to preferentially alter image signal components at high spatial frequencies, images with less signal information (or signal energy) in the high spatial frequency components (and thus more signal energy in the low-frequency components) will tend to be more highly compressible (i.e., can be compressed to higher ratios while maintaining acceptable image quality). In a study of ten images each from four different imaging modalities, variations were demonstrated in the fractional amount of image energy in low and high-frequency components [Erickson et al. 1998]. Digitized chest x-rays contained $99\pm2\%$ of their image energy in the lowest frequency wavelet subband. Corresponding measurements for CT, MR and ultrasound were $94\pm5\%$, $77\pm15\%$, and $74\pm15\%$, respectively. In our general experience, the SPIHT wavelet algorithm can be used to acceptably compress digitized chest x-rays, CT images, MR images and ultrasound images to ratios of approximately 20-40:1, 15:1, 10-12:1, and 10-12:1, respectively. The percentage of energy in the lowest frequency subband appears to be a good indicator of image compressibility.

Anatomy and Pathology. The specific structures in the field-of-view also have a bearing on the acceptability of the compressed image. The reasons for this also lie in the preferential alteration of high-frequency signal components by the quantization process, and the frequency content of the structures of interest. Figures 8 and 9 illustrate these concepts for computed radiographs showing a subtle lung nodule and the trabecular pattern in the bones of the hand. As shown in Figure 8, the nodule is quite robust with respect to the effects of compression, and is plainly seen in the 80:1 compressed image. This is because its subtlety is due to low contrast and not small size. Its edges are diffuse, and it consists primarily of relatively low-frequency spectral components which are well-preserved by the quantization algorithm, even at high compression ratios. The bone trabeculae are much finer structures and include significant high-frequency components. As a result, they begin to degrade at lower compression ratios. As seen in Figure 9, the structure of the bone is well preserved at 20:1, exhibits some blurring at 40:1, and is considerably blurred at 80:1.

Operations causing high-frequency weighting. This is actually a category of factors which includes any processing or alteration to the image which tends to increase the fraction of image signal energy in the high-frequency components. One example is the inclusion of alphanumeric text in ultrasound images [Persons et al. 1999]. Other examples include edge enhancement post-processing of computed radiographs, and detail or bone reconstruction algorithms in CT. For the same reasons explained above, all of these factors which tend to heavily weight the high-frequency components of the signal energy will also tend to decrease image compressibility.

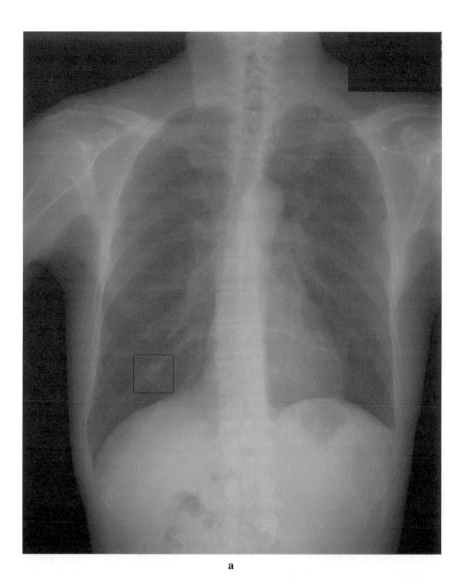

a

Figure 8. Effects of irreversible compression on the visibility of a subtle lung nodule in a computed radiograph. The original, uncompressed image is shown in (a), and a region of interest containing the nodule is indicated. A detail of the uncompressed image is shown in (b). The detail images in (c), (d) and (e) were obtained from images compressed with the SPIHT wavelet algorithm at compression ratios of 20:1, 40:1 and 80:1, respectively.

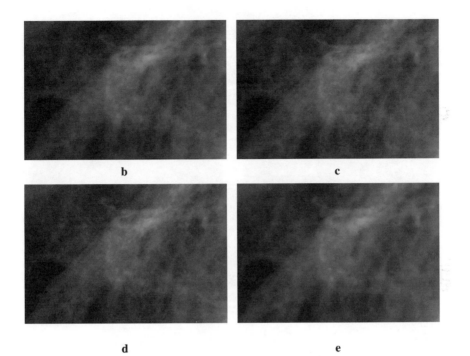

b

c

d

e

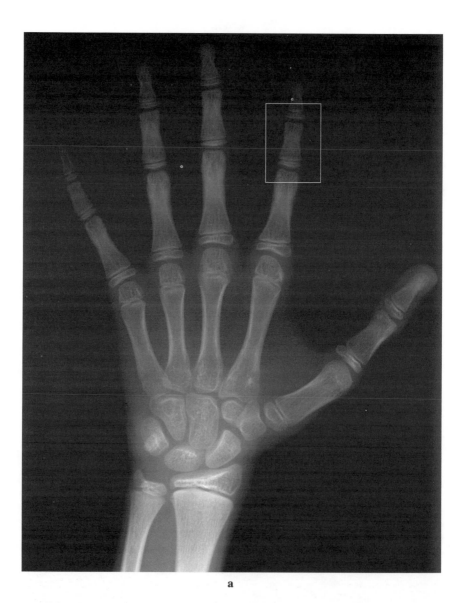

a

Figure 9. Effects of irreversible compression on the visibility of bone trabeculae in a computed radiograph. The original, uncompressed image is shown in (a), and a region of interest is indicated. A detail of the uncompressed image is shown in (b). The detail images in (c), (d) and (e) were obtained from images compressed with the SPIHT wavelet algorithm at compression ratios of 20:1, 40:1 and 80:1, respectively.

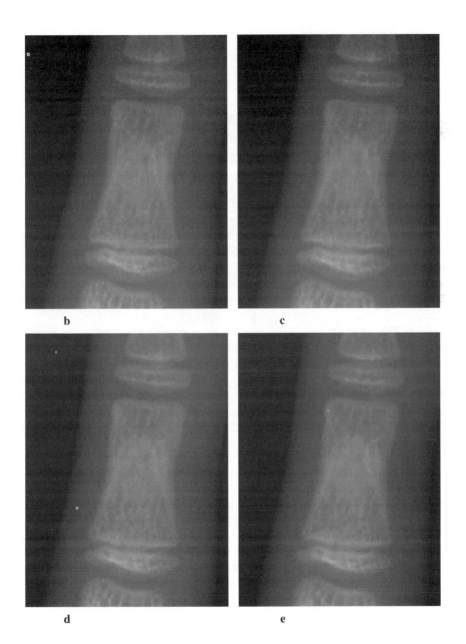

b

c

d

e

Image display task. This final factor simply points out that the acceptability of a compressed image will be strongly dependent on the task for which it is intended. We have found that computed radiographs compressed to between 100:1 and 200:1 are generally acceptable for secondary display on electronic medical record workstations in physician offices [Erickson et al. 1997-2]. Viewing conditions are often sub-optimal and the quality of the color cathode ray tube monitors is relatively poor. The highly compressed images are well suited to the rest of the imaging chain and the clinical task (often focused on patient education). These images would not be acceptable for primary diagnosis in radiology.

Methods for Quantifying Image Data Alterations

In the previous section we discussed qualitative differences between the original and compressed images, and factors affecting the magnitude of these differences. There is great interest in methods to demonstrate the diagnostic acceptability of irreversibly compressed images so that compression can be applied in practice and the potential practice improvements can be realized. There are several traditional metrics which have been used by image scientists to attempt to quantify image alterations caused by compression. These metrics include the mean square error, normalized mean square error, root mean squared error, average error, maximum pixel difference, and mean or peak signal-to-noise ratio [Huang et al. 1996, Persons et al. 1999]. These measures compute "error," "difference" or "noise" from pixel values in difference images computed by subtracting the original and compressed images (sample difference images are shown in Figure 6). None of these measures has been shown to correlate well with the image quality perceived by human observers and so their role in evaluating medical image compression techniques is limited.

Because of the shortcomings of traditional quantitative evaluation methods, the gold standard techniques for evaluating the acceptability of compression techniques are observer-based, with the most common approach being receiver operating characteristic (ROC) analysis. The literature includes many observer-oriented studies of image compression involving a variety of imaging modalities, body parts, and compression algorithms [Goldberg et al. 1994, Goldberg et al. 1997, Rebelo et al. 1993, Uchida et al. 1996, Wenzel et al. 1996, Sayre et al. 1992, Savcenko et al. 1998, Breeuwer 1995]. The discussion in the previous section of factors affecting image compressibility implies that it is inadvisable to freely extrapolate the findings of a particular compression study to other imaging modalities, body parts, and compression algorithms. This means that focused observer studies are required for each specific imaging application of interest. The time-consuming nature of observer studies is a clear disadvantage of these observer-based methods.

To address the practical difficulties with observer-based methods, quantitative techniques more sophisticated than the traditional mean square error (and related methods) have recently been proposed. One method employs the results of computer aided diagnosis (CAD) algorithms as a measure of the utility of compressed images [Chan et al. 1996]. Lower CAD accuracy is taken to indicate lower utility of the compressed image. The relevance of this measure with respect to radiologist performance is unknown because of the unknown correlation between the CAD algorithm and image interpretation by radiologists. Also, this approach is only applicable to imaging situations for which CAD techniques are well developed, such as in mammography and chest radiography.

Another new approach to quantitative evaluation of compressed images involves the use of model observers [Zhao et al. 1998, Eckstein et al. 1999]. Model observers are computer algorithms that are applied to two groups of images, one of which contains a signal of interest (e.g., a noduleshaped feature) and one which does not contain the signal [Barrett et al. 1993]. A signal-to-noise (or related parameter) is then computed. The signal-to-noise ratio derived from compressed images is compared with one derived from uncompressed images, and greater similarity between these measures is taken to indicate greater utility of the compressed images. This approach has the advantage that some model observers have been shown to correlate well with human observer performance. Human observer-based evaluations will probably always be considered as necessary. However reliable quantitative methods would be extremely useful in serving as a guide to indicate which image compression applications should be evaluated via human observer experiments. Reliable quantitative methods should also be valuable for extrapolating the results from one human-observer based study to other imaging situations. This is an important area for continuing research.

One caveat must be recognized when designing any compression evaluation experiment which requires generation of compressed images containing artificial features (e.g., phantom objects or simulated lesions). When phantom objects are used to evaluate the imaging capabilities of an imaging device (e.g., a CT or MR scanner), an implicit assumption is made that the system is linear and stationary. It is assumed, for example, that the frequency response measured with an edge or line phantom will reflect imager performance when a patient is in the bore of the device, and will apply in all important areas of the field-of-view. This assumption is not generally upheld in the strictest sense for real imaging devices, but is followed closely enough to allow phantom measurements to be useful predictors of patient image quality. The assumptions of linearity and stationarity are not closely upheld when compression is part of the imaging chain. In the JPEG algorithm, the organization of the image into 8×8 blocks is a nonstationary process, and the quantization is nonlinear. The coefficient ordering and refinement are nonlinear elements of the SPIHT wavelet algorithm. Experiments aimed at evaluating compression using artificial lesions or phantom objects must account for the nonlinear and nonstationery aspects of the compression process.

Implementation Issues

There are several important issues to address when considering implementation of irreversible compression in a clinical practice. These include the following.

Specific types of image data sets to be compressed must be identified in order to choose the compression algorithms for optimal performance. In this article, we have considered compression of only single frame, grayscale, 2D images. Three dimensional (3D) image data are becoming increasingly common. The third dimension may represent images acquired serially in time (e.g., ultrasound or fluoroscopy sequences), or at sequential slice positions along some axis of the patient (e.g., stacks of CT or MR images). Color images may be considered to consist of three independent images corresponding, for example, to the red, green, and blue components. The JPEG and wavelet techniques discussed can be utilized when dealing with such higher dimensional data through independent application to each individual image plane or frame. This is a very inefficient approach as it does not exploit the often large correlations between image planes. Algorithms geared to color or 3D data sets will usually give superior results. Also, as discussed in earlier sections of the article, different compression algorithms may be better suited for certain imaging modalities. Further, specific enhancements can sometimes be included in compression algorithms to optimize performance when working with images from certain modalities [Manduca et al. 1997].

Computational efficiency of the compression and decompression steps may make certain algorithms better suited to certain applications. Some algorithms are asymmetric in that the time it takes to perform the decompression step is much less than that required for the compression step. Such algorithms are well suited for use compressing images stored on a PACS (Picture Archiving and Communication System) server, where the images will be retrieved many times for decompression and display at workstations and speed is critical. For teleradiology applications on the other hand, the total time necessary for compression and decompression is probably most important performance figure of merit, regardless of how this time is partitioned between the compression and decompression operations.

Serial irreversible compression steps may be desired in some applications. For example, images irreversibly compressed using a moderate compression ratio prior to long-term storage in a radiology archive may be retrieved and compressed to an even greater degree for distribution in an electronic medical record environment. In general, it appears that the quality of the resulting image is determined primarily by the higher ratio compression operation, although increases in root mean square error may be introduced in later compression steps [Rabanni et al. 1991, Young et al. 1998]. The use of an embedded algorithm would be advantageous in this situation. This would allow a portion of the stored compressed image data to be directly utilized in the high ratio application, avoiding the need for another compression operation and the potential detrimental interaction between two compression algorithms.

Human visual system (HVS) weighting is another option which can often be included in both JPEG and wavelet compression algorithms to optimize the quantization of spectral coefficients. The aim is to quantize coefficients minimally where the human visual system is more sensitive, and to a greater degree where the HVS is less sensitive. Such weighting may consider different aspects of HVS performance including color sensitivity and frequency response. To best implement HVS optimization, assumptions must be made concerning the performance of the display device that will be used and the use of image enhancement tools at the display workstation (e.g., image zoom). Some imaging applications are inherently variable with respect to display devices and viewing modes (e.g., primary diagnostic interpretation, and long-term image archival), and the use of HVS weighting in these situations should be considered cautiously. Other applications are much more amenable to the use of HVS optimization (e.g., clinical image viewing on electronic medical record workstations).

Legal issues must also be considered. Irreversible compression presents an opportunity to trade off image quality for either lower cost or more timely patient care. The phrase "image quality tradeoff" means that in many cases, demonstrable image degradation with respect to the original image may be present (e.g., somewhat lower signal-to-noise ratio); however, this phrase does not imply that the diagnostic utility of the image will necessarily be compromised. Tradeoffs of this sort are common in radiology. Examples include the acquisition of MR data over some reasonable period of time although generally longer imaging times produce higher signal-to-noise ratio, and the use of computed radiography as a replacement for traditional screen-film systems. Another example is the diagnostic acceptability of relatively noisy (and blurred) radiographic images of thick patients as compared to images obtained of thinner patients, even though higher signal-to-noise could be obtained at the expense of higher patient dose.

In many teleradiology applications, the use of irreversible compression is clearly appropriate since a large measure of the value of the radiology service being provided is often directly related to the rapid access to specialty expertise enabled by the compression. When compression is used to lower archival costs in a PACS, it is often the case that the images originally reconstructed by the imaging modality are viewed by the radiologists during interpretation of the examination. Later, the images are irreversibly compressed and stored in the archive, and at some point the original images are deleted. At this point, the only "version" of the images that are available are compressed on the archive. It is interesting to consider the outcome of a legal challenge to the interpretation, and the possible consequences of the fact that the images viewed by the radiologist when the interpretation was rendered are not technically available (only the compressed "versions" may be retrieved and displayed). Assuming that valid experimental studies are done which support the diagnostic acceptability of the compression, it may be preferable that the compressed images (rather than the original images) be viewed by the radiologist during interpretation, and stored in the long term archive. In this scenario, the images could be compressed on the imaging modality itself. This measure of consistency would also be achieved in the teleradiology example if the transmitted images were stored at the receiving site after interpretation.

Another possible scenario for implementing irreversible compression in PACS that addresses the above consistency issues is the following. The original image data received from the imaging modality is stored on the PACS server and presented to the radiologist for the purpose of primary interpretation. These images are then reversibly compressed using an embedded algorithm and stored on the long-term archive. When the examination (consisting of the images and a diagnostic report) is later recalled for comparison purposes during a future episode of care, irreversibly compressed images would be provided by the archive. The level of compression would be that judged to be diagnostically lossless by the practice. If a legal challenge of the original examination were ever encountered, the original images viewed during interpretation would be retrieved from the full reversibly-compressed data set in the archive. This strategy allows the long-term per-exam archive costs to be reduced by a small factor (the reversible compression ratio), while the larger per-exam storage costs of the short-term PACS server are reduced by the larger irreversible compression ratio.

Irreversible image compression may be legally used for the delivery of patient care. The choices of compression algorithm and ratio are left to the judgment of the practitioner. It is required that, when an irreversibly compressed image is displayed, this fact be indicated by the display system to the viewer. To date there are no legal cases we are aware of which focus primarily on the use of irreversible image compression.

Compression standards allow images compressed on equipment provided by one vendor to be decompressed and displayed using equipment provided by another vendor. The DICOM standard does not supported the use of any compression algorithms other than JPEG (unless private attributes and syntax are employed). DICOM Working Group IV will act as a liaison to the group working to define the JPEG 2000 compression standard, with the intent to support this standard in DICOM when it is formally established. The JPEG 2000 standard is expected to be announced in November 2000, and wavelet-based algorithms are being considered.

Acknowledgments

The author would like to acknowledge helpful discussions regarding image compression with Armando Manduca, Ph.D., Bradley J. Erickson, M.D., Ph.D., and Kenneth R. Persons, as well as compression software tools provided by KRP.

Section II: Image Encryption

Introduction

The following briefly describes the four primary objectives of information system security.

1. Authentication. Are users or servers really who they say they are?

2. Authorization. What access privileges are available to users for creating, modifying or viewing information?

3. Confidentiality. Can an outside entity access and understand the information being shared?

4. Integrity. Can information or attributes be modified without detection?

Assuring the confidentiality and integrity of image data relies heavily on the use of encryption, and will be the focus of this section.

Encryption

Encryption involves the use of mathematical data transformations for mapping "plaintext" data into scrambled "ciphertext," while decryption involves the reverse process [Alexander 1996, Epstein et al. 1998]. The transformations are usually determined by specified algorithms and one or more keys. The two main approaches in current common use are symmetric key encryption and public key encryption.

Symmetric key approaches use a single key for both encryption and decryption. The transformations involved in encryption and decryption are computationally efficient. Knowledge of the key must be limited to only the parties involved in the communication. Each individual must have a secret unique key defined for each party (or group) with which secure communication is desired. Management of the keys (including storage of multiple keys in a secure manner, and secure distribution of keys to desired communication partners) is a weakness of symmetric key schemes. Key management is further complicated by the standard recommended practice of frequently changing keys to enhance security.

A common example of the symmetric key approach is the Data Encryption Standard (DES) developed by IBM and endorsed by the United States government. Security using this algorithm is often increased by applying the algorithm serially in three stages, using three different keys. This practice is called triple DES.

Public key approaches involve the use of two keys. One key is used for the encryption step, and the other is used for the decryption step. This method simplifies the key management problem by allowing the encryption keys for each particular receiving party to be made public. The public and private keys are mathematically related to one another (through the problem of factorization of large numbers). When they are created, they are identical in the sense that either could be selected to serve as either the public or private key. The public key is used by any party sending data to the receiver. The receiving party uses the private key to decrypt the transmitted ciphertext. The public key is useless for decryption (of data encrypted also using the public key), so the privacy of the transmitted data is assured. Each receiving party need only keep track of a single private key. The drawback of the public key approach is the relative computational inefficiency compared to symmetric key approaches. This performance penalty may be a factor of approximately 100 if the transformations are done in software, and may be as great as 1000-10,000 if dedicated hardware is used.

A common example of a public key cryptography system is RSA, named for the three inventors, Rivest, Shamir, and Adleman. RSA actually uses both public key and symmetric key approaches to leverage the strengths of each. A sender encrypts a message using a symmetric key approach (DES) and a key chosen at random. The randomly chosen key is sometimes referred to as a "session key" since it is used only for encryption during a short period (or session) of data exchange. The receivers public key is then used to encrypt the symmetric key. The plaintext public key, the cipher text symmetric key, and the ciphertext data are all bundled together into a "digital envelope" and transmitted to the receiver. The receiver uses their known private key to decrypt the symmetric key which is then used to (efficiently) decrypt the data. The computationally-inefficient public key approach is used to address the problem of symmetric key management, and the efficient symmetric key approach is used to encrypt and decrypt the data. PGP (Pretty Good Privacy) is another common (and free) public key crytographic system, and works in a manner similar to that described above.

Even in public key approaches, a receiver must keep track of at least one private key, which is a number that may be 200 or more digits in length. Secure storage of the key may be done through the use of a smartcard. To enhance security, the smartcard contains a computer that performs all of the necessary numerical calculation, so the private key is never made available to any external system (even those belonging to the receiving party). Decryption using the private key on the smartcard is enabled by a personal identification number (PIN) that is memorized by the user. If the smartcard is stolen, only three attempts to use the card with incorrect PINs are allowed before the card disables itself. The requirements of both a physical token (a card) and a PIN to assure security are identical to those employed for security by financial institutions for the use of automated teller machines (ATMs).

Digital Signatures

Digital signatures are a means of verifying the integrity of data. This includes assuring that data (e.g., images) have not been altered since they were "signed" by the originating device (e.g., an imaging modality), and assuring that the indicated signer (either a person or a device) was indeed the originator of the data.

Digital signatures rely on the use of public key encryption schemes. The process begins with the generation of a hash, which is a relatively short sequence of data derived from the data set to be signed. The mathematical algorithm used to generate the hash is such that the hash cannot be used to recreate the signed data set, the hash is essentially unique to a particular data set, and alteration of a single element of the data set will change ~50% of the bits of the hash (on average) [Epstein et al. 1998]. The hash is encrypted using the private key of the signing party and resulting ciphertext is used as the digital signature. Verification of the signature and the data set by the receiving party is performed by computing the hash of the received data set, decrypting the received digital signature, and comparing the two results. A match assures that the data set has been unaltered by a third party since it was signed, and authenticates the signer as the originator of the document. Digital signatures used along with certified time-stamps also assure that the signing party did not subsequently alter and re-sign a digital document or data set.

Radiology Applications

Security extensions to the DICOM standard have not yet been finalized. The use of both encryption and digital signatures are under discussion. Encryption will be implemented through the use of an existing standard technology such as SSL (secure sockets layer) or TLS (transport layer security) which is a later derivative of SSL. SSL or TLS operates at low levels of the network protocol stack, and provides secure communication over a nonsecure communication channel such as the Internet. These protocols provide authentication of both the data and the server and data privacy through the combined use of symmetric and public key encryption schemes as described above. The DICOM standard is currently focusing on secure interactive communications between devices, and at this time is not considering the security of data stored on individual devices. (The application of digital signatures to stored image data within the DICOM standard may be under discussion, however the initial draft of this proposal is not yet publicly available.) New regulations proposed by the Department of Health and Human Services concerning security standards for medical information [Meinhardt 1998] will almost certainly accelerate the incorporation of security extensions to the DICOM standard.

References

Alexander, M. *The Underground Guide to Computer Security.* Addison-Wesley Publishing Company, Reading MA. 1996.

Antonini, M., Barlaud, M., Mathieu, P., Daubechies, I. "Image coding using wavelet transform." *IEEE Trans Image Proc* 1:205-220, 1992.

Barrett, H.H., Yao, J., Rolland, J.P., Meyers, K.J. "Model observers for assessment of image quality." *Proc Natl Acad Sci USA* 90:9758-9765, 1993.

Boliek, M., Gormish, M.J., Schwartz, E.L., Keith, A. "Next generation image compression and manipulation using CREW." In IEEE international conference on image processing. Piscataway, NJ: IEEE, 1997.

Breeuwer, M., Heusdens, R., Gunnewiek, R.K., Zwart, P., Haas, H.P. "Data compression of x-ray cardio-angiographic image series." *Int J Card Imaging* 11:179-186, 1995.

Chan, H.P., Lo, S.C., Niklason, L.T., Ikeda, D.M., Lam, K.L. "Image compression on digital mammography: effects on computerized detection of subtle microcalcifications." *Med Phys* 23:1325-1336, 1996.

Eckstein, M.P., Abbey, C.K., Bochud, F.O., Bartroff, J.L., Whiting, J.S. "The effects of compression in model and human observers." *SPIE Medical Imaging 1999 Book of Abstracts:* 490, 1999.

Epstein, M.A., Pasieka, M.S., Lord, W.P., Wong, S.T.C., Mankovich, N.J. "Security for the digital information age of medicine: Issues, applications, and implementation." *J Digit Imaging* 11:33-44, 1998.

Erickson, B.J., Manduca, A., Persons, K.R., Earnest, F., Hartman, T.E., Harms, G.F., Brown, L.R. "Evaluation of irreversible compression of digitized PA chest radiographs." *J Digit Imaging* 10:97-102, 1997.

Erickson, B.J., Manduca, A., Palisson, P., Persons, K.R., Earnest, F., Savcenko, V., Hangiandreou, N.J. "Wavelet compression of medical images." *Radiology* 206:599-607, 1998.

Erickson, B.J., Ryan, W.J., Gehring, D.G., Beebe C. "Image display for clinicians on medical record workstations." *J Digit Imaging* 10 (Suppl 1):38-40, 1997.

Goldberg, M.A., Pivovarov, M., Mayo-Smith, W.W., et al. "Application of wavelet compression to digitized radiographs." *AJR* 163:463-468, 1994.

Goldberg, M.A., Gazelle, G.S., Boland, G.W., et al. "Focal hepatic lesions: effect of three dimensional wavelet compression on detection at CT." *Radiology* 202:159-165, 1997.

Harpen, M.D. "An introduction to wavelet theory and application for the medical physicist." *Med Phys* 25:1985-1993, 1998.

Huang, H.K. PACS: *Picture archiving and communication systems in biomedical imaging.* VCH Publishers, New York, NY, 1996.

Manduca, A. "Interactive wavelet based 2-D and 3-D image compression." *Proc SPIE* 1897:307-318, 1993.

Manduca, A., Said, A. "Wavelet compression of medical images with set partitioning in hierarchical trees." *Proc SPIE* 2707:192-200, 1996.

Manduca, A., Erickson, B.J., Persons, K.R., Palisson, P. "Histogram transformation for improved compression of CT images." *Proc SPIE* 3031:320-327, 1997.

Meinhardt, R.A., Tector, L.M. "New electronic security requirements for health information." *Group Practice Journal* Nov/Dec 1998: 22-26.

Persons, K.R., Palisson, P.M., Manduca, A., Charboneau, W.J., James, E.M., Charboneau, N.T., Hangiandreou NJ, Erickson BJ. "JPEG/Wavelet Ultrasound Compression Study." Presented at the SPIE Medical Imaging Conference. *SPIE Medical Imaging 1999 Book of Abstracts:* 438, 1999.

Rabbani, M., Jones, P.W. *Digital Image Compression Techniques.* SPIE Optical Engineering Press, Bellingham WA, 1991.

Rebelo, M.S., Furuie, S.S., Munhoz, A.C., Moura, L., Melo, C.P. "Lossy compression in nuclear medicine images." In: Proceedings of the 17th Annual Symposium on Computer Applications in Medical Care. New York, NY: McGraw Hill, 824-828, 1993.

Said, A., Pearlman, W. "Image compression using the spatial orientation tree. In IEEE international symposium on circuits and systems." Piscataway, NJ: IEEE, 279-282, 1993.

Said, A., Pearlman, W. "A new fast and efficient image codec based on set partitioning in hierarchical trees." IEEE Trans Circuits Systems Video Technology,6: 243-250, 1996.

Savcenko, V., Erickson, B.J., Palisson, P.M., Person, K.R., Manduca, A., Hartman, T.E., Harms, G.F., Brown, L.R. "Detection of subtle abnormalities on chest radiographs after irreversible compression." *Radiology* 206:609-616, 1998.

Sayre, J., Aberle, D.R., Boechat, I, et al. "Effect of data compression on diagnostic accuracy in digital hand and chest radiography." *Proc SPIE* 1653:232-240, 1992.

Schomer, D.F., Elekes, A.A., Hazle, J.D., Huffman, J.C., Thompson, S.K., Chui, C.K., Murphy, W.A. "Introduction to wavelet-based compression of medical images." *Radiographics* 18:469-481, 1998.

Shapiro, J.M. "Embedded image coding using zerotrees of wavelet coefficients." *IEEE Trans Signal Processing* 41:3445-3462, 1993.

Uchida, K., Nakamura, K., Watanabe, H., et al. "Clinical evaluation of irreversible data compression for computed radiography in excretory urography." *J Digit Imaging* 9:145-149, 1996.

Wallace, G.K. "The JPEG still picture compression standard." Comm of the ACM 34:30-44, 1991.

Wenzel, A., Gottredsen, E., Borg, E., Grondahl, H.G. "Impact of lossy image compression on accuracy of caries detection in digital images taken with a storage phosphor system." *Oral Surg Med Pathol Radiol Endodont* 81:351-355, 1996.

Young, S.S., Jones, P.W., Foos, D.H. "A study of multiple JPEG compression cycles in medical imaging." *Proc SPIE* 3335:336-347, 1998.

Zhao, B., Schwartz, L.H., Kijewski, P.K. "Effects of lossy compression on lesion detection: Predictions of the nonprewhitening matched filter." *Med Phys* 25:1621-1624, 1998.

Address all correspondence to:
Nicholas J. Hangiandreou, Ph.D.
Diagnostic Radiology, East-2
Mayo Clinic
200 First Street SW
Rochester, MN 55905
V: 507.284.3207
F: 507.266.4609
hangiandreou@mayo.edu

Teleradiology

Brent K. Stewart, Ph.D., DABMP
Professor of Radiology, Bioengineering and Medical Education
University of Washington School of Medicine
Seattle, WA 98195-7115
bstewart@u.washington.edu

Introduction

Simply put, teleradiology is the specialized use of computer technology to electronically transmit radiological images and supporting information from one location to another for the purposes of interpretation, consultation or education. According to this definition, teleradiology has been around for over 25 years [Steckel 1972], but the practical use of teleradiology has become more widespread due to several converging factors. The first of these is technological: more sophisticated and ubiquitous telecommunications infrastructures and more capable computer equipment. The second of these involves the reorganization of medical practice: the emergence of managed care, outsourcing of radiological services outside of the medical center and the coverage of multiple institutions from one or more centralized locations. Teleradiology can also be thought of as Picture Archiving and Communications System (PACS) [Huang 1996] on the wide area network, though typically without the archiving component.

The medical physicist is usually the chief technology vanguard in radiology departments, proficient with computer technology and usually tasked with the specification, selection, overseeing the installation and the QA/QC of highly complex and technical medical imaging equipment. Thus the medical physicist is usually requested to apply his technical aptitudes and understanding of complex systems toward the specification, selection, and oversight of QA/QC for teleradiology and PACS within his institution. This may require the medical physicist to expand his repertoire of technical knowledge of radiological modalities into the realms of networking, telecommunications, protocol standards, computer and database architectures, display technologies as well as image compression and data encryption. Sufficient base knowledge in all of these areas is required of the medical physicist to successfully complete this task.

Many of these topics are covered in greater depth elsewhere in this volume. It is the goal of this article to provide a basic, high-level overview of each of these areas, current trends, and requirements, and how they tie together in the guise of a teleradiology system. It is hoped that this medical informatics domain knowledge will allow the medical physicist to not only fulfill a limited obligation to assist in the implementation of a teleradiology system at his institution, but also that the medical physicist eventually become an essential element in the transformation of radiology departments from somewhat passive purveyors of diagnostic radiological information to proactive participants in the evolution of medical informatics at his/her institution.

Goals

Several chief functional goals of teleradiology include, but are not limited to the following, as teleradiology is an evolving and technologically fluid modality; additional future functions and goals may emerge. First is the provision of consultative and interpretative radiological services in areas of demonstrated need, for example, making radiological consultation service available to medical facilities without onsite radiology support. Teleradiology also involves the provision of timely availability of radiology images and radiological image interpretation in the support of emergent and non-emergent patient care (may overlap with the sphere of PACS). A further goal of teleradiology is the provision of radiological interpretation in on-call situations, such as night and weekend coverage from an attending physician home. Other goals involve the provision of subspecialty radiology support (primary interpretation and overreading). Teleradiology is also seen as enhancing the educational opportunities of practicing radiologists, promoting efficiency and quality improvement, sending interpreted images to referring providers, supporting broader telemedicine activities, and providing direct supervision of offsite imaging studies.

Teleradiology Zoo

There are a spectrum of teleradiology systems in existence, all implemented with specific goals in mind. As such, there are various ways of decomposing them into various categories (basis functions). They can be dichotomized into the various application environments or implementation architectures and models. There are generally three classes of teleradiology systems: on-call coverage, centralized off-site reading, and in-hospital. Those used in hospitals, generally referred to as mini-PACS, fall under the larger category of PACS and are covered by other articles in this volume. Scenarios for the on-call and off-site teleradiology systems are described below. The Handbook of Teleradiology Applications [RSNA 1997] published by the Radiological Society of North America (RSNA) offers descriptions of several teleradiology application environments: military [Crowther 1995], rural [Franken 1995], urban, large private practice, university, and international.

On-call systems are used for night/weekend (nighthawk) coverage of a medical facility's radiological service, typically for emergent cases that cannot wait for the next weekday morning interpretation and typically terminate in the radiologist's home. For example, the University of Washington Medical Center (UWMC) has had a teleradiology link with the Seattle Veterans Administration Medical Center (SVAMC) for the past five years. The purpose of this system is to allow the night/weekend radiology resident at the UWMC to provide radiology consultation to the SVAMC remotely. Prior to the implementation of this system, when radiology consultation was required at the SVAMC, this resident would drive ten miles to the SVAMC where the only hardcopy films existed, leaving the UWMC uncovered for the duration of the resident's absence.

Off-site systems usually refer to the outsourcing of radiology services, or the remote coverage of radiology services from another institution. Another example is the University of Washington Physicians Network. This is a constellation of nine primary care clinics throughout the Seattle-King County area that feed into the UWMC. Currently, only one of the ten clinics has a film digitizer that transmits images to a display workstation in the main radiology department at UWMC. The balance of the radiological films generated at the other sites is forwarded into UWMC with a laboratory specimen courier. This teleradiology system allows for much more rapid interpretation "turn-around" for radiographs. The current turn-around time for teleradiology interpretation/report generation is about 3-4 hours, versus the 18-36 hours for the films delivered via courier. It also allows for "stat" interpretation of some radiographs through paging of the attending radiologist. The primary care physicians greatly appreciate the rapid turn-around time for improved patient management.

Teleradiology Implementation Architectures

If teleradiology systems are examined according to their implementation architectures, there are three basic system types: dial-up [thick (or fat) client systems], web-based (thin client systems), and those that use DICOM (Digital Imaging and Communications in Medicine). Each of these has advantages and disadvantages based on the degree of accessibility, the dollar investment, functionality, and scalability.

Dial-up, thick client teleradiology systems have been and continue to be the mainstay of installed teleradiology systems (estimated to be over 7000 in 1995) [Perednia 1995]. These systems typically use proprietary file formats and communication protocols over public or private dial-up networks (e.g., POTS modem or DS-1 circuit) allowing fairly secure, point-to-point connectivity. Acquired images are either directly sent to a single location for interpretation ("pushed"), or to a central location for storage allowing the radiologist to "pull" to his display workstation. Images are transferred from the sending site to the receiving site and stored on the receiving site's hard disk. The display program on the receiving computer does all or most of the processing, hence the term thick client. The display software can cost upwards of $1-2K per station. Due to non-standardization and interoperability problems, equipment from a sole vendor is usually used throughout the network of teleradiology nodes. At present, there are no communication standards for image file formats in the teleradiology market place. Teleradiology technology is evolving toward standardization and it is hoped that greater product compatibility among vendors will take place in the near future.

This type of system operates efficiently unless one is trying to receive images from another location with a teleradiology system from a different vendor. For example, the

University of Washington School of Medicine serves a five-state region termed WWAMI (Washington-Wyoming-Alaska-Montana and Idaho) and naturally receives referrals from many physicians across this area (25% of the U.S. landmass and 2.3% of its population). Teleradiology networks from numerous vendors have been established throughout the WWAMI area. For the University of Washington Medical Center to receive images from various sites that are part of these independent networks requires the purchase of thick client software from each of the vendors represented running on multiple PCs.

With the advent of web technology over the past few years, thin client (e.g., web browser) software teleradiology systems have become available. The cost of teleradiology deployment has been reduced as the web browser software is free and vendors usually distribute any required browser plug-ins at no cost. Thus, the only costs associated with the display of images are the PC and any telecommunications charges. Acquired images are typically transmitted to a web server where the interpreting physician can retrieve (pull) them through their browser. Some vendors also push images to the web browser plug-in as they arrive at the web server. Commercial web servers to support this architecture typically cost $25-50K although numerous sites have developed their own systems in-house.

The third paradigm is that of utilizing DICOM throughout the entire teleradiology image acquisition, storage, and display chain. As new imaging modalities provide at a minimum Storage Service Class User functionality, they can be used to transfer DICOM images to a computer with a DICOM application entity that provides Storage Service Class User functionality. This software can be developed from various extant DICOM software toolkits (e.g., the UC Davis Medical Center DICOM Network Transport Library), or through fairly inexpensive ($1K) commercial software (e.g., Digital Jacket). Then a freeware DICOM image display program like Osiris or Dr. Razz can be used for image display.

The great thing about using DICOM is that it is nonproprietary (where shadow groups are not used) and that images are acquired in digital format (i.e., no film digitizers or video frame grabbers are necessary). The down side is that even though DICOM does have several adopted compression algorithms, most major vendors do not support them yet. Proprietary vendor systems typically offer 12-bit JPEG or wavelet compression, which is user selectable, that may be as high as 50:1-100:0 for projection radiographs. The lack of compression for transmission of DICOM images is a severe one, especially for low-bandwidth modem connections.

ACR Standard for Teleradiology

The American College of Radiology (ACR) is the principal professional society of radiologists and radiation oncologists in the United States. The primary purpose of the

ACR is to advance radiological sciences; improve radiological services to the patient, study the socioeconomic aspects of radiological practice; and promote continuing education for radiologists, radiation oncologists, and medical physicists. As part of its mission, the ACR periodically defines new standards for radiological practice. Existing standards are reviewed occasionally for revision or renewal as appropriate.

Each ACR standard represents a policy statement that has undergone a consensus process subject to extensive review requiring the approval of the Commission of Standards and Accreditation as well as the ACR Board of Chancellors, the ACR Council Steering Committee, and the ACR Council. The derived standards acknowledge that the safe and effective utilization of diagnostic and therapeutic radiology practices requires specific training, techniques, and technology as described in each document. The ACR standards documents attempt to define principles that, if practiced, should generally result in high-quality radiological care.

In 1994 the ACR published the first ACR Standard for Teleradiology [ACR 1994] which has subsequently been revised in both 1996 and 1998. The 1998 revision (Res. 35) document is available online in portable document format (PDF) at http://www.acr.org. The ACR Standard for Teleradiology document outlines the qualifications of personnel involved; equipment guidelines, licensing, credentialing, and liability; communication; quality control for teleradiology; and quality improvement and has a listing of up-to-date references. Relevant portions of the ACR document will be referred to in the balance of this article.

Teleradiology Equipment

The basic equipment used for teleradiology is generally the same as that used for PACS, except that as the workload is typically far less and the initial institutional investment is usually less, the teleradiology equipment uses standard personal computers with relatively inexpensive software. However, there is a natural synergy between teleradiology and PACS. In fact, at our institution, because we have standardized all radiological practice to the use of DICOM devices, our radiologists read PACS and teleradiology images from the same high-end diagnostic display workstations.

ACR Teleradiology Equipment Guidelines

The ACR Standard for Teleradiology contains both specific and general guidelines for teleradiology equipment when used for rendering primary interpretation of a radiological study. There is a caveat that less stringent guidelines for display systems apply when not used to product the primary interpretation. The ACR teleradiology equipment guidelines cover the following topics: acquisition or digitization, compression, transmission, display capabilities, archiving and retrieval, security, and reliability and redundancy. In each of the sections below on teleradiology equipment, the relevant

ACR Teleradiology equipment guidelines will be described before technical and functional descriptions are enumerated.

Image Acquisition or Digitization

Images for teleradiology can be received directly from the modality in digital format, or indirectly through analog film or video digitization [Horii 1996]. The advantage of direct digital capture is that it affords the radiologist access to the entire original digital data set without truncation of image matrix dimension, spatial resolution, and pixel bit depth. The latter gives the radiologist full capability in adjusting image window and level settings. There are image quality losses in the process of going from a digital representation to an analog medium and then digitizing the analog medium, but it is difficult to quantify whether these are significant. For example, analog video frame grabbing is still used at some institutions to print CT images to laser film printers and there is little visual loss of information aside from the inability to visualize the full 12-bit data set. Digitization of the laser printed multi-slice CT film can, however, cause a loss of spatial resolution, loss of contrast resolution and possibly Moire patterns or other artifacts.

The DICOM standard has become the predominant standard for the communication of medical images [Bidgood 1997] and allows for the direct digital transfer of images from scanner to teleradiology system. As there is a certain degree of flexibility and interpretation ambiguity in the implementation of DICOM, devices from different manufacturers are not necessarily interoperable ("plug and play") out of the box. Furthermore, there is the problem with legacy equipment that may or may not be upgraded to DICOM capability; if so, this upgrade will most likely carry substantial cost. Protocol converters were popular years ago before vendors had integrated DICOM capability into their modalities, but it is simpler and most likely less expensive to get the DICOM upgrade from the modality vendor, eliminating another box from the infrastructure.

ACR Teleradiology Guidelines for Image Acquisition or Digitization

Direct digital image acquisition is, of course, the most desirable method for primary diagnosis using a teleradiology system or PACS. It is highly recommended that the DICOM standard be used. For direct digital image acquisition, the inherent image data set produced by the radiological modality both in terms of image matrix dimension and pixel bit depth should be transferred to the teleradiology system.

Secondary capture image acquisition involves the digitization of an analog source, (e.g., radiographic film or video) to produce a digital output file. Secondary capture of radiological modality images is divided into small and large matrix systems. Small matrix systems are meant to encompass the following modalities: computed tomography (CT), magnetic resonance imaging (MRI), ultrasound, nuclear medicine, digital fluorography, and digital angiography. Large matrix systems include digitized projection radiography films, computed radiography (CR), and digital radiography (DR).

For small matrix images, the film digitizer or video frame grabber should digitize each image frame or slice to a matrix dimension at least as large as the inherent dimension for that modality (e.g., 512×512 for CT). The digitized bit depth should be at least 8 bits per pixel (256 digital values). For large matrix systems, the images should be digitized to a matrix dimension that corresponds to a spatial resolution of 2.5 line pairs/mm as measured in the original detector plane. The digitized bit depth should be at least 10 bits per pixel (1024 digital values). High spatial and contrast resolution film digitizers will generally be required to produce this level of fidelity.

Direct Modality Interface (DICOM – Storage SCU)

The essence of the DICOM standard is that it prescribes a uniform, well-understood set of rules for the communication of digital images. This has been accomplished through defining, as unambiguously as possible, the terms it uses and in the definition of object-oriented models for medical imaging information. The DICOM standard is extremely adaptable, a planned feature that has led to the adoption of DICOM by other medical specialties that generate images in the course of patient diagnosis and treatment (e.g., cardiology, endoscopy, and ophthalmology) [Bidgood 1996]. Thus, we should see DICOM used increasingly in future telemedicine applications. Please also see the expanded article by Richard L. (Skip) Kennedy *DICOM* in this volume.

The fundamental functional unit of DICOM is the service-object pair (SOP). Everything implemented in DICOM is based on the use of SOP classes. The elemental units that make up the SOP are information objects and service classes. As DICOM was founded on an object-oriented design philosophy, things such as images, reports, and patients are all objects in DICOM and are termed information objects. The definition of what constitutes an information object in DICOM is called an information object definition (IOD), which is simply a structured list of attributes. An example of a DICOM IOD is that of a CT image (CT Image IOD). Once the attributes (e.g., patient identification number) are "filled in," the object then becomes an information object instance.

The second elemental unit of DICOM is the service class. Information objects and the communications links between devices are not sufficient in and of themselves to provide functionality, it is necessary that these devices perform some operation (service) on the information objects. Some of the many DICOM services are: Storage, Query/Retrieve, Print, and Modality Worklist Management. Due to the object-oriented nature of DICOM, services are referred to as service classes. In part, this is because a given service may be applied to a variety (or class) of information objects (e.g., Storage Service Class). A distinction is also made based on whether the device acts as a user or provider of a given service.

The service classes and information objects are then combined to form service object pairs (SOPs). The process of DICOM communication involves the exchange of SOP instances using DICOM messages. For example, the transfer and storage of a specific CT image on the DICOM web server represents a CT image storage SOP instance. If the device is accepting the image object for storage (e.g., the DICOM web server), it is termed a Storage Service Class Provider (Storage SCP). The device that requests the image to be stored (e.g., the CT scanner) is termed a Storage Service Class User (Storage SCU). For teleradiology systems, therefore, each digital imaging modality should act as a DICOM Storage SCU for its specific image object (e.g., CT IOD).

Film Digitizers

The most common teleradiology device for image acquisition is the film digitizer. Film digitizers convert to digital format the still ubiquitous conventional projection radiographic films captured using screen-film technology or laser printed multi-format films from digital modalities (e.g., a CT scanner) that do not provide DICOM Storage SCU. There are two major competing technologies in the film digitizer marketplace. Laser film digitizers, the past and current gold standard of film digitization, offer superior contrast and spatial resolution, but with an expensive price tag. Current generation charged coupled device (CCD) digitizers offer comparable (or greater) spatial resolution than laser film digitizers, but in many cases manufactured systems employing CCDs fall somewhat short with respect to contrast resolution [Hangiandreou 1998]. CCD digitizers are typically smaller, lighter, and less costly than laser-based digitizers. CCD digitizers may also be easier to maintain as there is no rotating or vibrating mirrors to adjust periodically. The optical components in a CCD digitizer are also much simpler than those found in laser digitizers [Forsburg 1995].

Laser film digitizers use a highly focused, intense, and phase coherent beam of light to scan the film. In almost all systems used today, the film is transported using pinch rollers and high-precision stepping motors across an area where the laser beam is swept in raster fashion across the film using either a rotating polygonal mirror or vibrating galvanometer mirror. A photomultiplier has typically been used to convert the transmitted laser light into an electrical signal. This signal is then amplified either linearly or logarithmically. An analog to digital converter (ADC) then converts this signal to a digital value.

> Ideally, the range of optical densities the film digitizer is capable of capturing should span the entire range encountered clinically. For all applications with the exception of mammography this equates to a dynamic range of $10^{3.5}$ (optical density range 0.0 to 3.5). The choice of amplifier and digitization method for the transmitted light signal will determine the digital value distribution function and the contrast resolution. Use of a linear amplification results in digital values represented by equal increments in transmitted light and unequal optical density increments. Use of a logarithmic amplifier results in digital values represented by equal optical density increments, which is preferred.

Film digitizers vary as to the spatial resolution (usually assumed to be the digitization spot size, typically 200 microns down to 25 microns), the contrast resolution (number of useable bits, typically 8-16), the film size handled, whether multiple film sizes are handled, whether the digitization spot size is variable and whether only single sheets are handled or multiple sheets can be batch loaded using a sheet feeding mechanism. Laser film digitizers are typically twice the cost of CCD digitizers, but exact cost depends not only on the spatial and contrast resolution capabilities and features of the system, but also the workstation and software used to drive the digitizer. In order to adhere to the ACR Teleradiology equipment guidelines, a 200-micron digitization element must be used (2.5 lp/mm) and a bit depth of at least 10 bits per pixel. For a 14" × 17" radiographic film, this equates to a digitization matrix of 1780 × 2160 and using 12-bits per pixel, but stored along 16-bit (two byte) boundaries results in a file size of 7.4 megabytes.

Linear CCD scanning systems consist of a collimated light source, film pinch rollers with stepping motors, a fixed focus lens, and a CCD linear array. CCD systems suffer from the limited visible light sensitivity range of most solid-state detectors and the reduction in radiographic contrast through inclusion of light scattered in the film and the focusing lens (flare). Spatial resolution is determined by the number of CCD elements on the linear sensor and the characteristics of the focusing lens.

The digitization matrix for film digitizers is a tradeoff between the number of pixel elements that are necessary to adequately represent the analog film, the film digitization speed, and the digital file storage requirements. Please also see the expanded article by *Film Digitizers and Laser Printers* by J. Anthony Seibert in this volume.

Video Frame Grabber

If an imaging system has video output signal, such as an ultrasound scanner or fluoroscopic system with a vidicon camera, a video frame grabber can be used to digitize these temporally varying one-dimensional signals into a two-dimensional digital image. In the recent past, video frame grabbing has accounted for the largest proportion of installed teleradiology acquisition devices for CT and MR imaging. This has been a reflection of economic considerations as well as the dearth of DICOM capable imaging scanners. Even though today all new vendor equipment installed at your institution should provide at a minimum DICOM Storage SCU, the long amortization schedules for previously purchased (pre-DICOM) high-ticket radiological scanning equipment and expense to retrofit DICOM into existing scanners means that the video frame grabber may be around for some while yet.

The video frame grabber utilizes ADCs and vertical and horizontal blanking detection circuitry to capture the digital equivalent of the analog video image. Usually there are hardware or software switches to denote the video input as interlaced or progressive. High-resolution video systems, like those for fluoroscopy and angiography, may have

1024 lines scanned progressively, which produces a high frequency bandwidth and requires high-speed ADCs of the flash type. Some frame grabbers are capable of adapting to different bandwidth video signals (like multi-sync video monitors), whereas others utilize potentiometers that must be "tuned" for the specific video signal to be digitized correctly. Frame grabbers typically digitize to 8 bits as most video signals for display use 8-bit digital to analog converters (DACs). Depending on the amount of memory resident on the frame grabber board, computer bus clock rate, and disk write speed, real-time video digitization can be stored to disk in real-time, although this requires very large data storage requirements for even short video clips (as is described in the telemedicine section).

One major problem with the use of video is that contrast resolution is curtailed to 8 bits. This is not really a problem with ultrasound images that only have a useful data bit depth of 6 to 8 bits, but poses problems for modalities like CT and MRI where the ability to adjust the window and level settings of the images is severely compromised and thus useful diagnostic information is lost. While it is possible to video frame grab at various window and level settings (exactly as in the case where being printed to film with say soft tissue, lung, and bone windows for CT), this requires additional work on the part of the radiology technologist, more data to be transmitted, and a greater number of images for the radiologist to manage and interpret on the display workstation.

Computed and Digital Radiography

Computed radiography employs reusable storage phosphor plates in cassettes that take the place of the conventional screen-film cassette imaging [Sonoda 1983]. The storage phosphor plate is typically made of a barium fluorohalide crystal matrix with a lanthanide-series dopant such as europium. When exposed to x-rays, electrons from the dopant ion are trapped in potential wells ("traps") in the vicinity of the fluorine atoms and just below the conduction band. When exposed to laser light of sufficient energy to liberate these electrons from their traps into the conduction band, and upon reuniting with their dopant ions, visible light is released that can be captured by a fiber-optic light guide and digitized through Photomultiplier Tube (PMT) and ADC. The dynamic range of CR imaging plates is in excess of 10^4. Commercially available pixel dimensions are currently either 200- or 100-micron square. A contrast resolution of 10-12 bits is used. Please see the expanded articles by Katherine P. Andriole and Charles E. Willis on Computed Radiography in this volume.

Digital radiography is essentially synonymous with flat-panel detectors, which were in vast abundance at the past RSNA meeting. Flat-panel detectors have an active element of thin amorphous silicon, or a silicon-selenium layer on which millions of photodiodes are etched. Silicon-based detectors use thin films of silicon integrated with two-dimensional photodiode arrays. Each element in this array is connected to a field effect transistor. These thin film transistors (TFTs) use a series of data and gate lines to control the readout of the collected charge. Scintillating material overlays the photodiode array. This scintillating material acts to absorb incident x-rays and converts these to light in the visible or near-visible range for photodiode detection. The resulting electrical charge registered at each element is proportional to the x-ray energy deposited in the scintillator coating. Both cesium iodide and gadolinium oxysulfide scintillators are being used.

For selenium-based flat panel detectors, the TFT array is combined with a conversion layer of amorphous selenium. This coating acts to directly capture and convert x-ray energy into electron-hole pairs. These charges migrate along strong electric field lines in the selenium. The TFT array is used to store and gate the collected charge to readout electronics as with the scintillator flat panel systems described above.

Most manufacturers offer 14" × 17" or 17" × 17" arrays. The dynamic range of DR detectors is on the order of 10^4. Other factors that distinguish systems include pixel resolution, speed of image acquisition, and whether or not the array is tiled into multiple areas. DR image sizes are typically 2-3K in each dimension and use 12-bit contrast resolution. Although it would seem obvious that the conversion of x-rays directly into charge carriers and the tight and parallel electric field lines would favor selenium-based systems, most manufacturers are offering flat panel systems using scintillators. There are conflicting claims being made for the detective quantum efficiency (DQE) as a function of spatial frequency for both types of systems. In all cases, the image quality will be superior to CR where the analog imaging plate must still be scanned with a laser as in a film digitizer as described above. There are other claimed benefits, including enhanced productivity through more efficient workflow with DR. Please also see the expanded article by Martin Yaffe on Digital Radiography in this volume.

Telemammography

Although not yet a mainstream application and there is no explicit ACR standard, telemammography remains a challenge because of its unique spatial resolution requirements. Given the magnitude of the public health problem being addressed (breast cancer affects 1 in 8 women in the United States), there has been considerable research activity and funding devoted to investigating both digital mammography (i.e., the direct digital acquisition of mammograms) and telemammography. However, given the current low reimbursement rate for the acquisition and interpretation of mammograms, it may be some time before widespread telemammography is realized in all but grant-funded trials and pilot programs. Please see the expanded article by Martin Yaffe on Digital Mammography in this volume.

Compression

Medical image data sets are relatively large and image compression has a valuable role to play. A computed radiograph (CR) of 1760 × 2140 pixels and a 10-bit pixel depth runs about 7.5 megabytes. A CT examination consisting of 150 images runs 75 megabytes. Obviously, image compression must be used judiciously as it generally trades image quality for compression ratio. This is especially important when low bandwidth connectivity (e.g., a 33.6 kbps modem) is used. With lossless (reversible) compression the original images can be exactly reconstituted (bit for bit), so there is no degradation in image quality unless there is an error in the transfer of the image data. Lossy (irreversible) compression techniques cause a varying amount of degradation in image quality, depending on image feature characteristics and the degree of compression.

Lossless compression schemes typically permit between 2:1 and 3:1 (in some extreme cases, up to 4:1) reduction in the number of bytes required to represent an image. Techniques that claim compression factors exceeding 4:1 are almost certainly lossy. Vendors euphemistically term this "visually" lossless (*caveat emptor*). Compression ratios closer to 10:1 or 20:1 are required to have a significant practical and economic impact. Although the concept of lossy data compression was not readily embraced initially by the medical community, there is growing evidence that such schemes can be implemented without compromising the diagnostic content of images [Aberle 1993; Bolle 1997; Good 1994].

Even though compression may cause a loss of image quality, images compressed by as much as 10:1 to 20:1 may still be clinically acceptable. In the current health care environment, which stresses cost-effectiveness, a slight reduction in image quality may be offset by financial considerations such as increased capacity of the image storage media and reduced image transfer and transmission times. Compression may be performed either through software or special hardware. There is a trade-off between the speed of compression and decompression and the monetary cost of the compression mechanism. Software-based compression methods are usually slower than special hardware compression boards but cost much less than the hardware solutions and are typically more flexible.

Compression is a flexible technology because the degree of coding complexity and the compression factor can be varied to suit the application. Medical images contain redundancy, areas in which many pixels have similar values. The actual information in the image is known as the entropy, which is the unpredictable part of the signal, and the remainder is redundancy, which is the part of the signal that is predictable. The sum of the two is the original (uncompressed) data file size. Once the entropy is known, a decision can be taken about how much of the entropy is to be preserved. It is therefore important to determine the entropy statistics of the particular image as well as how varying the entropy in a destructive way affects the image quality of the received and decompressed images.

Compression algorithms can be modeled as a sequence of three operations: transform mapping, quantization (bit allocation) and entropy coding. The transform mapping operation transforms the input data from the pixel domain into another domain where the quantizer and entropy encoder can be used more efficiently in the sense that fewer bits are required to encode the mapped data than would be required to code the original input data. For example, using the discrete cosine transform (DCT) as the transform mapping function recasts the spatial domain of an image into the spatial frequency domain where a vast majority of the image energy is resident in and around the DC coefficient. The majority of the remaining spatial frequency domain coefficients contain values several orders of magnitude smaller. The quantizer rounds off each mapped data value to one of a smaller number of possible values so that fewer code words (represented with as few bits as possible) are required. The entropy encoder assigns a code word to each quantizer output.

Once transformed, there are various techniques that can be used in the quantizer to reduce the data needed to carry the coefficient information. This is where the majority of the data compression occurs. The simplest reduction method involves a simple threshold magnitude for coefficients. Coefficients below the threshold are discarded. The coefficients may also be weighted according to various criteria. Psycho-visual knowledge may be used to weight the coefficients. Psycho-visual coding takes advantage of the eye's falling sensitivity to noise by dividing each coefficient by a different weighting factor as a function of its spatial frequency, reducing the magnitude of high-frequency coefficients disproportionately. If a coefficient threshold is used, the weighted coefficients failing to exceed the threshold are discarded and the results will be more acceptable than in the absence of weighting. The effect of weighting is that the coefficients are individually requantized with quantizing step sizes that increase with frequency. Larger step sizes increase the quantizing noise at high frequency where it is less noticeable.

ACR Teleradiology Guidelines for Compression

Both reversible (lossless) and irreversible (lossy) data compression may be utilized only when there is no demonstrable reduction in clinical diagnostic image quality as determined by and under the direction of a qualified physician. There are no mandates regarding the use of specific compression algorithms or compression ratio limits. If lossy compression is used, the compression ratio must be labeled clearly on each image so that the interpreting radiologist realizes the degree of compression applied to ensure appropriate clinical image quality. To ensure appropriate clinical image quality, The selection and periodic review of the compression algorithms and compression ratios used for the various imaging studies transmitted and stored by a teleradiology system are the obligation of the responsible physician. In this responsibility, the radiologist will undoubtedly consult the medical physicist.

Lossless Compression Algorithms

Lossless (reversible) compression algorithms only use the first (transform mapper) and last (entropy encoder) elements of the generalized compression algorithm, as the quanitization step is usually irreversble in order to provide a relatively large compression ratio. As such, the entropy encoder provides all of the compression capability, which is then limited usually to around 2-4:1. There are various transform-mapping functions that can be used. The lossless JPEG (Joint Photographic Experts Group) algorithm [Pennebaker 1993] used for DICOM utilizes a differential pulse code modulation (DPCM) algorithm where each adjacent pixel in a row is subtracted from its previous neighbor. This is also known as linear prediction. This acts to remove a majority of the redundancy and reduces the histogram variance, but does not result in image compression, as the resulting file is the same size as the original. The second stage, entropy encoding, is a process to assign binary symbols to the pixel prediction values. The Huffman entropy encoding technique is widely used in PC commercial software and freeware (and is utilized in the lossless JPEG compression algorithm specified in DICOM).

Other lossless entropy encoding processes can be used; for example, Run Length Encoding (RLE), arithmetic coding, and dictionary-based techniques like LZW (Limpel-Ziv-Welch). Arithmetic coding can reduce the redundancy as close to zero as desired by increasing the length of the coding sequence, i.e., ganging pixel values in series. However, this approach is only more efficient than Huffman coding for images with highly skewed probabilities like faxes, but not so in general for medical images. LZW is used in commercial/freeware PC software compression packages, in V.42bis modems and GIF (Graphics Interchange Format), however, dictionary-based compression techniques are most useful when structural constraints restrict the frequently occurring patterns to a small sub-set of all possible patterns. This is the case with text as well as computer-to-computer communication, but not the case with images.

Lossy Compression Algorithms

Lossy (reversible) compression algorithms employ all three elements of the generalized compression algorithm. The entropy encoders are usually the same ones used in the lossless compression algorithms. The transform mapping functions can also be those used in lossless compression algorithms, but the DCT and the wavelet transforms are the ones used most frequently for teleradiology. Wavelets have been used with great success over the past five to six years in radiological image compression, from digital thoracic x-ray images [Goldberg 1994] and mammograms [Laine 1994] to ultrasound video [Andrew 1998, 1999]. As mentioned previously, the component that provides the majority of the data compression is the form of quanitizer that performs the bit allocation for the transform coefficients.

DICOM and Compression

The DICOM standard currently provides a mechanism for supporting the use of JPEG and RLE image compression. For JPEG [Wallace 1991] the following coding processes are supported (transform mapping processes in parentheses): the first-order horizontal prediction of JPEG Process 14 (DPCM), the 8-bit lossy Baseline Compression of JPEG Process 1 (DCT), and the 12-bit lossy Extended Compression of JPEG Process 4 (DCT). All these processes utilize Huffman coding and non-hierarchical storage. RLE is an 8-bit lossless compression scheme. Although DICOM Working Group IV has been considering the adoption of wavelet image compression to the standard, it has not yet been ratified.

Practical Limits for Teleradiology Compression

Even though JPEG is the most widely employed algorithm today, there is increasing evidence that alternative approaches, such as wavelets, may have advantages for the compression of radiological images. Although both 8- and 12-bit lossy JPEG are supported by DICOM, its inclusion was not intended as an explicit endorsement of JPEG as the technique of choice for compressing medical images. JPEG was not expressly created for medical applications. Its principal advantage is that it is widely available on a variety of computing platforms and is inexpensive. JPEG, however, suffers from blocking artifacts that become annoyingly apparent at higher compression ratios [Ho 1993]. These blocking artifacts arise from the 8×8 pixel block subdivision of the image for DCT transformation. With increasing compression ratio, artificial edges are created between blocks to which the human visual system is acutely sensitive. Compression techniques that utilize the entire image frame (e.g., wavelets) do not generate the same type of artifacts, and as a result, higher levels of compression can be achieved before easily visible image degradation becomes apparent. Using JPEG, generally accepted safe levels of image compression are in the range of 6-8:1 for MR and CT images and 20:1 for radiographs.

Under extreme compression ratios wavelets generally degrade more gracefully than JPEG compressed images. As the compression ratio increases for wavelets, the images typically appear more and more highly smoothed and eventually small "bricks" or "rice grains" appear irregularly throughout the image. A rule of thumb for wavelets is to double the maximum JPEG levels: 12-15:1 for MR and CT images and 40:1 for radiographs. However, as specified by the ACR, each radiologist must use his own informed judgment when electing to incorporate image compression in a teleradiology system. Please also see the expanded article *Compression and Encryption* by Nicholas J. Hangiandreou in this volume for further discussion on image compression.

Transmission of Images and Related Data

Teleradiology nodes connect to other teleradiology nodes through either point-to-point (connection-oriented) methods, or through Intranets (local area networks—LANs) or the Internet (wide area network—WAN) which are typically packet-switched. The descriptions below are not meant to be exhaustive, but rather briefly describing how these telecommunication and networking technologies are used in practical teleradiology systems. Please also see the expanded article *Networks, Pipes and Connectivity* by Brent K. Stewart in this volume for further detail. Other excellent network references are provided by Blaine 1996 and Stewart 1993.

POTS

POTS stands for "plain old telephone system." Unless one is using ISDN (see below), the handset and modem one uses every day are analog instruments. However, the telephone network uses a very high-speed and hierarchical fiber-optic digital switching matrix between central offices. The rate for digital traffic of the phone line to your home is 64 kbps; but because of the analog modem, the throughput is limited to a fraction of this, depending on the condition of the phone wiring in your home and to the central office. For example, I have a 56 kbps modem on my laptop, but only connect into my Internet Service Provider (ISP) at between 26.4 and 31.2 kbps. POTS is inexpensive and is ubiquitous in this and many other countries. POTS service is connection-oriented and entirely circuit-switched with dedicated access.

Analog modems are used for teleradiology in two ways. The first is simple and direct point-to-point (modem-to-modem) connection. The other is through the Internet or an Intranet. For the Internet, one dials into an ISP modem pool. An Intranet is a fairly well self-contained local area network, which will have its own modem pool. The Intranet may or may not be tied into the wider Internet. PPP is the Internet standard for serial communications and defines how your modem connection exchanges data packets with other systems on the Internet. However, typically due to the large number of users accessing modem pools, dynamically allocated Internet Protocol (IP) addresses are assigned to users as they log-in from their locations. If the connection is terminated through logout or timeout (ISPs are getting rather aggressive about this), and the connection re-established at a later time, a different IP address will be assigned from the pool.

This makes it difficult to use DICOM to transfer images from a radiological scanning device to, for example, an on-call teleradiology display computer at a radiologist's home. DICOM requires three pieces of information to transfer images: IP address, port number and the DICOM application entity title (AET). If the IP address is not permanent, the technologist will have to get the current IP address from the radiologist at home once the PPP link has been established and an IP address has been assigned, and then transmit the images. This would not be a problem for a radiologist's DICOM application at home if it acts as a Query/Retrieve service class user. The radiologist can simply query the scanner over the network and retrieve the studies he wishes to examine.

Integrated Services Digital Network (ISDN)

ISDN is a network standard evolved from the telephony integrated digital network that provides end-to-end digital links to support a spectrum of applications, including voice, data, and compressed video services, to which users have access by a limited set of standard multipurpose user-network interfaces (60). ISDN provides end-to-end customer services with access through a limited number of standard network interfaces. ISDN provides a basic rate interface (BRI - two B channels at 64 kbps each and one D channel at 16 kbps) and a primary rate interface (PRI - 23 B channels at 64 kbps each and one D channel at 32 kbps). The cost for an ISDN BRI is about $80/month for unlimited usage. ISDN has been used widely for telemedicine, but less so for teleradiology.

Switched Dial-up Lines

The T-1 carrier point-to-point service is equivalent to 24 voice-grade channels, each with a bandwidth of 4,000 Hz or 8,000 samples per second [Dwyer 1992]. Each sample may be 7 bits (8,000 samples per second × 7 bits per sample = 56 kbps) or 8 bits (64 kbps). The signaling rate for 24 voice-grade channels is 1.544 Mbps (64 kbps) or 1.344 Mbps (56 kbps). The T-1 carrier service is provided for designated point-to-point locations, 24 hours per day. Cost for T-1 service after installation consists of a monthly access charge and a distance cost.

DS-1 switched, dial-up digital service is based on 24 digital voice-grade channels, each channel being 56 or 64 kbps, for a signaling rate of 1.344 or 1.544 Mbps, respectively [Dwyer 1996]. DS-0 dial-up service is a 56 (aka switched 56) or 64-kbits/sec digital voice-grade channel. Whenever image transmission is desired, the Ethernet data packets are formatted by the bridge into a standard, high-speed, serial bit stream of 1.344 Mbps. This bit stream is applied to the n × 56 kbps multiplexer, which dials up the desired number of 56 kbps switched digital voice-grade channels and which transmits the serial data in parallel to the selected destination. The system carries full duplex traffic in a serial stream between any two dial-up points equipped with an equivalent multiplexer.

Cable Modem

As the name implies, cable modems use a converter box (the cable modem) to impress Ethernet traffic (TCP/IP) onto the cable video infrastructure where it is eventually tied into the Internet. The network interface card (NIC) sends Ethernet packets to the cable modem. The cable modem modulates the data and transmits radio frequency (RF) signals over coaxial cable to the receiving modem at the other end of the connection that is tied into the Internet. In the opposite direction, your modem converts the RF signals it receives back into Ethernet packets before sending them to the Ethernet card in your computer. Cable modems generally use about a 30 Mbps channel swath of the video cable service. This bandwidth is shared with others using cable modems in your neighborhood, so depending on their usage, your bandwidth will vary in time. Depending on your local cable infrastructure, the downstream (to your location) data rate is usually many times faster than the upstream (from your location) rate. This is of course fine for teleradiology if one is only receiving images. Typically a hard IP address is given for use by the NIC which makes teleradiology using DICOM much easier to implement as was explained in the POTS section above. General cost is about $40/month.

Digital Subscriber Line (DSL)

Stated simply, DSL provides high-speed multimedia services, such as video-on-demand and super-fast Internet access (for teleradiology) to anyone with a standard, copper telephone line. DSL technology represents one solution to the well-publicized last-mile problem, although DSL deployment to date is not going as smoothly as carriers originally hoped and is getting heavy competition from cable modem service. DSL is run over existing copper phone wires, so carriers do not have to run new cable to and within your location. However, users will need to install a DSL modem that communicates with a DSL access muliplexer (DSLAM) at the telco central office. The DSL modem connects to the 10BaseT Ethernet card on your PC.

DSL service operates in frequencies outside those used for voice. Voice or analog transmission typically falls in the 0 to 3400 Hz range and transmits at speeds from 9.6 to 56 kbps. By extending the top frequency boundary, DSL can operate on the same line without interfering with the analog signal. However, to support DSL, the copper wiring from the central office must meet certain criteria. For example, the line must be free of load coils, which are often added to long local loops to improve voice quality. Thus for DSL, one typically has to be less than three miles from the central office and the longer the local loop, the slower the DSL rate.

Two of the most common flavors of DSL are high bit-rate DSL and asymmetrical DSL (ADSL). Rates in multiples of 256 kbps up to 10 Mbps are available. For 256 kbps DSL service through a local carrier, the rate is around $30-40/month. Again, typically a hard IP address is given for use by the NIC, which makes teleradiology using DICOM much easier to implement as was explained in the POTS section above. General cost is about $40/month.

ACR Teleradiology Guidelines for Transmission

Digital data transmission must provide effective error checking capability and not cause a loss of clinically significant information. The form of the transmission infrastructure utilized is left to the user as dictated by the environment of the studies to be transmitted.

Display Capabilities

Image display capabilities include the video monitors used and the image display and enhancement software used. Important video display characteristics include: screen size, resolution, bit depth, luminance, dynamic range, noise, and distortion [Stewart 1993]. Typical screen resolutions for PC video monitors can be adjusted from 640×480 through about 1600×1200 depending on the amount of video RAM installed. Bit depths per pixel may range from 8 to 32 bits for color display cards and between 8 to 16 bits for monochrome display cards. The digital-to-analog converters (DACs) used for driving the display are usually only 8 bits.

Luminance describes the amount of visible light emitted by the CRT display surface and is expressed in units of foot-Lambert (ft-L). Luminance affects the human eye response through two important characteristics, the acuity of the eye and the detection of luminance differences [Wang 1997]. While this information is rarely given in vendor specifications, it is important when comparing teleradiology-viewing stations. Brighter monitors (with high ft-L measurements) are better for viewing because the brightness differential between the shades (just noticeable differences) is greater and thus easier for the human eye to detect. Standard PC color monitors (20-40 ft-L maximum luminance) will most likely not provide adequate brightness for primary interpretation of radiographs as in the ACR guidelines. Monochrome video monitors (50-200 ft-L maximum luminance) with special display boards may be used in PCs for primary interpretation. Monitor screen sizes generally range from 15 to 21 inches. Larger monitors typically provide a better viewing environment. High luminance monitors typically have a short lifetime (2-3 years). Several spectacular five megapixel, 200 ft-L flat panel displays were demonstrated at the past RSNA with a projected five-year fluorescent tube lifetime.

In designing user interfaces for display stations, the goal is to create an intuitive tool that rapidly becomes transparent to the user, allowing complex task performance with a minimal amount of technical training. Most current interactive computer systems rely on underlying graphical tools used for display, often referred to as graphical user interfaces (GUIs). Although there are some hybrids, GUIs consist of three major components: a windowing system, an imaging model, and an application program interface (API). Most window-based user interfaces provide a rich environment designed to facilitate display and manipulation of images, text, and graphics in windows that may overlap.

Presentation functions provide for the interactive selection, positioning, and sequencing of image data on the display screen, including: (1) patient exam selection, (2) selection of presentation on the display monitor; and (3) multi-modality and composite image display. Auxiliary text information (identification of clinical problem, relevant patient history, previous reports, specification of time constraints, and radiology requisition) should be provided to orient the user of the suspected patient problem. Three major modes of presentation are the stack, tile and cine modes. The tile mode allows side-by-side presentation of images of an examination. The stack mode allows sequential presentation, one at a time, with overlapping windows. The cine mode provides dynamic sequential viewing of either spatially or temporally contiguous images.

With the wealth of different imaging modalities and the possible large number of images for a single patient, it is important to have two additional viewing modes: survey and pictorial index. In the survey mode, images are displayed at lower resolution than acquired in order to allow more images to be displayed simultaneously; for example, viewing four CR images on a system with only two monitors. The pictorial index presents all available image modality examinations available for a patient case, conveyed as minified versions of the actual diagnostic images.

Gray level optimization is especially important for displaying images that have greater than 8-bit contrast resolution (dynamic range of cathode ray tube displays; 8-bit DACs are used). For example, a 12-bit (4096 discrete gray levels) CT image typically contains CT numbers in the range of 200-1800. Thus, a blind 12- to 8-bit conversion will result in a displayed image with sub-optimal contrast. Window and level operations must then be performed manually. Pre-determination of optimal look-up tables (LUTs) is desirable for bone, soft tissue, lung, etc. The LUT for CR and MR might be based on a histogram of the image, the image type (anatomy, modality, etc.), and an estimation of the signal-to-noise ratio.

Interactive manipulation operations should enhance the visibility of anatomical and pathological features (lesions, nodules, bone fractures, etc.). The basic tools required include intensity transformation tables (automatic preset windows, manual independent window and level control, and image reversal) and image enlargement and translation (zoom and pan). Adjustment of the intensity transformation tables will undoubtedly be the most frequently used image processing operation. In all probability, adjustment will be performed on each displayed image. In addition, the ability to add graphic overlays (text annotations and pointers), as well as rotation and flip capabilities is important. Although there are a plethora of image processing functions available for use at the display stations (e.g., adaptive histogram equalization or unsharpmasking), we have found that radiologists either do not have the patience for them or do not realize their utility.

ACR Teleradiology Guidelines for Display

Display workstations used for primary interpretation must have a video monitor luminance of at least 50 ft-L and the reading environment lighting conditions (e.g., low ambient lighting and elimination of reflections) should be controlled as much as possible. The user interface must provide: accurate association of the patient and study demographic information with the study images, image sequence selection, window and level adjustment, magnification and pan functions, image reorientation (rotation and flip) providing that patient orientation labeling is preserved, and calculation and display of accurate linear displacement measurements and pixel value representation appropriate to that modality (e.g., CT Hounsfield units). In addition, the matrix size, bit depth, total number of images in the acquired study, as well as the image compression ratio should be displayed.

The display workstations must be capable of meeting the guidelines outlined in the image acquisition section for large and small matrix images. Less stringent guidelines may apply for display systems when not used for primary diagnosis. Please also see the expanded articles on workstations by Kenneth M. Spicer and Janice C. Honeyman in this volume.

Archiving and Retrieval

Images transmitted for off-site interpretation need not be permanently stored at the off-site location and will typically be archived at the sending institution. Only a sufficient level of disk storage at the receiving site to store images until interpreted or overread is required. Considering the rapid pace of digital storage media densities of late, this is usually not a problem, even without image compression. However, new and historical images should be accessible through a query/retrieve process over the teleradiology link to the interpreting physician.

ACR Teleradiology Guidelines for Archiving and Retrieval

A difficult requirement for teleradiology systems to adhere to under the ACR guidelines is that prior examinations should be retrievable in a time frame appropriate to the clinical needs of the facility and medical staff. Also that teleradiology systems should provide storage capacity capable of complying with facility, state, and federal regulations regarding medical record retention. However, there is the stipulation that images interpreted off-site need not be stored at the receiving facility if they are archived at the transmitting site.

These requirements seem to fall more into the realm of PACS. As most teleradiology systems employ display workstations of limited disk space capacity and a first-in-first-out disk management algorithm, the burden of archiving examinations then falls to the originating organization in sufficient digital or hardcopy formats. Each facility should have policies and procedures for the archiving of digital image data equivalent to the policies that currently exist for the protection of hard-copy storage media to preserve imaging records. Most institutions will still have film-based radiographic archives in addition to teleradiology until the full transition to PACS is achieved. In this way the storage requirements at the receiving site are obviated through the original hardcopy film if no digital archive is available.

Required database fields for each examination must include patient name, identification number, exam data, type of examination, and the facility at which the examination occurred. Specific instances of these database entries must accurately correspond with the associated examination. In addition to the above fields, it is desirable to include a free-text field for a brief clinical history note.

Security

As our society relies more and more on the Internet to communicate and do business, healthcare is also taking advantage of the "information superhighway." As healthcare information, including teleradiology, shifts further and further from private networks and Intranets to the Internet, enhanced security of individually identifiable patient information becomes a prime concern [Baur 1997]. Please also see the expanded article *Compression and Encryption* by Nicholas J. Hangiandreou in this volume.

ACR Teleradiology Guidelines for Security

Teleradiology systems should provide network and software security protocols to protect the confidentiality of patients' identification and imaging data. There should be measures to safeguard the data and to ensure data integrity against intentional or unintentional corruption of the data.

HIPAA and HCFA Requirements

A national debate about how and how much to protect the privacy of personal health data entered and stored in computers and transferred electronically has simmered for approximately 25 years without resolution. The Health Insurance Portability and Accountability Act of 1996 (HIPAA) [NRC 1997] is forcing resolution and compromise quickly because Congress has set an August 1999 deadline for itself to enact privacy protections. President Clinton stated in his 1999 State of the Union Address that he would sign the HIPAA legislation into law if Congress does not act by that time. The health privacy rules in the HIPAA legislation are a requisite to implementing the Administrative Simplification provisions of HIPAA, which mandate use of a uniform, electronic data set for financial and administrative transactions along with a unique identifier for every participant in the health system.

Along with this, the Health Care Financing Administration (HCFA) has until October 1998 had a long-standing policy of banning the Internet for the communication of individually identifiable patient information. HCFA has come to recognize that its ban on the use of the Internet is inconsistent with technology trends, economics, and new federal policies and rules, not the least of which are the forthcoming HIPAA mandated security regulations. HCFA drafted a new policy in October 1998 that provides HCFA contractors with guidelines for the appropriate use of the Internet. HCFA policies only officially apply to the information protected under the Privacy Act of 1974, which is a mandate on federal agencies. In the healthcare context, this Act protects information about patients covered under Medicare, Medicaid, and Federal Child Insurance programs. However, the HIPAA legislation will, almost assuredly, increase the scope of this policy to apply to all patient information.

As more and more teleradiology systems move toward client-server and web server operation over the Internet from the point-to-point dial-up modem model, the HCFA policy guidelines and HIPAA legislation will have great impact on future teleradiology transactions. It will be permissible to use the Internet for transmission of individually identifiable patient information or other sensitive healthcare data, as long as an acceptable method of encryption is utilized to provide for confidentiality and integrity of this data. Also required is the employment of authentication or identification procedures to assure that both the sender and recipient of the data are known to each other and are authorized to receive such information. Neither the HCFA policy statements nor HIPPA legislation spell out the exact mechanisms to be used for these functions as encryption and authentication technologies are moving targets.

Encryption

Encryption is the transformation of data to conceal its information content, prevent undetected modification, and/or prevent its unauthorized use. Encryption uses a key or keys. Key management will be required when encryption is used. There are two main types of encryption: asymmetric encryption (also called public-key encryption) and symmetric encryption (also called private-key encryption). Encryption may be employed using hardware or software. Currently, teleradiology systems employing encryption use software. Two methods are Secure Sockets Layer (SSL) and Secure MIME (S/MIME).

SSL is a protocol developed for transmitting private documents via the Internet. SSL works by using a private key to encrypt data that is transferred over the SSL connection. SSL is a protocol to authenticate server to client and (potentially) client to server, to establish a "session" and to negotiate parameters for the encryption of messages exchanged during that session. These parameters include a shared "symmetric" encryption key and chosen encryption algorithm. SSL does not require any particular choice of these parameters. Both the Netscape Navigator and Internet Explorer browsers support SSL, and many web sites use the protocol to obtain confidential user information. By convention, web pages that require an SSL connection start with https: instead of http:. SSL comes in multiple strengths using various length (e.g., 40, 56, 128, and 168-bit) encryption keys. SSL using greater than a 40-bit encryption key is termed "strong" encryption. Using "default" SSL configurations in browsers and servers will likely result in no client authentication and 40-bit DES (Data Encryption Standard) encryption.

MIME (multipurpose Internet mail extensions) is a specification for formatting non-ASCII messages so that they can be sent over the Internet. S/MIME is a protocol for the cryptographic enveloping of MIME messages. Because e-mail is asychronous, the sender determines algorithm/key length prior to sending the S/MIME message. S/MIME itself does not determine key length, merely how to securely exchange keys and algorithm information. S/MIME implementations usually support a number of algorithms but the standard only requires support for relatively weak algorithms (due to the federal export restriction and patent concerns). The sender choosing relatively strong encryption may find some recipients unable to decipher the message, while relative insecure messages will routinely be received and decrypted. For example, Netscape's domestic S/MIME implementation's default configuration calls for 168-bit DES.

Authentication

Authentication is the process of identifying an individual, usually based on a username and password, but is extending now into biometric (fingerprint and retinal) identification as well as "smart cards." A smart card is a small device the size of a credit card that displays a constantly changing user ID code. A user first enters his/her password into the computer and then the card displays a user ID that can be used as authentication. Typically, the user IDs change every 1-5 minutes. In security systems, authentication is distinct from authorization, which is the process of giving individuals access to system functions based on identity. Authentication merely ensures that the individual is who he or she claims to be, but says nothing about the access rights of the individual.

A certificate authority (CA) is a trusted third-party organization or company that issues digital certificates used to create digital signatures and public-private key pairs. The role of the CA in this process is to guarantee that the individual granted the unique certificate is, in fact, who he or she claims to be. Usually, this means that the CA has an arrangement with a financial institution, such as a credit card company, which provides it with information to confirm an individual's claimed identity. Certificate authorities are a critical component in authentication security on the web because they guarantee that the two parties exchanging information are really who they claim to be. Every SSL server must have an SSL server certificate. When a web browser connects to a web server using the SSL protocol, the server sends the browser its public key in an X.509 certificate.

Reliability and Redundancy

The reliability of a teleradiology system of course relies chiefly on good computer hygiene which includes the consistent use of disk and virus scanning software, periodic system backup and use of an uninterruptable power supply (UPS), preferably one with a serial line to the computer for graceful shutdown of the system near the end of the stored UPS charge. It may seem obvious, but an alternate backup computer system or components with alternate communication connection (e.g., low cost 56 kbps modem to back-up a DS-1 line) will help ensure maximum uptime, as well as 7×24-maintenance contract or help desk support from the vendor.

ACR Teleradiology Guidelines for Reliability and Redundancy

Quality patient care depends on availability of the teleradiology system. Written policies and procedures should be in place to ensure continuity of care at a level consistent with those for hard-copy imaging studies and medical records within a facility or institution. This should include internal redundancy systems, backup telecommunication links, and a disaster plan.

Quality Control and Improvement

The major quality control issue for teleradiology is image quality assurance [Forsberg 1995]. The laser film digitizer mirrors should be adjusted approximately every 2 to 3 months. There are also test patterns printed on laser film that can be used to check the quality of the digitized image. Video systems like frame grabbers and display monitors can be checked using SMPTE [Gray 1992] test patterns. Some video monitors also come with an attachable photometer that interacts with the display card to adjust the overall brightness and black level. Some also calibrate the display for perceptual linearization as specified in DICOM supplement 28 (Grayscale Standard Display Function), maximizing the number of just noticeable differences [Blume 1997].

ACR Teleradiology Guidelines for Quality Control and Improvement

Facilities using teleradiology should have documented policies and procedures for monitoring and evaluating the effective management, safety, and proper performance of system components. These component functions include image acquisition, digitization, compression, transmission, archiving, and retrieval. The QC program's goal should be to maximize the quality and accessibility of diagnostic information. Utilization of teleradiology does not reduce the responsibilities for the management and supervision of radiological medicine.

A phantom image, such as the SMPTE test pattern should be captured, transmitted, archived, retrieved, and displayed at appropriate intervals, but at least monthly, to test the overall operation of the teleradiology imaging chain under conditions that simulate the normal operation of the system. As a spatial resolution test, the phantom image should be at least 512×512 for small matrix primary interpretation, and 2.5 lp/mm resolution for large-matrix primary interpretation. As a test of the display, SMPTE pattern data files sized to occupy the full area used to display images on the monitor should be displayed. The overall SMPTE image appearance should be inspected to assure the absence of gross artifacts (e.g., blurring or bleeding of bright display areas into dark areas or aliasing of spatial resolution patterns). Display monitors used for primary interpretation should be tested at least monthly. As a dynamic range test, both the 5% and the 95% areas should be seen as distinct from the respective adjacent 0% and 100% areas.

Synergism with PACS and Telemedicine

Synergism with PACS

There is obviously a natural synergism between teleradiology and PACS. Teleradiology systems may be thought of as PCS (picture communication systems), or PACS sans archive systems. As the investment in a digital archive can be fairly prohibitive, teleradiology may be the first step for most radiology departments before moving to mini-PACS and then department-wide PACS (filmless or "less film" radiology). PACS usually have some kind of teleradiology component with, for example, a film digitizer at a remote primary care clinic. In this case, it behooves institutions to invest in teleradiology components that provide DICOM capabilities so that protocol and file format converter computers are not necessary. This will be easier once lossy compression algorithms ratified as part of DICOM become more available. Please also see the articles by Larry J. Filipow and G. Donald Frey on PACS in this volume.

Synergism with Telemedicine

Telemedicine has been variously defined, but can be broadly described as combining telecommunications technology with medical expertise for the remote delivery of medical care or education. Several telemedicine subspecialty applications have evolved: teleradiology, telepathology, teledermatology, telepsychiatry, telecardiology, medical consultations, continuing medical education, and others. Teleradiology is by far the most mature of these telemedicine subspecialties, and is therefore an obvious component of many telemedicine systems [Goldberg 1996, Franken 1996]. As the telemedicine system usually has a fairly high bit data stream made available to it (e.g., 384-1544 kbps), the teleradiology component shares this bandwidth for fairly rapid transmission in a "stat" mode, or in the background using unallocated bandwidth when a video telemedicine session is ongoing.

Compressed Streaming Video and Video Clips

One area where teleradiology and telemedicine intersect is in the use of video compression. Moving, real-time medical imagery, from x-ray fluoroscopy and angiography, diagnostic ultrasound, echocardiography, and video endoscopy make use of video compression to transmit to another site for viewing. The video can be compressed, transmitted, and reviewed in real-time. This mode is termed synchronous video telemedicine. An example of this is in obstetric ultrasound, which typically relies on real-time involvement by the radiologist [Fisk 1995]. The video can also be compressed and stored. This video clip can then be transmitted and reviewed at a later time. This mode is termed asynchronous video, or store-and-forward video. An example of this is echocardiography where the video is commonly videotaped and subsequently reviewed off-line by a radiologist or cardiologist [Karson 1995].

The first question is how much data is there in video? The current standard for component color video digitization is CCIR 601, which prescribes a spatial resolution of 720 samples horizontally and 480 samples vertically. Sampling rates are based on multiples of 3.375 Msamples/second. Sampling rate multiples can vary for the luminance and chromanance signals, usually given by sampling ratios: luminance:chromanance (red channel - C_r):chromanance(blue channel - C_b). The green chromanance can be reconstructed from these three signals. The 4:2:0 sampling rate scheme is adequate for most applications where video compression is to be employed. The luminance is sampled at every sample point, but C_r and C_b are sampled every other sample point and every other sample line. The undersampling of color can be justified based on extensive studies of the psychophysics of color vision. If 8-bit sampling is used for intensity and chromanance, the data rate to store this real-time digitized video is 20.25 Mbytes/sec. This is equal to 1.2 Gbytes/min or 73 Gbytes/hour! If only the intensity (monochrome) component is considered through discarding the color components, these data rates are reduced by a factor of one-third.

How can this digital video stream be compressed? Various methods are employed. Using the 4:2:0 schema already introduces the concept of sub-sampling, which can be performed spatially and temporally (periodically dropping adjacent frames). Essentially we want to remove the redundancies and leave only the entropy (non-stationary) signal to be transmitted to the remote location. There are a number of extant standards for video compression which are extensions of the JPEG intraframe compression standard: Motion-JPEG (no still frame redundancies removed, thus limiting the compression ratio), ITU-T (International Telecommunication Union - Telecommunication Standardization Sector) Recommendations H.261/H.263 and MPEG-1 and MPEG-2.

In order for the 162 Mbps of the 4:2:0 sampled CCIR 601 digitized video to be compressed down to a DS-1 rate requires a compression ratio of just over 100:1. Additional investigation is required to recommend specific guidelines for applications that require real-time, full-motion video. Requirements will vary depending on the imaging modality and the type of information being sought. Ultrasound video has been found to be compressed down to 384 kbps and yet retain sufficient information for diagnosis [Stewart 1998].

References

Aberle, D.R., Gleeson, F., Sayre, J.W., et al. "The effect of irreversible image compression on diagnostic accuracy in thoracic imaging." *Invest Radiol* 28:398-403; 1993.

ACR - American College of Radiology. ACR Standard for Teleradiology: diagnostic radiology standard no 12. Reston, VA: American College of Radiology, Res 21; 1994.

Andrew, R.K., Stewart, B.K., Langer, S.G., Stegbauer, K.C. "Wavelet compression of ultrasound video streams for teleradiology." IEEE International Conference on Information Technology Applications in Biomedicine ITAB98:15-9; 1998.

Andrew, R.K., Stewart, B.K., Langer, S.G., Stegbauer, K.C. "A 3-D wavelet-based codec for lossy compression of pre-scan converted ultrasound video." *Proc. SPIE* 3658:(in press); 1999.

Baur, H.J., Engelmann, U., Saurbier, F., et al. "How to deal with security issues in teleradiology." *Comput Methods Programs Biomed* 53:1-8; 1997.

Bidgood, W.D., Horii, S.C. "Modular extension of the ACR-NEMA DICOM standard to support new diagnostic imaging modalities and services." *J Digit Imaging* 9:67-77; 1996.

Bidgood, W.D., Horii, S.C., Prior, F.W., Van Syckle, D.E. "Understanding and using DICOM, the data interchange standard for biomedical imaging." *J Am Med Inform Assoc* 4:199-212; 1997.

Blume, H., Hemminger, B.M. "Image presentation in digital radiology: perspectives on the emerging DICOM display function standard and its application." *Radiographics* 17:769-77; 1997.

Bolle, S.R., Sund, T., Stormer, J. "Receiver operating characteristic study of image pre-processing for teleradiology and digital workstations." *J Digit Imaging* 1997; 10:152-57; 1997.

Crowther, J.B., Poropatich, R. "Telemedicine in the U.S. Army: case reports from Somalia and Croatia." *Telemedicine Journal* 1:73-80; 1995.

Dwyer, S.J., Stewart, B.K., Sayre, J.W., Honeyman, J.C. "Wide area network strategies for teleradiology systems." *Radiographics* 12: 567-76; 1992.

Dwyer, S.J. "Imaging system architectures for picture archiving and communication systems." *Radiol Clin North Am* 34:495-503; 1996.

Goldberg, M.A., Pivovarov, M., Mayo-Smith, W.W., et al. "Application of wavelet compression to digitized radiographs." *AJR* 163:463-8, 1994.

Goldberg, M.A. "Teleradiology and telemedicine." *Radiol Clin North Am* 34:647-65; 1996.

Gray, J.F. "Use of the SMPTE test pattern in picture archiving and communication systems." *J Digit Imaging* 5:54-8; 1992

Fisk, N.M., Bower, S., Sepulveda, W., et al. "Fetal telemedicine: interactive transfer of realtime ultrasound and video via ISDN for remote consultation." *J Telemed Telecare* 1:38-44; 1995.

Forsberg, D.A. "Quality assurance in teleradiology." *Telemedicine Journal* 1:107-14, 1995.

Franken, E.A., Berbaum, K.S., Smith, W.L., et al. "Teleradiology for rural hospitals: analysis of a field study." *J Telemed Telecare* 1:202-8; 1995.

Franken, E.A., Berbaum, K.S. "Subspecialty radiology consultation by interactive telemedicine." *J Telemed Telecare* 2:35-41; 1996.

Good, W.F., Maitz, G.S., Gur, D.: "Joint photographic experts group (JPEG) compatible data compression of mammograms." *J Digital Imaging* 7:123-32; 1994.

Hangiandreou, N.J., O'Connor, T.J., Felmlee, J.P. "An evaluation of the signal and noise characteristics of four CCD-based film digitizers." *Med Phys* 25:2020-6; 1998.

Ho, B.K.T., Tseng, V., Ma, M., et al. "A mathematical model to quantify JPEG block artifacts." *Proc SPIE* 1897:269-74; 1993.

Horii, S.C. "Image acquisition: sites, technologies, and approaches." *Radiol Clin North Am* 34:469-94; 1996.

Huang, H.K. *PACS: Picture Archiving and Communication Systems in Biomedical Imaging.* New York, NY: VCH; 1996.

Karson, T.H., Chandra, S., Morehead, A.J., et al. "JPEG compression of digital echocardiographic images: impact on image quality." *J Am Soc Echocardiogr* 8:306-18; 1995.

Laine, A.F., Schuler, S., Jian, F., Huda, W. "Mammographic feature enhancement by multiscale analysis." IEEE Transactions on Medical Imaging 13:725-40; 1994.

National Research Council. For the Record: Protecting Electronic Health Information. Washington, DC: National Academy Press, 233-46; 1997.

Pennebaker, W.B., Mitchell, J.L. *JPEG Still Image Data Compression Standard.* New York: Van Nostrand Reinhold; 1993.

Perednia, D.A., Allen, A. "Telemedicine technology and clinical applications." *JAMA* 273:483-8; 1995.

RSNA – Radiological Society of North America. Handbook of Teleradiology Applications. St. Joseph, MI: IPC Communication Services; 1997.

Sonoda, M., Takano, M., Miyahara, J., Kato, H. "Computed radiography utilizing scanning laser stimulated luminescence." *Radiology* 20:833-38; 1983.

Steckel, R.J. "Daily x-ray rounds in a large teaching hospital using high-resolution closed-circuit television." *Radiology* 105:319-21; 1972.

Stewart, B.K., Aberle, D.R., Boechat, M.I., et al. "Clinical utilization of grayscale workstations." *IEEE Engineering in Medicine and Biology* 11:86-102; 1993.

Stewart, B.K., Carter, S.J., Langer, S.G., Andrew, R.K. "Compressed ultrasound video image quality evaluation using a likert scale and kappa statistical analysis." *Proc. SPIE* 3335:365-77; 1998.

Wallace, G.K. The JPEG Still Picture Compression Standard. Comm. ACM 1991; 34(4): 30-44.

Wang, J., Langer, S. "A brief review of human perception factors in digital displays for picture archiving and communications systems." *J Digit Imaging* 1997; 10:158-68.

The Radiologist's Workbench— Critical Features for Image Review and Reporting

K. M. Spicer, M.D., Ph.D. and Ehsan Samei, Ph.D.
Department of Radiology
Medical University of South Carolina

Introduction

Considering the time spent at image interpretation stations, radiologists seem amazingly passive about their requirements. The radiology literature scarcely addresses this topic. By and large, radiologists have been slow to appreciate how a modicum of forethought can produce significant changes in their work environment and display instruments that dramatically improve their performance. Mammographers have devoted considerable thought to workplace issues to improve their deficiency for screening mammograms and to decrease errors of omission. Hopefully, digital reading rooms will take advantage of the mammographers' experience. One only has to throw off the "if it ain't broke, don't fix it" mind set and closely observe a medium-sized reading room to appreciate the potential for improvement.

The ambition of this presentation is to identify some of the critical functional features of a radiologist's workstation, to contrast them with the film-based counterpart, and to recommend improvements, taking into account cost-effectiveness and current technical capabilities. All recommendations are based on the daily softcopy interpretation experience at Medical University of South Carolina (MUSC) for four years department-wide (all modalities) and for six years in nuclear medicine and ultrasound.

Workstation Environment

The big five reading room environmental variables are light, noise, motion, temperature and humidity, and space. With planning, all of these variables can be readily controlled.

Light

Ambient light has a significant impact on the quality of soft-copy displays. This is particularly important since the luminance of monitors is variably one-tenth to one-third that of light boxes and current display devices [such as CRTs (cathode ray tubes)] readily reflect ambient light. Ambient light hinders the diagnostic performance at three different levels. First and foremost, the light from other sources can be directly reflected from the monitor's face-plate (Flynn 1999). The reflected light can signifi-

433

cantly interfere with diagnostic interpretation. Secondly, the diagnostic reflection of ambient light in the face-plate can reduce image contrast (Flynn 1999, Wang 1997). And last, but not least, optimum light adaptation and contrast sensitivity of the human eye requires uniform lighting within the room.

Obviously, overhead ceiling lights must be extinguished and the overall light level in the room should be kept as low as possible. If electronic medical record or order-entry systems are not integrated with your Picture Archiving and Communication System (PACS), then the radiologist must work with paper/requisitions. Accordingly, an indirect light source for examining the paperwork is necessary. Monitors should be positioned so that they receive little or no reflective light during normal operation. This includes light from other workstations, light boxes, and table-top light sources. Ceilings and walls reflect lights as well, and this can be minimized by painting them a dark color with a non-glossy surface. Only an indirect light source should be used in the room. Computer screens should be black when not in use. All images should be bordered and all icons shaded in a dark color to facilitate ocular adaptation and to minimize distraction by non-image light.

Noise and Motion

Noise and motion cause distractions. Reading room noise levels decrease significantly when multi-viewers are removed. Soundproofing partitions between workstations, carpeting, and high ceilings with sound-absorbing tiles (painted black) all help and are inexpensive to implement. When a multi-viewer leaves your reading room, so do the file clerks and technologists. For large centralized reading areas people entering and leaving the room can be shielded from view by sound-absorbing partitions to further diminish distractions. Incorporating these recommendations at minimal expense produces a paradigm shift in the reading room environment. Some visitors have questioned how we tolerate working in what appears to them to be a tomb-like environment. In reality our reading rooms' quiet and darkness facilitate concentration. Further, our radiologists leave work at the end of the day much less frazzled and weary than in the pre-PACS days.

Temperature and Humidity

The undesirable effect of high temperature and humidity in a radiology reading room is obvious. Heating and air conditioning requirements and their associated expenses increase with PACS. CRT monitors running 24 hours a day are the chief culprit. Planning ahead for these needs is critical, especially since reading room space is usually decreased in PACS viewing rooms.

Space

While decreased reading room space in a PACS operation is probably justified, due to a smaller number of required workstations, the space needed for a workstation usually equals that for a multi-viewer station. That is especially necessary at present, since few PACS workstations can simultaneously run the RIS (Radiology Information System), HIS (Hospital Information System), and/or RadLAN or Rad NET (e-mail, scheduling, etc.) applications. Furthermore, display stations must be accompanied by a dictation unit or a voice recognition computer.

Workstation Ergonomics

Position of Radiologist

As CRT monitors have considerably less luminance than view boxes, the need to decrease ambient, extraneous light is readily recognized; however, overlooked but equally important can be the need to position the radiologist comfortably in the path of maximum light emission. Off-axis viewing or viewing from a large distance alters the effectiveness of the display presentation (Wang 1997). An ideal display device would have a Lambertian distribution, similar to film, for which perception of brightness does not change with the viewing angle. CRT monitors do not as closely follow the Lambertian distribution and thus brightness may vary as a function of viewing angle. The display(s) must be positioned so that multiple-sized radiologists can readily make adjustments to place themselves facing the display's face-plate. Consequently, the radiologist's chair should be orthopedically supportive and wear-resistant (adjustable height with thick castors to roll over sound-deadening carpet). Active matrix liquid crystal flat panel displays (AMLCDs) are replacing CRTs in some viewing applications. Advanced AMLCDs have greater luminance than CRTs, occupy less space, and generate much less heat, while providing long-term stable viewing. However, they are much less tolerant of off-angle viewing, and should be positioned taking that into account.

If multiple viewing stations are used, monitors should be placed to face the viewer(s) dead on (Strickland 1995). Placing multiple monitors for diagnostic viewing by more than one radiologist at a time is a complex challenge, a task that has not been fully addressed in current commercial products.

Commonly, a radiologist uses more than one computer to do his/her tasks. In such cases, the viewing area will need to accommodate considerable physician movement, potentially placing a premium on physical conditioning for the usually sedentary radiologist (the authors recognize that this is a "sweeping" generalization and hence provide no references). Needless to say the optimal solution will be to run multiple radiologist work-related applications on the same workstation.

Hardware

Monitors

The number of monitors required for a PACS diagnostic viewing station is inversely proportional to the speed and intelligence ("user-friendliness") of the PACS display station. As networks' bandwidth increases and servers grow more powerful, the ability to operate multiple software applications on a single computer is fast approaching. Without this "thin client" functionality, a minimum of four computers (five or more monitors) must be immediately available to the diagnostic radiologist (PACS—two or more monitors, RIS, HIS and dictation stations). At present most specialized image processing (e.g., off-plane reconstructions of computed tomography (CT), nuclear medicine, magnetic resonance (MR) angiographic, maximum intensity pixel rendering, virtual CT endoscopy) is performed on separate, dedicated workstations. Having these capabilities on a radiologist workstation would improve efficiency as well as quality. However, enhanced functionality should not increase the complexity of using the workstation. The workstation for the radiologist has the potential to vary from one emulating a nuclear reactor control center or the security guard's monitoring station at the Sears Tower to that of Bill Gates' home personal computer (sleek, elegant and simple, but incredibly powerful, one might imagine).

Systems with slow, cumbersome graphical user interfaces (GUIs), for example those that do not display images in the radiologist's preferred format, or those that do not display the old study on one CRT and the current one on the other, will benefit from additional monitors. If RIS, HIS, etc., are not fully integrated and displayed on the PACS monitor, then additional CRTs are essential.

Table 1 lists some of the most important variables of CRT performance, which have been widely discussed in the literature (Dwyer 1997, Muka 1995, Roehrig 1990, Otto 1998). For the diagnostic radiologist, maximum luminance, resolution, and size should be as great as one's budget can tolerate. Refresh rates (flicker), distortion, and other diagnostic detractors have been successfully minimized for the much more reasonably priced CRTs sold during the last two years.

The question of whether to buy 2K or 1K monitors is arguable and probably moot. During the last four years that our department has been entirely "soft-copy," 1K displays have won out over the 2K's. The higher utilization of 1K monitors has been due to the fact that they are brighter, their image size is considerably larger, they screen feed the images faster, and they are more stable over time. The 2K workstations have decreased in number and remain as workstations dedicated to reading large numbers of CR (computed radiography) images and high resolution studies (e.g., 4K bone detail imaging). At this point, the relative merit of the 2K and 1K monitors, as far as diagnostic quality, is not fully substantiated.

Table 1. Important Display Monitor Performance Variables.

1. Maximum and minimum luminance

2. Dynamic range

3. Luminance response

4. Resolution

5. Flicker

6. Stability (changes in performance over time)

7. Geometrical distortion

8. Image size at full resolution

9. Color tint

10. Viewing angle

CPU

A variety of computers are used to drive radiologist's diagnostic display stations, from PCs (IBM, their clones, or Macintosh) to the faster, more powerful, but significantly more costly RISC (Reduced Instruction Set Computers) stations (Sun SPARK, Silicone Graphics, etc.). These instruments, guided by user-interface hardware (mouse, trackball, keyboard, etc.) acquire image data into very fast video driver boards [often associated with accelerator processors and extensive video RAM (random access memory)] for rapid display, and basic computational manipulations (window and level, image inversion, zoom, etc.). Hence, they all have in common very rapid internal bus circuitry, multiple processors, and powerful video drivers. In the last few years, the physical size of computers has decreased, as has their heat production to the point that placement in work environments is usually not a problem.

Expansion of a workstation image storage capacity is usually accomplished by external hard drives, offering two practical double benefits. The first is the obvious improvement in display speed performance when a desired study is "local" on the workstation hard drive. Secondly, the light and sounds emanating from an external hard drive reassure the radiologist that the study requested (current, old, or correlative) is soon to arrive, i.e., that the system is working. This is especially important since radiologists as a whole are used to "being in control" and don't suffer well its loss. Lightboxes and multi-viewers were rather simple devices, such that even the most technologically impaired radiologist could detect malfunctions and arrange for repair. In contrast, computers, especially workstations that offer the user very limited feedback, are apt to generate considerable physician frustration. Sounds and lights emanating from the external hard drive immediately after initiating a retrieval request is reassuring and averts a "control crises". Likewise, absence of these clues can quickly prompt an ulcer-reducing call to the radiology department help desk.

User Interface Hardware

The mouse and keyboard are ubiquitous and efficient tools for directing the operations of a workstation. User-friendly GUIs minimize keyboard interaction. Future complete replacement of the keyboard will be some time coming, and this is unfortunate as few radiologists count typing as a skill about which they wish to boast. Ideally, the interface hardware would be simpler, matching the on/off key and toggle (move right/move left) switch of multi-viewers. As workstations are pushed to provide greater functionality, it is unreasonable to expect such simplistic interface. Track balls, scratch or touchpads, and joysticks have received attention, but have failed to displace the mouse. Perhaps fingerprint identification devices may, in the not too distant future, eliminate the need for logging in via the keyboard, and with voice recognition capabilities, it is conceivable that the user may interface in the future without any hardware. At least future radiologists may only be required to use a few mouse clicks to carry out their daily work.

Software

Graphical User Interface (GUI) Principles

Corporations around the world are competing furiously to sell more and more powerful computers. Consequently, display hardware may be expected to continuously improve for many years to come. On the other hand, software dedicated to facilitating the radiologist's function receives many orders of magnitude less attention and corporate support. As a result, GUIs are not progressing to keep pace with computer hardware improvements or with clinical demand. Discerning, constructively critical radiologists will need to press their case in open forums to stimulate corporate competition to meet their needs.

There are three critical but essential requirements for good workstation display. The GUI must be: 1) intuitive, 2) efficient, and 3) user-friendly (Gay 1997, Erickson 1992, Lou 1996). Unfortunately, few PACS software engineers have a parent or close relative who is a radiologist and few have spent even one full day with a radiologist at work, and hence there is ample room for improving diagnostic radiology GUIs.

An **intuitive** GUI 1) anticipates, 2) emulates, and 3) teaches. It anticipates the work steps each radiologist routinely undertakes for each modality area. The result is the fewest manipulations of the image data, the fewest clicks, and the shortest time lag between tasks that a radiologist routinely undertakes. The GUI should emulate other popular software programs, such as standard Windows operational features so that minimal or no user training is required to carry out basic tasks. Finally, intuitive GUIs optimally utilize the hardware interface, including shortcuts that the radiologists may learn to improve their efficiency.

An **efficient** GUI manages the workflow of the radiologist with the fewest possible mouse clicks by anticipating the routine operations which most radiologists would use to complete their work. Obviously, these types of image manipulations will vary from modality to modality and the GUI must be written to account for these differences. For example, when a radiologist logs on to read MRI (magnetic resonance imaging) studies, the first view of the patient data should be an overview which illustrates all of the pulse sequence series obtained. The next click might position the first two series to be observed on each of the two display monitors in stack (one on one) mode. Some radiologists might prefer that after identifying the study for interpretation, it immediately be displayed on one monitor while the patient's most recent, prior like study be automatically placed on the other monitor in the same format. Both studies should be in the overview mode to begin with and then rapidly move to the stack view format. The GUI should know from the system log-on how the individual radiologist prefers to read his/her studies and provide the appropriate manipulation of images to meet the needs. Reading an ultrasound study, the radiologist may be more likely to prefer four images on each monitor, again with the current study on one monitor and the previous or correlative image study on the other monitor. Individual preferences for image formatting and manipulation need to be operational and easily changed.

Hopefully, more efficient GUIs will evolve over the next few years to accomplish all of the tasks that a radiologist performs during a common work day. One good example of a current deficiency for most display programs is the inability to accommodate interruptions in the radiologist's interpretation session, which are a common occurrence. For example, the radiologist may have called up an eight-sequence MRI study of approximately 300 images and have displayed it on the left monitor while the most recent previous MRI is displayed similarly on the right monitor. The tumor may be localized to the appropriate slice and the radiologist is just at the point where he is measuring the tumor size on the current study and in walks the liver transplant surgeon who urgently needs to review another patient's ultrasound. Leaving the present MRI study and being able to return to it at exactly the point it was on the monitors before the interruption is extremely important, but it is not a feature found at this time on the major vendors' display programs.

There are four major attributes of a **user-friendly** GUI. First, the screen should be dark with the majority of the screen at a light intensity level (usually in the grey range) which approximates that found for most of the features of the radiographic images reviewed and, in particular, the contrast and intensity of the pathology which must be detected. Obviously, screens with significant portions of their pixels at the contrast extremes are annoying and prevent the human eye from adapting appropriately, thereby potentially masking pathology.

Second, the non-image field should contain targets (icons) which are large and use a big pistol (cursor) to hit them.

Third, the non-image portion of the display field viewed should contain only the most pertinent and relevant information, yet provide quick access to additional fields as needed. Corporation logos and designs, as well as numerous non-relevant icons and other patient information, provide unwarranted distraction.

Finally, the fourth important attribute of the user-friendly GUI is to provide the "control-conscious" radiologist feedback. Short of discovering too late that you've paid more taxes than you need to, nothing makes one feel more foolish or generates more frustration for the time-constrained physician than sitting and gazing at a frozen computer screen—only to discover 20 minutes later that it is locked up and hasn't even requested the old correlative scan from the archive as you wanted. All the while, of course, the patient has been pacing anxiously in the waiting room for the radiologist to return or to call the physician with a "verdict."

Radiologist's Tasks

A radiologist's workstation should facilitate all of the tasks that a radiologist routinely performs. Table 2 lists these tasks in chronological order, comparing the means by which they are accomplished in the film-based world, in the current digital world, and in the future, hopefully more efficiently.

Upon arriving at work the radiologist first must determine what his/her clinical responsibilities are for the day, and this may either be from a centralized bulletin board or from a paper schedule. Many radiology departments have their own departmental computer network (RadNET or RadLAN) which can be logged onto at any site in the department to determine the schedule. Future workstations should facilitate this step by presenting the information as the radiologist logs on, or at least having it readily available through a single icon.

The radiologist must generate a work-list, composed of all the patients for whom he/she will be expected to provide diagnostic services. The requisitions for these patient studies should be reviewed by the radiologist to determine appropriateness of the requested study to plan any special interventions that might be required. Though not available at present, future workstations should be intimately linked with the RIS and thereby able to rapidly summarize this information. After reviewing the requisitions, the radiologist in many modality areas (nuclear medicine, angio, MRI, CT, and even ultrasound) will frequently write prescriptions for image data acquisition to tailor the study to meet the patient's clinical problems. Again, while not available on current systems, future workstations should possibly, through a web interface to the modality computer, facilitate delivery of these instructions to the technologist. Likewise, while the studies are being acquired, future workstations should provide a window where the incomplete study can be seen on the radiologist's workstation sequentially as it is acquired prior to being completed, i.e., "work-in-progress images." This window should be easily turned on and off, and also should allow the radiologist to carry on a teleconference with the technologist and thereby point out technical problems and prescribe adjustments.

Teleconferencing with the patient during the acquisition (CT, MRI, nuclear medicine) would also improve the quality of radiologic care given and be of benefit to the patient, as well as the technologist, who is striving to maintain throughput.

Prior research has been directed toward defining how radiographic images can be best displayed and formatted on workstations (Strickland 1995). Future thin-client PACS displays may be anticipated to have such blazing speed that one to two second delivery of images may eliminate the need for pre-fetching and auto-routing (Ghosh 1997).

After the interpretation is complete, report generation remains a task that has only been marginally improved by computers. As voice recognition software improves, and as it is integrated into the workstation, major improvements in the efficiency and speed of delivery of this information to the referring physician and patient may be expected.

Editing, signing, and associating codes with the patient study are all tasks which the radiologist's workstation should facilitate, and these tasks should all be available on a single, multi-tasking workstation. As electronic medical records mature and become intimately interfaced to PACS, referring physicians will be more efficiently and timely notified of study interpretations. Similarly, the progressive utilization and implementation of web technology in the next few years will make it much easier for the radiologist to consult with referring colleagues and thereby review current and past studies through teleconferencing. Finally, a weak link in most systems at present is that the radiologist is unable to easily collate and then subsequently address interesting and educational study results. An electronic teaching file function will be a most important element of future workstations.

Table 2. Radiologist's Workstation Tasks.

Function	Film Based Solution	Digital Solution Current	Digital Solution Future
Radiologist work schedule	Paper mail/ bulletin board	RadNet/ LAN PC	WorkStation avail. by icon click
Patient request review	Clerk delivers stack	RIS gives individual pt. info	WS by icon
Work list formed from sched. pts. list	None or modality log book	RIS-list	WS by icon
Study protocols	Written on request/Sneaker Net	None at present	WS-Web link to modality
Image review	Slave CRT + phone/intercom	CRT + phone	Window on WS + teleconf. (web)
Patient discharge	Sneaker Net	Sneaker Net	Teleconf from WS
Review prior studies	Clerk loads MV if found	Pre-fetched	Retrieved with patient selection
Image interpretation	Clerk loads MV/Lbox	Auto-routed WS	Retrieved as work list activated
Report/transcribe	Tape/ transcriptionist	Digital/sep computer	Voice recognition integrate
Edit/sign/code	Paper	RIS/sep computer	WS integration
Notify/consult review	Phone/Lbox, MV & hall light	Fax	EMR/Web
E-teach files	Film, photo, write, type, file	——	WS icon

Abbr.: WS = workstation; MV = multiviewer; Lbox = lightbox; EMR = electronic medical record; RIS = radiology information system; LAN = local area network; CRT = cathode ray tube

Security

Loss of patient confidentiality can potentially harm the patient(s) and will ultimately damage the institution. Recognizing that the government will eventually force security measures upon PACS users if they do not incorporate them first, then how can one optimally implement system protection from unauthorized users and deliberate abuse? Constraining network firewalls are an effective method to deal with external security. Internal security, however, has received little attention. We recommend large quantities of carrots and very little stick.

First the stick. User log-on screens have the ability to obstruct unauthorized access; however, they require typing and place a time delay on the user. If not designed and applied carefully, the log-on screen can become a significant irritant. As with radioactivity (also very beneficial when used appropriately) the ALARA principle should be followed when applying access restrictions, i.e., keep their intrusiveness As Little As Reasonably Allowable. The log-on screen, while allowing only authorized access: 1) should not glare at the viewer (i.e., should minimize disruption of user's light adaptation), 2) should require minimal or no typing (just a couple of mouse clicks would be best), 3) should respond rapidly (one second or less), and 4) should result in or provide the user the perception of significant benefit.

The carrot is the key. If the user associates significant benefit with logging on to the system, he/she will be unlikely to attempt to thwart the system. For example, if the PACS is fully integrated with a RIS and the department's RadLAN/RadNET, then the first screen displayed should be the radiologist's personal work list. In addition, the radiologist's individual preferences for "hanging" or formatting images by modality should occur automatically. This anticipation of the radiologist's interpretation preferences should extend to how prior and/or correlative studies are displayed as well. Once the radiologist has taken the time to personalize and fine-tune display features for all modalities, he/she will become so accustomed to (spoiled by) the time saving and benefits that when confronted with a display someone else logged on to, he/she will log out and then log back in to obtain the preferred display features. This has been our experience in the last few years as the personalized display feature (user-profile) has become more tailored. The frequent confrontations between residents, faculty, and attending radiologists to determine whose log-on is used to drive the display during an interpretation session is an indirect indication of the magnitude of perceived benefit which we witness daily. Similarly, sitting through interpretation sessions with someone else driving, frequently results in discussions on how the "user's profile" could be changed to more efficiently review images. Interestingly, complaints about log-on delays have been nonexistent, even when radiologist display screens are set to time out at three minutes. Our remote consulting display stations do not have user-profiles associated with the logon and hence we have been reticent to require non-radiologists to log-on to these displays.

References

Flynn, M.F. and Badano, A. "Image quality degradation by light scattering in display devices." *J Digital Imaging.* In press, May 1999.

Wang, J. and Langer, S. "A brief review of human perception factors in digital displays for picture archiving and communications systems." *J Digital Imaging.* 10(4):158-168; 1997.

Strickland, N.H. and Allison, D.J. "Default display arrangements of images on PACS monitors." *Br J Radiol.* 68:252-260; 1995.

Dwyer, S.J. "Copy displays and digitizers." *The Expanding Role of Medical Physics in Diagnostic Imaging.* AAPM Monograph No. 23, American Association of Physicists in Medicine, College Park, MD; 1997.

Muka, E., Blume H., Daly, S. "Display of medical images on CRT soft-copy displays: a tutorial." SPIE. 2431:341-359; 1995.

Roehrig, H., Blume, H., Ji, T.L., Browne, M. "Performance tests and quality control of cathode ray tube displays." *J Digital Imaging.* 3:134-145; 1990.

Otto, D., Bernhardt, T.M., Rapp-Bernhardt, U., Ludwig, K., Kästner, et al. "Subtle pulmonary abnormalities: detection on monitors with varying spatial resolutions and maximum luminance levels compared with detection on storage phosphor radiographic hard copies." *Radiology.* 207:237-242; 1998.

Gay, S.B., Sobel, A.H., Young, L.Q., Dwyer, S.J. "Processes involved in reading imaging studies: workflow analysis and implications for workstation development." *J Digital Imaging.* 10(1):40-45; 1997.

Erickson, B.J., Ryan, W.J., Gehring, "D.G. READS: a radiology-oriented electronic analysis and display station." *J Digital Imaging.* 10(3):67-69; 1997.

Lou, S.L., Huang, H.K., Arenson, R.L. "Workstation design: image manipulation, image set handling and display issues." *Radiol Clin North Am.* 34(3):525-544.

Ghosh, S., Andriole, K.P., Avrin, D.E., Arenson, R.L. "Optimization of a low-cost truly preemptive multitasking PC diagnostic workstation." *J Digital Imaging.* 10(3):171-174; 1997.

Workstations: Acceptance Testing and Quality Control Considerations

Janice C. Honeyman, Ph.D.
Department of Radiology
University of Florida

Abstract

A Picture Archiving and Communication System (PACS) can only be effective if high quality workstations are used to display images. To assure that workstations perform correctly and display images properly, a quality control program must be used both at installation and then periodically.

Aspects of workstation quality assurance include PACS input and output, functional testing of the workstation software, and tests to ensure that the display characteristics accurately reflect image data. The program described in this paper should serve as a starting point for practical PACS workstation quality assurance.

Introduction

The PACS workstation is the physician's window into digital radiology. Many times, the workstation is the defining measure of whether or not a PACS is acceptable. All PACS workstations must be able to receive and display images properly, apply the correct functions and measurements to the images, display reports when available, and correctly send output to appropriate archives or hardcopy devices. The workstation must be judged acceptable when it is deployed or whenever a change in the PACS occurs and must be checked using periodic quality control measurements.

This paper attempts to set some guidelines for a practical quality assurance program that examines the workstation from a number of perspectives, then evaluates the quality of the images on a routine basis. Although some of the measurements are time consuming, the routine quality control can be performed quickly and will help assure that the workstation does not become the breaking point of the PACS.

PACS Input/Output (I/O)

The interaction of the workstation with other PACS components is absolutely necessary for softcopy viewing. If the workstation cannot receive images from or send images to other devices, it cannot be used. In radiology, only Digital Image Communication in Medicine (DICOM) standard network communications should be used, if a workstation is not DICOM compliant, it should not be considered. Specifically, the workstation needs to be a DICOM storage class provider and user and a DICOM print class user.

The obvious first step toward acceptance testing of the workstation from a DICOM I/O perspective is to review the DICOM conformance statements. Unfortunately, even when two devices appear to be compatible because the DICOM conformance statement indicates that they will be able to communicate, in reality the connection must be tested. This connection test must be performed every time new equipment is added to the system and every time an upgrade or service is performed.

To be assured all interactions are tested, a DICOM environment form should be created. This form contains a list of all other equipment with which the workstation will need to communicate and includes the type of equipment, the expected interaction, the manufacturer, and the model or version number. Figure 1 shows a sample DICOM environment form for a PACS workstation.

Workstation Name: MRI1		Manufacturer: WS-R-US		
Date: Feb. 14, 1997		Location: MRI RR		
Required Interactions				
Type of Equip.	Interaction	Manufacturer	Model/ Version	Comments
MRI	DICOM Send from MRI to workstation	GE	Signa	Must display GE-MRI images correctly as well as CT, DF, FD, US, CR, SC
Archive	Query/Retrieve using custom SQL Interface to database	UF	Vs. 1.1	Must display GUI to database
Archive	Receive DICOM image from archive	UF	Vs 1.1	Must receive DICOM CT, MRI, US, DF, FD, CR, SC objects
Paper Printer	Send formatted print to printer	Softwerks		
Laser Camera	Send formatted print to laser camera	Kodak	2180	

Figure 1. Sample DICOM environment form.

This sample workstation will be used primarily in a magnetic resonance imaging (MRI) area and the MRI studies will be routed directly to it. Since radiologists use companion or comparison studies during study interpretation, the workstation must be able to move any DICOM study from the archives for display. Tests designed for this installation include routing studies from the MRI modality to the workstation and pulling a representative sample of all studies from the archives, validating that they can be moved and displayed correctly, and printing the studies to the paper printer or laser camera. The studies used in the archive/print tests should be documented so the test can be reproduced. The configuration and types of images involved in the routing communication should also be documented so a similar test can be performed when the workstation or modality devices are changed.

Input Testing

Prior to installation, it must be determined what types of images will be associated with a given PACS component. Since workstations need to be able to receive and display many different types and sizes of images from multiple manufacturers, a comprehensive test group needs to be assembled. It is important to be sure that all the images that can be generated or used are identified so the installation can be tested prior to introduction into clinical use. A detailed list of images to be used for testing should then be made and acquisition of the appropriate images should be performed. For example, Table I lists the image types and patient position that must be tested for an interaction with an MRI unit. A table or form like this should be created for each modality based on the DICOM conformance statement along with the image protocols used in the institution. It is important to determine that all types of images that can be generated in a specific institution can be successfully communicated to the workstation. For example, if the institution uses a unique coil for MRI, the communication and display of the resulting images must be fully tested.

Table I. MR and general image types with all patient positions for an MRI installation.

Original	Primary		
	Secondary	Screen Save	
Derived	Primary	Projection	Collapse
			Vascular
			IVI
	Secondary	Reformatted	
		Screen Save	
Head First Prone		Head First Supine	
Feet First Prone		Feet First Supine	
Head First Right Decubitis		Head First Left Decubitis	
Feet First Right Decubitis		Feet First Left Decubitis	

During the test, records should be kept of the identifiers, types, and numbers of images sent to the workstation from all modalities using automatic routing as well as all images retrieved from the archive. Timing of image transfers should be recorded to serve as a benchmark measure of DICOM communication efficiency, storage performance, and any observed delays. Correct and complete receipt of all images must be determined and recorded. A record of the studies used for the test will assure reproducibility.

The number of concurrent DICOM associations that are allowed should be determined and tested. With too few allowed associations, an operation involving the network can fail with a time-out while waiting for resources to continue. From the user's point of view, this would act as if a requested study from the archive failed to arrive. To test this, a number of studies from different locations should be queued to be sent to the workstation and the time required to send all the images measured. All images should arrive correctly and completely.

Output To Hardcopy

Testing the output from the workstation will include all DICOM storage class and print class providers that will be used. To test the print ability, all possible formatting options should be exercised including the number of images that can be formatted on a page, the inclusion of annotations and graphics, and using different levels of text display. If the user has printing options such as the selection of media type or size, each option must be tested. The workstation and printer or camera can be compatible from a DICOM perspective, but the size of the memory on the output device may not be adequate for formatting many large images on a sheet of film. The output characteristics of the hardcopy image should match that of the workstation softcopy display so the user can adjust settings and expect them to be transferred correctly to the chosen media.

Records should be kept so these tests can be reproduced. These include the identifier for the studies being printed, as well as window/level, magnification, annotation level, and format used. Visual correlation between the resulting hardcopy images and the softcopy display should be performed to determine that the settings have been accurately reproduced.

A quantitative test of the correlation between the hardcopy and softcopy image can be performed using a digital phantom. The optimal system will accurately reproduce the workstation grayscale on the hardcopy. Digital phantoms for PACS can be created for an institution or purchased from a vendor. In order to measure transfer characteristics of the grayscale curve, the phantom should have enough sample points to accurately reflect the representation of the pixel value on each type of media and the area to be measured must be large enough to perform accurate measurements. The end points of the curve should represent the limits of brightness and darkness achievable by the workstation. A discussion of measurement techniques and phantom examples are presented later in this paper.

Output To Archive or Other DICOM Storage Class Provider

Workstations may also be able to move images to other locations in the PACS network, such as the archive or other workstations. If this function is available, it must be tested. One of the options available on many PACS workstations is the ability to annotate relevant images and send the reduced set of images to the archive for clinical review purposes. If this option is available, a representative set of images should be selected, annotated, and transferred to the archive. These images must then be retrieved from the archive to a workstation for clinical display/review and verified as correct and complete.

Hospital Information System (HIS) and Radiology Information System (RIS) Input and Output

Most PACS workstations have the ability to interact with the HIS and/or the RIS. Reports for studies are retrieved from the HIS or RIS and displayed on the workstation. If worklist management has been implemented, a worklist of studies to be interpreted may be downloaded from the RIS and as studies are dictated, a message indicating completion of the task can be sent back to the RIS. If these functions are available, they should be tested using a representative sample of historical reports and a realistic worklist.

Periodic I/O Quality Tests

If all the input systems work correctly, it is reasonable to expect that they will continue to work correctly unless a change is made. Changes can be made at the modality, network, archive, or workstation level. Whenever an upgrade or maintenance change is made at any level, the appropriate tests for the change should be repeated. For example, if an MRI unit is upgraded or maintenance performed, the tests associated with the MRI transfers should be repeated. If the workstation software is changed, all tests should be repeated. For a daily check of input as well as the interaction with imaging modalities, it is recommended that a simple test pattern or representative image be sent to the primary workstations and examined for completeness of transfer and image appearance.

Since laser cameras and printing devices can exhibit changes over time, periodic quality control should be performed to assure that hardcopy images remain within the acceptable range in comparison with the benchmarked acceptance testing results. The digital test pattern can be periodically printed from the workstation and measured to determine that the hardcopy images remain acceptable.

Functional and Application Tests

Another group of tests confirms that all the functions of the workstation operate correctly. When new software is installed or a display workstation is installed for the first time, each function should be tested using a combination of images that might be encountered in a clinical environment. Table II contains a test set of images used during installation of a PACS workstation. Table III lists the workstation functions to be tested during the installation (Honeyman et al. 1997).

The images to be assembled for these tests may be quite extensive. For example, images from computed tomography (CT), MRI, digital fluoroscopy, ultrasound, digitized film, and computed radiography from all manufacturers must be successfully displayed on a workstation. In addition to images from each modality and manufacturer, each type, size, and resolution that can be produced must be tested as well as all possible patient orientations. The workstation must correctly display the orientation of the patient with special attention to the right and left sides being accurately shown. After the display requirement is satisfied, the functionality of the workstation must be tested. The studies in Table II are typical of the types that must be reviewed for a typical patient encounter. Using the image sets, the operation of the workstation when handling single image studies, multi-image studies, and multiple studies (of the same or different types) for a patient should be evaluated.

Table II. Sets of images used to test a workstation installation

Test set number	Test set description
T1	Digitized chest study—two views, PA and Lateral, normal portrait orientation.
T2	Digitized chest studies, three single view AP landscape orientation on the same patient to be used for comparison. Typical for ICU application.
T3	One digitized orthopedic study, several views on different sized films, all on the same patient.
T4	Three digitized radiographic studies, each with more than one film, all on the same patient, to be viewed together for comparison.
T5	Two CT studies, each with 50 or more images, for the same patient to be viewed together for comparison.
T6	Two MRI studies, each with 200 or more images, for the same patient to be viewed together for comparison.
T7	One secondary capture study (ultrasound or digital fluoroscopy).
T8	One CT study with 50 or more images and one digitized chest study with two views, both on the same patient.

A check list should be prepared to test each display function of the workstation, based on the tests suggested in Table III. Some of the more advanced features of the workstation, measurement, annotation, layout options, and navigation should be tested for accuracy and correct operation. In the case of MRI and CT images, the measurement tool should accurately denote the actual size of an object based on the pixel size as specified in the DICOM packet. For all others, the accuracy of the measurement should be evaluated and a recommended use of the measurement tool be posted for users.

Table III. Suggested functional tests for a workstation

Functional Tests—Image Transfer
Query/Retrieve
Print Format—Print to selected printer
Send Formatted composites/annotated studies to archive
Functional Tests—Image Manipulation
Window/Level; Zoom/Roam
Magnification; Flip/Rotate
Measurement; Annotation
Image Processing
Image Layout, Navigation
Functional Tests—General Operation
Correct information (patient, study, date)
Appropriate display
Controls working correctly

The workstation should be able to display multiple studies for a patient for comparison or collaboration. The workstation should allow the selection of multiple studies for the same patient and refuse to show images from different patients to avoid mistakes in comparison. There is a universal problem with PACS databases when patient identifiers are entered manually. For example, if a patient's name is entered differently on two different examinations, the computer will not recognize that they are the same person and should refuse to allow the examinations to be viewed together. The workstation should have a facility to "merge" two patient entries when the user desires so they can be viewed together; however, this function should display a warning that the merge is occurring.

After the acceptance test of the functionality is completed, it should not be necessary to repeat the test on a periodic basis. If a change in the workstation software occurs, the test should be repeated in its entirety. If a change in a modality occurs, the functional tests should be repeated using studies from that modality.

Disk Space Management

The management of the disk and database space should be part of the application functionality. When disks or databases are allowed to fill to capacity, no more images can be handled by the workstation and, in fact, the workstation may no longer operate correctly at all. If the workstation refuses studies, the entire PACS network can become clogged with rejected studies and performance will suffer. Most workstation manu-facturers have a mechanism for deleting older studies automatically to eliminate this problem. To test disk space and database management functions, it is necessary to attempt to over-fill the workstation by retrieving more studies than the capacity of the disk or database and observing the behavior of the workstation.

Display Quality Control

The display monitor is one of the most important parts of the workstation and the one most vulnerable to failure and performance degradation. Initial and periodic quality control is necessary to assure that diagnostic images are displayed. When multiple monitors are associated with a workstation all monitors should appear identical and the quality control task becomes more complex. As PACS replaces film with softcopy viewing, the number of workstations in use may become very large and quality con-trol can rapidly become unmanageable.

Several authors have described complex methods for determining the optimal perfor-mance of monitors (Muka et al. 1995, Eckert 1995, Reimann et al. 1995, Keller 1997). In a large institution, these methods may become impractical and beyond the capability and budget limitations of a department. The American Association of Physicists in Medicine (AAPM) has formed a task group to provide guidelines for monitor/work-station quality control, but these recommendations will not be available immediately, so the tests recommended in this paper are meant to serve as a practical step toward assuring high quality displays until the formal recommendations are published. At that time, the quality control program should be altered to meet the AAPM guidelines.

It is generally agreed that grayscale monitors should be used for diagnostic display. Color monitors do not provide the quality required for diagnostic display; however, they will probably be used for clinical viewing. A quality assurance program should also be available for these monitors in spite of the reality that there may be many more to check.

Parameters of image quality for diagnostic quality include resolution, luminance, grayscale fidelity, linearity, uniformity, and glare. Most of these can be measured using a combination of subjective and objective measures and should be performed both at setup and periodically.

Display Monitor Setup

The acceptance test or initial monitor setup will determine the benchmarks that will serve as the goal of periodic quality control measurements. Since most diagnostic workstations will have multiple monitors, it is important to guarantee that the monitors have the same display characteristics.

The tools required to perform basic quality control of monitors are digital phantoms and a photometer. There are several digital phantoms available to be purchased, or they can be created in software. The Society of Motion Picture and Television Engineers (SMPTE) test pattern, widely used to show resolution, grayscale response, and linearity can be used for many tests (SMPTE 1986). Digital phantoms with different patterns and possibly more measurement capability are also available (Halpern 1995, Halpern et al. 1991). In order to set up monitors correctly, patterns with a range of grayscales are necessary. The ones described below have been used successfully at the University of Florida for monitor quality control.

Photometers measure the luminance or light output from monitors. Several are available at a wide range of prices. Some use a suction cup attachment to the monitor that allows a direct measurement of luminance, eliminating much of the contribution by ambient lighting. Spot photometers are used at a distance, usually a viewing distance, and include the luminance of the monitor in the presence of room lighting. The comparative value of each type is still being hotly debated; however, one of them must be used for these tests. Since the objective of the luminance test is to measure the light emanating from the monitor, it makes sense to use a photometer that eliminates the contribution from ambient light. The photometer with a suction cup or light mask measures only the light from the monitor. If a spot photometer is used, measurements should be made in a dark room.

Since each monitor will have different luminance capability, all monitors on the workstation must conform to the one with the least luminance. If all monitors are set to the brightest possible luminance and measured, the luminance of all can initially be set to match that of the lowest one. To perform this measurement, set the monitors to display either no image at all or a phantom with command levels set as high as the monitor will display. Measure each monitor with the photometer and tune all monitors using the brightness control to the level of the lowest one. The contrast control needs to be set so each monitor displays the same grayscale curve. One or more phantoms with command levels set at measured values between brightest and darkest should be used to measure the grayscale response of each monitor, then the contrast control on each monitor set to the same curve. This is an iterative process that may take significant time. After the brightness and contrast have been adjusted, they should be checked against the SMPTE test pattern or some other test pattern that tests low contrast discrimination using at least the 5% square within the 10% square and the 95% square within the 100% square. These patterns must be visible. It is highly recommended that after the brightness and contrast settings are set correctly, the manual controls be removed so users cannot adjust them. Record the phantoms used and readings so the test can be reproduced.

To accurately represent the grayscale response to digital values, a series of command levels should be measured and graphed. An adequate curve can be generated with 32 gray levels; more will improve the accuracy of the curve. A practical way to do this is to construct a series of phantoms, each with a different command level, stored as a series in a DICOM study that can be retrieved from an archive. The phantom should cover a large area of the monitor to allow the photometer to measure a representative sample of values while measuring the same level without another gray level overlap. The photometer can then be aimed at or attached to the monitor and the series stepped through while readings are recorded. The baseline curve readings should be recorded for future reference when the test is repeated.

Although the grayscale response of the monitor can be correct according to digital phantom readings, the look-up-table (LUT) used by different modalities must also be accurately represented by the workstation. For some modalities (Computed Radiography and Digital Fluoroscopy), a step wedge can be imaged and the workstation display compared with the modality display. In other cases, a grayscale phantom available with the modality can be compared with the workstation. If the LUT is not interpreted correctly, nondiagnostic images can result.

In addition to luminance levels and grayscale response, uniformity over the face of the monitor is important. Photometer measurements at the center of the monitor and in each corner should demonstrate uniformity.

Spatial Resolution

Spatial resolution is a description of the limits of viewable detail. A monitor can have an addressable space indicating the number of pixels in the horizontal and vertical dimensions. This addressable space is commonly referred to as the "monitor resolution"; however, this measure does not accurately reflect the viewable detail. A "high resolution" monitor capable of displaying 2048×2048 pixels may have such poor focus that the viewable resolution is very much lower. In order to measure the resolution of monitor, it is necessary to use a point or line phantom or a phantom with repeating points or lines. Methods that can be used to evaluate resolution are visual inspection, microscope trace width measurements, aperture/slit-scan measurements, and diode array charged couple device (CCD) scanning.

Visual Inspection

Of all the methods for evaluating spatial resolution, visual inspection uses the least instrumentation but relies on subjective observation. A digital phantom, such as the SMPTE pattern, is displayed on the monitor and the smallest resolvable lines noted. If a quantitative measurement is not required, this is by far the fastest and easiest evaluation method. The phantom can be magnified to identify the resolution desired, then decreased in magnification until the lines no longer appear clearly. The SMPTE pattern measures lines in horizontal and vertical orientations, but does not measure diagonal lines. Other test patterns are available to demonstrate the resolution in a diagonal orientation. (Halpern 1995, Halpern et al. 1991) A small hand-held microscope with a calibrated reticle can measure spot or line width, but again this method is highly subjective. If the brightness level is set very high, the line or spot will "bloom" making the measurement of line width larger. The window and level should be adjusted to achieve the smallest possible line or spot width.

Aperture/Slit-scan Measurements

The aperture or slit-scan measurements can be more accurate than a visual inspection, but are more complex and require greater operator skill, as well as more instrumentation. Using this method, a detector scans across a line or spot and displays the profile characteristics on an oscilloscope. Although this method could be used initially to evaluate the characteristics of a display monitor, it is probably impractical to use on a routine basis.

Diode Array Scanning

Diode array CCD scanning methods are recent advances and again require a high level of instrumentation. A two-dimensional array can allow a complete beam profile to be measured. These methods again may be beyond the practical application of quality control in a typical PACS installation.

Geometric Distortion

A variety of factors can cause geometric distortion in display monitors. The presence of a magnetic field may cause the display to tilt with respect to the faceplate sides. It is important that the monitor has a tilt adjustment to correct this problem. Pincushion and barrel distortion cause the sides of the projected image to bulge or draw in at the edges. This distortion may require monitor adjustment when the defect is slight or a factory adjustment if the distortion is severe. Nonlinearity can distort straight lines or bunch pixels, usually toward the edge of the display.

Geometric distortion should be easy to detect using a digital phantom with straight lines in both the horizontal and vertical directions. During system acceptance and setup the phantom can be visually inspected and measured, then checked on a regular basis.

Artifacts

Artifacts in the display monitor can occur as the monitor ages, or be present in a new monitor. An improperly seated video card can cause some artifacts. Artifacts can usually be identified by a regular (daily) visual inspection.

Color Monitors

In general, color monitors cannot provide the resolution usually required in diagnostic workstations; however, they may be widely used for teleradiology, clinical review, and Internet-based applications. Since radiology images are displayed in a grayscale mode, which on a color display is a mixture of red, green, and blue color patterns, some of the quality control mentioned above can be used. The DICOM input/output, HIS/RIS interface, and functional tests should be performed on clinical review software before deploying. Display characteristics can be checked during the acceptance tests, but routine quality control may be less rigorous, mainly due to the practical limitations of trying to check what may be hundreds of workstations throughout an institution.

The display of grayscale images on a color monitor, especially when the computer is used for tasks other than radiology image display, can be severely compromised by actions of users. Monitor brightness and contrast can be easily altered, ambient room light may be uncontrolled, and the use of other software may change the grayscale response of the monitor. One way to attempt to assure that high quality images are displayed is to provide a digital phantom to be viewed prior to radiology images. This is difficult to enforce; however, it provides a way for a conscientious user to check his or her display characteristics.

Summary

The quality assurance program outlined in this paper provides a reasonable effort to provide a properly working PACS workstation. Although the initial setup of the workstation involves substantial time, periodic quality control need not be a burden to a PACS manager. Visual daily checks of a digital phantom can assure that the monitor display is devoid of artifacts, that the display has no geometric distortion, that the grayscale response and the resolution remains acceptable. In addition, the monitors can be cleaned of fingerprints and dust.

Monthly checks of the luminance and grayscale response can be performed quickly using the grayscale phantoms and compared to the baseline readings.

Some practical aspects of room layout should be observed. The monitors should not reflect glare from bright lights or view boxes placed opposite the workstations and the room lighting should be low and indirect. Workstations should be placed on comfortable furniture that can be moved to allow access to the back of the computer and monitors. Since reading rooms are busy and sometimes chaotic places, it is recommended that the computers be placed on a shelf rather than on the floor to reduce dust in filters and to protect them from feet. Periodic cleaning of the computer's filters and surroundings is recommended to assure correct operation.

It is important to remember that the AAPM has formed a task group to recommend a complete quality assurance program for workstations and/or displays. When the recommendations of the task group are released, a quality assurance program should be altered to comply with the recommendations. Until that time, the program suggested in this paper should form a basis for a program that will assure properly working workstations and high-quality displays.

References

Eckert, M.P. "Video display quality control measurements for PACS." *SPIE* 2431: 328-340, 1995.

Halpern, E.J., Esser, P.O. "An improved phantom for quality control of laser scanner digitizers in picture archival and communications systems." *Journal of Digital Imaging* 4(4): 241-247, 1991.

Halpern, E.J. "A test pattern for quality control of laser scanner and charge-coupled device film digitizers." *Journal of Digital Imaging* 8(1): 3-9, 1995.

Honeyman, J.C., Frost, M.M., Staab, E.V. "PACS component testing: beta and acceptance testing." *SPIE* 3035: 405-412, 1997.

Honeyman, J.C., Jones, D., Frost, M.M., Staab, E.V. "PACS quality control and automatic problem notifier." *SPIE* 3035: 396-404, 1997.

Keller, P.A. *Electronic Display Measurement.* New York, NY: John Wiley and Sons, Inc, 1997.

Muka, E., Blume, H., Daly, S. "Display of medical images on CRT soft-copy displays: A tutorial." *SPIE* 2431: 341-359, 1995.

Reimann, D.A., Flynn, M.J., Ciarelli, J.J. "A system to perceptually linear networked display devices." *SPIE* 2431: 316-326; 1995.

Society of Motion Picture and Television Engineers (SMPTE). Specifications for Medical Diagnostic Imaging Test Pattern for Television Monitors and Hard-Copy Recording Cameras. SMPTE Recommended Practice RP: 1986.

PACS Economic Issues and Justifications

David Avrin, M.D., Ph.D.
Vice Chairman, Clinical Services
Clinical Professor
Department of Radiology
University of California at San Francisco

Objectives

This presentation will help you to understand how to present the economic issues and the advantages of PACS (Picture Archiving and Communication System) and to understand how your particular environment affects your approach. Positive and negative experiences elsewhere for justifications give guidance in avoiding pitfalls, and provide a formula for what works well, both as persuasive arguments and in practice. Financial tools that empower you for battle with your hospital administrators will be explained. These tools will also give you a framework for internal analysis. In summary, the goal of this presentation is to help you develop a formula for success in obtaining the support of the two key constituencies, administration and medical staff, for your PACS project, as well as to understand the critical factors for having an economically and clinically successful project.

Introduction

Most of this presentation will focus on administrators, following Sutton's law: "Because that's where the money is," an answer given in response to the question: "Mr. Sutton, why would a man of your intelligence choose to rob banks?" Administrators sign the purchase order and write the check.

There are some key issues regarding radiologist and non-radiologist physician support that will be explored. The most important one is the practice model and strength of bonding between the medical staff and the institution.

Staff support inside and outside of the diagnostic imaging department is more important for successful implementation in radiology and critical care areas, than in the plan approval process.

Administrators

Financial

In my experience, including tales related by others, PACS is a polarizing issue for hospital administrators. These folks tend to fall into one of two categories, with very few sitting on the fence: (1) NO WAY and (2) Don't preach to the choir because I am convinced that this is something our institution needs to do. PACS is a tough sell if you have the misfortune of dealing with a member of the first group. They will make you, your diagnostic imaging medical director, and your manager go through all kinds of hoops to prove a positive economic return in your business plan (which we will discuss in detail later). For the second group it becomes a matter of capital priorities, vendor selection, successful rollout, and dealing with the physician contingent, all difficult but not obstructionist.

Integrated Delivery System (IDS) Needs

Most administrators in a growing multiple hospital, integrated multi-specialty group environment are more sophisticated in general regarding information technology, and understand the benefits of diagnostic images being available anytime, anywhere they are needed, with little or no human intervention. Simply stated, the IDS needs dominate the financial considerations. This is an easier sell.

Quality of Care

Unfortunately, quality of care is one of those intangible factors that is difficult to quantify. It is challenging to demonstrate a direct financial benefit, although many of us believe that in reality there is a hard value as well as significant indirect benefits to the organization. These arguments tend to take second place behind the MD and staff efficiency issue, which will be explored later. Vendors relate that the focus of the discussion with administrators and non-radiologist MDs changes dramatically after a visit to a successful implementation site.

The Business Plan

The business plan is a financial document (spreadsheet) that compares the costs of continuing the traditional radiology department film system with the cost of implementing a digital department. Costs include capital investment (equipment and software), operating costs, and should include direct costs (those assigned to the imaging department) and indirect costs (those outside the department but attributable to diagnostic imaging). Some operating costs are fixed, and some are variable. You need to understand all of these terms.

The most important message is that financially PACS is a tradeoff of decreased supplies and disposables (film and chemicals), and personnel costs, for depreciated computer and network equipment (Arenson et al. 1986, 1996). The cost of the media for digital archiving is now so low (less than the cost of a postage stamp per case) that archive media cost can effectively be ignored. In other words, to the degree that film is not produced, there are essentially no variable direct supply costs.

The second most important message is that there is a huge cost of continuing traditional film methods, including future commitment of personnel and space resources to maintain for seven or more years the archive of the film you create today. The Mayo Clinic has conservatively estimated these costs at $15.82 per exam! The components of these costs are contained in Figure 1 (King et al.). Continuing to use traditional film methods is "cost commitment by omission." Economically successful implementation of PACS requires limitation of production and storage of film, and aggressive control of associated personnel costs by intelligent folder manager or workflow software. Clinicians must have an easy and efficient way to review imaging studies and reports. Intranet tools (server/browser technology) are one way to meet these needs.

Mayo Study: Total Estimate
per Exam: $15.82!

- Film $6.25

- Supplies $1.46

- Personnel $5.91 and $2.20

- "Our estimated cost of film per exam per year is most likely an underestimation of real costs when compared to other institutions."

Figure 1. Mayo data for cost of traditional film method (King et al.).

Types of business plans include break-even analysis using depreciation costs, diagrammed in Figure 2, IRR (internal rate of return) which the accountants love, and an incremental or phased approach. IRR calculations provide a measurement of the effective rate of return from investing capital to save on operating costs, and is shown in Figure 3. These various approaches will be explained in detail.

A warning regarding CIOs (Chief Information Officers): CIOs also tend to be polarized, but with a control orientation. They can be a significant source of obstruction, but their support is valuable. Often they control the networks required for your system. Unfortunately, they sometimes do not understand that there are no good demonstrable PACS that are integrated components of a commercial Hospital Information System (HIS). They may not understand the data quantities and bandwidth required in PACS. They may want control of the project implementation, even though they do not understand the needs of radiology.

Break-Even Analysis Diagram

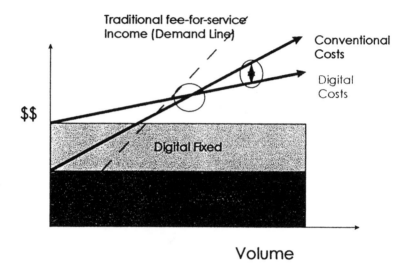

Figure 2. Break-even analysis.

NPV and IRR Examples:

NPV Example		IRR Example: $1250 to $1000 investment			
Rate:	8%	Guess:	1%	5%	5%
	250	Year 1	-1000	-1000	-750
	250	Year 2	250	250	250
	250	Year 3	250	250	250
	250	Year 4	250	250	250
	250	Year 5	250	250	250
		Year 6	0	250	0
NPV	998.18	IRR	0.0%	7.9%	12.6%

Figure 3. Net present value (NPV) and internal rate of return examples (IRR).

Physicians

For the acute care clinician, PACS provides rapid access to image data where and when it is needed. In addition, for an IDS, image data are available across the enterprise geography. PACS tends to be an easier sell where the medical staff is tightly bonded to the institution; for example, an academic institution compared to a community hospital where most of the medical staff cares for patients at two unrelated institutions. Bonded staff tend to be more supportive and less critical of change. Image distribution is also technically easier.

One potential source of opposition is service line competition for capital. For example, a PACS investment may be weighed against a new cardiac cath lab. You need to make persuasive arguments regarding competing priorities.

OR and clinic problems: Image access in the operating room (OR) remains problematic. Experiences of others in placing monitors or workstations in the OR have been less than satisfactory; flat panel displays appear promising and are coming down in cost. In some environments, producing film selectively for surgery can be a temporizing approach. We believe that web access via intranet will be a viable solution for the outpatient clinic.

From the radiologists' perspective: A successful PACS implementation can improve radiologist and group efficiency, as well as improve the standard of care. Studies can be delivered to the subspecialist expert for interpretation, and a geographically constrained inefficient group practice environment can be converted into an efficient "virtual" department. Efficient workstation user interface is crucial.

Whose money is it? Institutional financial analyses may or may not include radiologist or other physician efficiency. This is related to the binding issue discussed above. It is possible that PACS can result in sufficient radiologist savings that the concept of co-investment in the PACS project by a radiology group could be a sound business decision. Furthermore, it may form the basis for a healthy joint venture (win/win).

The Most Important Weapon

A PACS "champion" other than the imaging department chairman is invaluable. This person could be from administration or a non-radiologist member of the medical staff. This person should preferably not be a "techie" or "propeller head."

There can be value in carefully retaining an outside independent consultant, with specifically assigned tasks.

Conclusion

You want to sell a vision of an extended virtual department with no walls, where image data are available anytime, anywhere it is needed. Pre-fetch needs are anticipated with no human intervention. There are no lost studies. Certainly for digital modalities, the institution saves money on film, chemicals, and personnel in excess of the investment cost of the system. There is potential for increased radiologist efficiency. These two economic benefits can form a basis for partnership between the radiology group and the institution. Most important, there are intangible but significant benefits to quality and efficiency of care. It is simply a better way to practice diagnostic imaging in medicine.

Note: Portions of this presentation are derived from my presentations to the AHRA in October 1997 at Lake Tahoe, and the UCSF PACS Conference, April 1998.

Acknowledgments

Ron Arenson, M.D.
Chairman, Radiology, UCSF

Mercy Healthcare Sacramento

First Consulting Group
    Sam Barley
    Mark Moffitt

Jim Green, CPA
Sacramento Radiology Medical Group

References

Arenson, R.L et al. "Cost-effectiveness of PACS" (1986).

Arenson, R.L., Burnside, E.S., Avrin, D.E. et al. "Cost benefits of picture archiving and communications systems (PACS)." International Symposium on Costs & Benefits of Radiology. St. Johns College, Oxford University, England. August 3-5, 1995. Published in supplement to Academic Radiology, 1996.

King, M.D. et al. "Cost of film: purchasing, processing, packaging, storing and disposal over the lifetime of a film examination in a large radiology department." *SCAR* 96 pp 152-157.

An RFP for a PACS
(or)
A Request For Proposal for a Picture Archiving and Communications System

Larry J. Filipow, D.Phil.
Department of Radiology
University of Alberta
Edmonton, Alberta, Canada

Introduction

I would like to begin this chapter by first acknowledging an excellent source for information on PACS and how to develop an RFP. John H. Perry has had a website operational since February 1996. Its address is: http://www.xray.hmc.psu.edu/dicom/rfp/RFP.html#Top, and it's titled "A PACS RFP Toolkit." It contains virtually everything anyone would need to know about RFP development, and a lot about PACS and its components as well. It is very much worth a visit.

The development and release of an RFP marks the transition from the beginning phase: planning of a PACS initiative to the second phase: implementation. Or so one would hope. Before release of an RFP, appropriate work should have been done to have:

1. Funding secured.

2. All stakeholders involved in the planning of the PACS identified.

3. Operational and functional reviews completed.

4. A business plan/cost justification prepared.

5. A timeline created.

In real life, however, and especially where PACS is concerned, responses back from an RFP will likely disrupt or invalidate most, if not all, of the above five undertakings. Budget funding may not be accurate, additional stakeholders may have to be (should have been) involved, operational reviews may not have not been sufficiently comprehensive, the business plan may need to be readjusted, and the timeline may need to be extended. And it is nobody's fault.

The reason for this scenario is simply this: PACS is fundamentally dependent on computer hardware and software, and it primarily replaces and/or changes existing process and function. Nothing changes with respect to performance, price, and functionality faster than computing hardware and software, and process changes get people's attention very quickly and intensely. What I'm trying to say is that during the 3 to 6 months required for: vendors to respond to an RFP, the buyer to evaluate the responses, the site visits to be completed, the decision to be made, the final negotiations to be completed, the contract to be awarded, the site(s) to be prepared, the equipment to be delivered, configured, and finally commissioned, a lot can have changed. And usually has. And the entire process can take much more than 6 months.

The main issue in creating an RFP is, I believe, to be sufficiently detailed in the document so that "surprises" are minimized. Surprises, in this context, are things that nobody thought of, nor were included or discussed in the RFP process. Things such as essential renovations to "site" the equipment. Surprises such as delivered hardware being two platform levels below current technology. Nobody likes "surprises"—neither the customer nor the vendor, and nothing can poison a business relationship faster. An RFP, therefore, should, if anything, be comprehensive and account (as much as possible) for the dynamic nature of the PACS environment.

Most RFPs are public domain, (e.g., see J.H. Perry, above), and it is very easy to get sample RFPs from any of the vendors that will be asked to respond. I present here the RFP jointly developed by myself (specifications) and the Purchasing Department of the Capital Health Authority (front-end documents).

Beforehand, though, I would also like to talk a bit about the purchasing process, which I believe is quite different between facilities and institutions. I offer a reasonable, comprehensive process that should ensure a smooth acquisition of an appropriate system.

The Purchase Process

The acquisition of a PACS (or, in fact, any item of diagnostic imaging equipment) will include most, if not all, of the following 25 steps. The order is logical, and has worked very well for us in acquiring everything from mobile x-ray units to MRIs to PACS.

1. Petition for equipment (i.e., confirmation/justification of need).
2. Commitment of funds.
3. Review of vendor material (just to acquaint oneself with the most current technology).
4. Appointment of Technical Evaluation Committee (TEC). This involves the technically adept personnel and the relevant stakeholders who will be using the equipment. This does not need to include administration or financial people.
5. Preparation and release of RFP (usually done by or with the collaboration of the TEC, in collaboration with the purchasing department).
6. Development of timeline (done in collaboration between TEC and administration).
7. Return of RFPs.
8. Removal of pricing information (pricing information goes to administration; the TEC is burdened only with selecting based on performance, without the bias of cost).

9. Spreadsheet of specifications responses (to allow for straightforward comparison).
10. Vendor experts/TEC meetings (to scrutinize the responses and provide any additional information).
11. Short List (based on perceived performance of equipment from RFP response and vendor meetings).
12. Site visits (factory, clinical, as required).
13. Recommendations to Selection Committee (Selection Committee includes administration, financial personnel).
14. Final discussions, negotiations (timelines, payment schedules, upgrades, works-in-progress, renovations).
15. Award of contract.
16. Downpayment (if required).
17. Manufacture/configuration of equipment.
18. Site preparation.
19. Systems Administrator(s) training.
20. Delivery and installation.
21. Interim payment.
22. Acceptance Testing.
23. Applications training.
24. Final payment.
25. In-house service training (if applicable).

Facility Overview, Preview of Facility

A well-written facility preview will go a long way in clarifying a number of items. First, it will help the purchasers to elucidate in their own minds what type and extent of PACS equipment they really need. Second, it will clearly inform vendors what extent of equipment is really needed. Based on the facility preview, vendors may be able to suggest equipment or software more appropriate for the need, rather than what is simply asked for. The facility preview should include a comprehensive and accurate table of exam statistics, detailing exam volumes, recall rates for exam review, user numbers, image sizes. This will enable the vendors to correctly size the RAID (redundant array of independent discs) and the archive required. Examples of a Facility Preview and a CT Exam Volume Analysis are contained in the RFP which follows.

The order of the RFP may seem a bit turned around, because digital image production devices [Film digitizers, CR (Computed Radiography), DR (Direct Radiography)] are located at the back of the RFP specifications. The reason for doing this is so that these sections can easily be removed, leaving an intact RFP that would be appropriate for a PACS for CT (Computed Tomography), MRI (Magnetic Resonance Imaging), US (Ultrasound), or NM (Nuclear Medicine). This, for most institutions, is the first phase of a PACS initiative, with general radiology to follow sometime later. I leave the final order of the equipment specifications to the discretion of the reader, should you wish to use any or all parts of this RFP.

References

Perry, J.H. A PACS RFP Toolkit—Version 3. Presented to the 5th RIS-PACS School, Georgetown University Medical Center. Website: http://www.xray.hmc.psu.edu/dicom/rfp/RFP.html#Top ; 1996.

Clark, R.P. Request for Proposal—Regional PACS. Greater Vancouver Health System. Private communication; 1997.

Honeyman, J.C., Frost, M.M., Huda, W., Loeffler, W., Ott, M., Staab, E.V. "Picture Archiving and Communications Systems (PACS)." *Current Problems in Diagnostic Radiology;* 23(4): 101-160; 1994.

Strickland, N.H. "Review article: Some cost-benefit considerations for PACS: a radiological perspective." *British Journal of Radiology;* 69: 1089-1098; 1996.

Abiri M., Kirpekar, N. "Designing a Request for Proposal for Picture Archiving and Communication System." *Journal of Digital Imaging;* 10(3): 20-23; 1997.

Filipow, L.J. "MRI Equipment Purchase Specifications and Applications." AAPM Monograph 21; *The Physics of MRI; AIP Publishing;* 673-698; 1992.

Image Management and Communication System

For

CHA Referral Hospitals System

For

General Radiology, Computed Tomography, Magnetic Resonance Imaging, Ultrasound, Nuclear Medicine

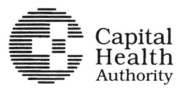

CHA-CAP-01-23-456

Request for Proposal

Table of Contents

14.0 Dry Laser Film Printer

Statement of Service Support

The Capital Health Authority

Referral Hospital System

IMACS / PACS Network for Diagnostic Imaging

Introduction and Overview

The Capital Health Authority Referral Hospital System is a tertiary care facility located on two sites in the City of Edmonton. They are the University of Alberta Hospital site and the Royal Alexandra Hospital site. Each site operates two large radiology departments, providing the majority of diagnostic imaging exams done for the CHA Region. Total procedures number approximately 500,000 a year for the two sites, distributed more or less equally.

Since regionalization, it has become apparent that a means of transmitting diagnostic images between the two referral sites, as well as having images readily and conveniently available for referring medical disciplines (Emergency, Neurosciences, ICU's), and also providing image review capabilities for on-call radiologists at their homes is essential to patient care.

This proposal will establish an image management and communications system (IMACS) within the Capital Health Authority, to address constantly increasing demands for diagnostic image service and performance. The IMACS network will be designed to provide an infrastructure to referring physicians and radiologists to enable them to communicate in a timely and helpful fashion with respect to diagnostic imaging requirements for their patients. The network will serve to significantly enhance patient care.

The long term goal of the Diagnostic Imaging Service of the CHA is to become fully digitized among all imaging modalities, with a full-region IMACS/PACS network. This implementation will be done in phases.

Diagnostic Imaging is committed to an evolutionary approach to digital image information management. Because of this it is important that all systems and devices conform as much as possible to current and future DICOM standards, including information objects, commands, and service classes.

1.0   FORM OF PROPOSAL AND PRICING

1.1   Prices offered must be met and must be held until goods are delivered and installed. **No escalator clauses will be accepted.**

Response:_____

1.2   Complete the pricing summary sheet enclosed and return with your proposal. The pricing summary sheet is attached at the end of the "Instructions to Vendors" section.

Response:_____

2.0   ADDENDA

2.1   The Owner reserves the right to amend or revise the Proposal Documents prior to the closing date. Vendors shall be informed of all such changes by means of written Addenda issued up to five (5) days prior to Proposal closing date. Verbal instructions given in person or by telephone are null and void and shall not be accepted by the Vendor. Receipt of all Addenda must be acknowledged.

Response:_____

2.2   Addenda or clarification will be sent in writing (or by FAX) to all Vendors by:

The Capital Health Authority
c/o Materiel Management Services
Hospital Site 1
12345 – 6th Avenue
Fax: (123) 456-7890

Attention: Purchaser

Response:_____

2.3   Addenda to submitted proposals must be sent in writing (or by FAX) to:

The Capital Health Authority
c/o Materiel Management Services
Hospital Site 1

12345 – 6th Avenue
Edmonton, Alberta
Fax: (123) 456-7890

Attention: Purchaser

Response:_____

3.0   SCOPE OF WORK

3.1   Vendors submitting proposals shall be responsible for design, fabrication, supply and installation of all equipment offered.

Response:_____

4.0   TRADE-INS

4.1   Vendors shall itemize trade-in value of existing equipment offered. Vendors shall be responsible for dismantling and removal from site.

Response:_____

5.0   DELIVERY/INSTALLATION TIME

5.1   The Vendor shall indicate time required for installation (specify in weeks and days).

Response:_____

5.2   Vendors must state the earliest possible delivery date of the equipment proposed.

Response:_____

6.0   SPECIAL ELECTRICAL REQUIREMENTS

a)   All services and installation requirements shall be identified including details of power requirements, voltage, current phase and operational limitations.
Response:_____

b) Any special requirements such as dedicated circuits, "clean" electrical supplies, line conditioning shall be identified.

Response:_____

c) The Vendor must state the total heat generated from the equipment proposed, expressed in BTU's per hour.

Response:_____

d) It will be the responsibility of the Vendor to evaluate the existing power supply for each location and make appropriate recommendations to ensure that the power supplies meet the requirements for installation and optimal operation of the equipment. If the quality of the existing power supply is not adequate, Vendors are required to include supplementary equipment recommended, as well as associated costs, in their proposal.

Response:_____

e) The effect of power outages or transitional discontinuities experienced upon transfer to emergency power generators shall be stated, together with the significance of interruption of any other supplies.

Response:_____

7.0   PROGRESS SCHEDULE

7.1 A progress schedule will be established for the benefit of the successful Vendor once final Health Authority approval to purchase has been granted and delivery dates have been established. It will be the responsibility of the successful Vendor to notify the Owner of any deviation from this accepted schedule.

Response:_____

8.0   SITE VISIT

8.1   As part of the final equipment selection process, each vendor may be requested to arrange for a site visit by representatives of the Capital Health Authority.

                        Response:_____

8.2   The necessity of a site visit; the date; and the number and names of representatives to be involved in the site visit will be determined following analysis of each proposal.

                        Response:_____

CAPITAL HEALTH AUTHORITY

PRICING SUMMARY SHEET

1.   This form must be completed by Vendor.
2.   Signature of authorized person must be legible.
3.   Unless otherwise stated, prices will remain firm for a **period of 120 days** from the closing date.
4.   We reserve the right to accept all or any part of your proposal.
5.   We reserve the right to cancel any purchase order or contract issued should the terms stated on this request for proposal be ignored.
6.   Pricing must be F.O.B.
        Capital Health Authority
        Edmonton, Alberta, Canada

This proposal is subject to all conditions as specified by:

        A.   Instructions to Vendors

        B.   General Conditions of Contract

        C.   System Specific Requirements

        D.   Drawings Numbered

        E.   Addenda Numbered (list addenda received)

COMPANY NAME:_____

DATE:_____

TELEPHONE NUMBER:_____

FAX NUMBER:_____

SIGNATURE:_____

COMPANY REPRESENTATIVE:_____

        (PLEASE PRINT)

Date:_____   Our Ref No:_____

Your proposal must be received **NO LATER THAN**:

_____
Day / Month / Year

ITEM	QUANTITY	DESCRIPTION	UNIT PRICE	EXTENDED PRICE

1.0   CONTRACT DOCUMENTS

1.1   The Contract Documents will consist of an executed Agreement and Purchase Order, as well as the General Conditions of the Contract, Specifications, Instructions to Vendors, Shop Drawings, and all addenda issued to the Request for Proposal.

Response:_____

1.2   The fact of the Vendor submitting a proposal shall be construed by the Owner to mean that the Vendor agrees to carry out all the conditions set forth in the drawings and these specifications. **ANY PROPOSED VARIATION FROM THESE SPECIFICATIONS MUST BE CLEARLY IDENTIFIED.**

Response:_____

1.3   In the event of conflicts between Contract Documents the following shall apply:

a)   Documents of later date shall govern.

b)   Figured dimensions shown on the Drawings shall govern even though they may differ from scaled dimensions.

c)   The General Conditions of the Contract shall govern.

d)   The Contract shall govern over all documents.

Response:_____

2.0   SHOP DRAWINGS

2.1   The term "shop drawings" means drawings, diagrams, illustrations, brochures and other product data which are to be provided by the Vendor to illustrate details of the Work.

Response:_____

2.2   The Vendor shall arrange for the preparation of clearly identified shop drawings, to be prepared from accurate drawings provided by the Owner. The approved shop drawings will then be used as the basis for preparation of the installation site (production drawings).

Response:_____

2.3   It is distinctly understood that the Vendor is responsible for the accuracy of the information of which such shop drawings are prepared. Any cost for changes to the work resulting from inaccuracies in production drawings will be the responsibility of the Vendor.

Response:_____

2.4   The Vendor shall make any changes in shop drawings which the Owner may require and resubmit unless otherwise directed by the Owner. When resubmitting, the Vendor shall notify the Owner in writing of any revisions other than those requested by the Owner.

Response:_____

2.5   Shop drawings shall be submitted in standard metric drawing sizes.

Response:_____

3.0   TECHNOLOGICAL ADVANCEMENTS

3.1   Should any of the equipment proposed be superseded by a newer model during the period of time between the signing of a contract and the delivery date, the successful Vendor is required to make this information available to the Capital Health Authority, together with any price information. It will be the Owners option to make changes by altering, adding to, or deducting from the equipment list with the contract price, and progress schedule being adjusted accordingly.

Response:_____

4.0 COMPONENT DETERIORATION

4.1 In instances where equipment contains components which deteriorate with time, the Vendor shall insure that these components are scheduled to be shipped and installed at the latest possible time to ensure Owner receives maximum life of such components.

Response:_____

5.0 SETTLEMENT OF DISPUTES

5.1 In the case of any dispute arising between the Owner and the Vendor as to their respective rights and obligations under the Contract, either party shall be entitled to give to the other notice of such dispute.

Response:_____

5.2 In the event that an acceptable solution is not reached, the laws of the Province of Alberta related to arbitration and settlement of disputes shall apply.

Response:_____

6.0 HOSPITAL INSPECTION/ACCEPTANCE TESTING

6.1 New equipment must pass a hospital inspection for safety, performance and compliance with manufacturer's specifications prior to acceptance for clinical use. Such testing will constitute "Acceptance Testing". In all instances where published standards or specifications are not available the acceptance criterion shall be the demonstration, in the Owner's opinion, of good engineering practice and equipment performance.

Response:_____

7.0   CANADIAN STANDARDS ASSOCIATION APPROVAL (CSA)

7.1   All items will be Canadian Standards Association approved. Workmanship and fabrication of all items must be of the best quality and where these conditions are not met, the Owner reserves the right to reject these items for replacements.

Response:_____

8.0   SERVICE AFTER INSTALLATION

8.1   The supplier shall maintain a completely staffed service department with a complete stock of replacement parts. A qualified engineer shall be available in Edmonton to make service calls as required at the Owners location. The above service shall be guaranteed and maintained for a period of not less than ten (10) years. **All technical data to be left on site after warranty expires.** The Vendor must update servicing and technical manuals on an ongoing basis. In addition, the Vendor must notify, in writing, of any recommended design changes or functional upgrades during the life of the equipment (10 years). Any deviation from the above shall be approved by the Capital Health Authority.

Response:_____

9.0   OPERATOR TRAINING

9.1   Upon completion of the installation the Vendor will be expected to provide **"product specialists"** for a comprehensive [one-week minimum] training program to operators. The Vendor will also supply the Owner with a list of present users of equipment purchased in order that the Owner may arrange orientation for operation, if so desired. A three-day revisit, by the Product Specialist, shall occur during the warranty period.

Response:_____

9.2   The Vendor shall provide on-site demonstration and instruction in system operation by application specialists. In addition, the Vendor shall arrange for availability of training at other established sites as requested.

Response:_____

10.0   <u>SERVICE PERSONNEL TRAINING</u>

10.1   It is understood that the Owner's resident service personnel will be in attendance during the installation phase and during warranty service, in order to enhance their overall knowledge of the systems and component parts.

Response:_____

10.2   Vendor will be required to give service instruction to the Owner's service engineer(s) during the warranty period; and agrees to cooperate with the Owner by ensuring timely access to company service training programs for resident in-house engineers.

Response:_____

10.3   The Vendor shall supply a complete "related" service training program, which is equal to training programs available to the Vendor service representatives. The training program shall include, but not be limited to; theory of operation, operation of all service and calibration tools, operation of all diagnostic and calibration software and actual servicing and calibration of all components of the unit as supplied by the Vendor.

Response:_____

The Vendor shall supply all service, diagnostic, and calibrating software for all systems and components of the unit. In addition the Vendor shall provide all updates and revisions to this software for the life of the system.

Response:_____

a)   Incorporate in your proposal , as a separate unit price, the estimated all inclusive cost for same. The cost and specifications for any required laptop service computer must also be included.

Response:_____

b)   Please provide details of the Service Training Program with actual class dates.   Actual class date must be established within the warranty period and prior to final equipment payment.

Response:_____

10.4   Service Support. The resident service personnel shall have access to free telephone service support from the Vendor's corporate service support program office.

Response:_____

11.0   OPERATING AND MAINTENANCE INSTRUCTIONS/MANUALS

11.1   The coordination of the compiling and delivery of the operating manuals and maintenance instructions shall be the responsibility of the Vendor.

Response:_____

11.2   Prior to final payment the Vendor shall provide **one (1) set** of operating and maintenance manuals.   The manuals shall be coordinated in style, arrangement, indexing, etc. providing a complete index in the front of the binder.

Response:_____

11.3   Maintenance manuals shall be kept current for the life-time of the equipment, and shall contain the following:

a)   Maintenance and operating instructions for each piece of major equipment requiring maintenance.

Response:_____

b)   Descriptive and technical data.

Response:_____

c)   Control and schematic drawings.

Response:_____

d)   Wiring diagrams.

Response:_____

e)   A listing of specialized test and service tools, calibration devices, software and diagnostics required for servicing and performance assurance.

Response:_____

f)   A list of spare parts recommended for the Owner to carry.

Response:_____

g)   Copy of all factory and field tests.

Response:_____

h)   Names and addresses of service representatives and parts locations.

Response:_____

11.4   All product data information and instructions for use to be in the English language.

Response:_____

11.5   Only instructions as approved by manufacturer will be given to operating staff. All costs incurred due to any dysfunction caused by the operation of equipment contrary to approved instructions shall be the responsibility of the Owner.

Response:_____

12.0   GUARANTEE AND WARRANTY

12.1   All equipment is guaranteed to be free from defects in workmanship and material and this guarantee shall remain in effect for a period of one (1) year from the date of first availability for clinical use. Any work that has to be carried out, or parts installed during this one (1) year period shall be carried out without charge to the Capital Health Authority.

Response:_____

12.2   The Vendor shall correct, at his own expense, any defects in the Work due to faulty products and/or workmanship appearing within a period of one year or the time period specified in the individual sections from the date of first availability for clinical use.

Response:_____

13.0   EXTENSION OF WARRANTY

13.1   Should any component of a total system fail to function, and this breakdown causes a dysfunction of the total system, the warranty period of the total system shall be extended beyond the expiry date for a period equal to the length of time the total system was inoperable.

Response:_____

13.2   Should any single component dysfunction, but not render the total system inoperable, warranty on the specific component shall be extended beyond the expiry date for a period equal to the length of time of the dysfunction.

Response:_____

13.3 All performance parameters, as listed by the Vendor in the proposal and specifications , will be tested. Modification and/or repair to any parameters not met as originally stated, will be the responsibility of the Vendor at no charge to the Owner.

Response:_____

13.4 If the equipment does not perform as stated, and the Vendor is unable to meet the original specifications following adjustments and/or repair, the equipment will be returned to the Vendor. The Owner will receive a full refund or any payments made to date, and the Vendor will bear the expense of removal.

Response:_____

13.5 Downtime, defined as "total system failure to function" in excess of 10% per annum (18-25 days per annum) during the warranty period shall be considered unacceptable performance. The owner reserves the right to return the unit under the terms described in Item 13.4.

Response:_____

14.0 TERMS OF PAYMENT

14.1 A schedule of payments will be established pending final authorization of funding. The actual schedule of payments will be arrived at by negotiation between the successful vendor and the owner.

Vendors are required to submit proposed terms of payment for information/consideration with their proposal.

Response:_____

14.2 The Request for Proposal, must include separate pricing for each unit/system described in Section C, as well as discounted pricing for purchase of multiple systems from a single Vendor.

Response:_____

PACS / IMACS Project Timeline

Task	O			N			D				J				F				M				A
	13	20	27	3	10	17	24	1	8	15	22	29	5	12	19	26	2	9	16	23	2	9	16	23	30
Prepare Draft RFP - *Completed*																							
Appoint Committees * - *Completed*																							
Review / Finalize RFP - *Completed*																							
Release RFP - Oct 6th																							
Arrange Vendor presentations																							
Vendor Responses																							
Create spreadsheet of responses																							
Vendor presentations																							
Summarize and create Shortlist																							
Holiday Break																							

Site visits with shortlisted vendors													
Final negotiations													
Award contract - issue P.O.													
Manufacture, delivery, installation													
Applications training—offsite													
Acceptan testing													
Applications training—onsite													
clinical use													

* (1)Technical Evaluation and (2) Selection

Diagnostic Imaging Examinations Statistical Data

| **EXAMPLE – COMPUTED TOMOGRAPHY EXAM DATA** |

Site 1 Statistics – Computed Tomography

Number of exams per year (96/97): **18,953**
Average Number of images per exam (512^2):

Chest:	1,679 x 41 images	=	68,839
Abdomen:	3,565 x 65 images	=	231,725
Head:	10,767 x 36 images	=	387,612
Spine:	2,586 x 43 images	=	111,198
Extremity:	356 x 40 images	=	14,240
	Total Images:		**813,614**

Recall rates:
- On average, techs are asked to retrieve exams 3 times per day from prior studies up to 2 weeks old.
- With current use, CTi scanner only holds 4 days worth of exams.

Transfer volumes:
- Currently all abdomen/pelvis, chest, CT angio are transferred daily to the Advantage Windows workstation.

Raw Data:
- 40 % of raw data is required to be saved for 1) Trauma, 2) CT angio, 3) Reconstructions.

Site 2 Statistics – Computed Tomography

Number of exams per year (96/97): **15,769**
Average Number of images per exam (512^2):

Chest & Abdomen:	6,612	x	50	images	=	330,600
Head & Neck:	7,847	x	30	images	=	224,610
Spine & Extremity:	1,629	x	40	images	=	65,160
Interventional:	41	x	20	images	=	820
		Total Images:				**621,190**

Recall rates:
- On average, techs are asked to retrieve exams 2 times per day from prior studies up to two weeks old.
- With current use, CTi scanner only holds 4 days worth of exams.

Transfer volumes:
- Currently abdomen/pelvis, chest, CT angio images from the CTi scanner are transferred daily to the Advantage Windows workstation. The High Speed Advantage images go to the independent console.

Raw Data:

0 % of raw data is saved. All post processing occurs immediately after exam is finished. There is no subsequent additional reconstruction.

GENERAL RADIOLOGY EXAM DATA
(continue with similar analysis as provided for CT example)

MRI EXAM DATA
(continue with similar analysis as provided for CT example)

ULTRASOUND EXAM DATA
(continue with similar analysis as provided for CT example)

ANGIOGRAPHY EXAM DATA
(continue with similar analysis as provided for CT example)

NUCLEAR MEDICINE EXAM DATA
(continue with similar analysis as provided for CT example)

Major Equipment List / Summary of Major Components

The proposed network will include, but may not be limited to the following components:

- Twenty Four (24) Primary Diagnostic reporting stations[1] (12 at each hospital site).
- Thirty (30) Mid-range diagnostic / clinical review stations[1] (20 at Site 1, 10 at Site 2).
- Sixty (60) PC review stations (40 at Site 1, 20 at Site 2).
- Twenty-five (25) PC review stations - software only (for home review).
- Network RAID device(s) of sufficient size for one (1) month current exams plus all prior exams.
- Network Archive device(s) of sufficient size for two (2) years current exams plus all prior exams.
- All required switches, routers, hubs appropriate for the efficient and clinically useful running of the network[2].
- Appropriate hardware and software to enable film printing to two laser cameras at each site.

1. Vendors are required to include all monitor configurations as optional quotes in their responses. Monitor configurations may be mixed, to address functionality on a modality by modality basis.

2. It is likely that these network devices will be supplied through CHA Information Systems. Nevertheless, vendors are required to optionally price these devices, should a "turn-key" solution be requested.

N.B.:   The final numbers of reporting and review stations purchased may change from the quantities listed above, depending on the capabilities of the devices proffered by the successful vendor. **Vendors therefore are required to unit price the above components**.

A brief description of minimum expectations of the above devices follows, but it should under no circumstances be considered as limiting or exclusive, and the vendor is invited to substitute freely.

Device Descriptions (Minimum Requirements)

Primary Diagnostic Quality Reporting Station

- Full Analysis software (ROI, window/level, roaming zoom, pixel read-out, edge enhance, smooth, distance, angle, multi-display, "page format save")
- A minimum of two (2) $1.5K^2$, 100 Foot-lambert intensity display monitors.
- $1.5K^2$ video display controller
- 256 MB RAM
- Local Hard Drive (~ 6 GB)
- Local Hard Drive to be sized appropriately for minimum 48 hour storage capacity of estimated film volumes.
- P-300 CPU or better or equivalent
- IMACS software
- Network interface
- Print capabilities

Mid-Range Reporting Station

- Analysis software (ROI, window/level, roaming zoom, pixel read-out, edge enhance, smooth, distance, angle, multi-display, "page format save")
- A minimum of one (1) $1.5K^2$, 100 Foot-lambert intensity display monitors.
- $1.5K^2$ video display controller
- 128 MB RAM
- Local Hard Drive (~ 4 GB)
- Local Hard Drive to be sized appropriately for minimum 48 hour storage capacity of estimated film volumes.
- P-300 CPU or better or equivalent
- IMACS software
- Network interface
- Print capabilities

PC Review
- PC based
  P-300 CPU or better
  64 MB RAM
  4 MB Video RAM (1280 x 1024 x 32 bit true color) or high contrast gray scale

Cache memory
17" or larger monitor, non-interlaced colour or high
resolution gray scale
4.0+ GB Local Hard drive (EIDE or SCSI)
Network Interface
IMACS Software

- Local Hard Drive to be sized appropriately for minimum 48
  hour storage capacity of estimated film volumes
- Very simple, intuitive software:
  File Directory - Fetch, Display
  Brightness/Contrast
  Window width/level presets
  Roaming zoom
  Region of interest
  Distance, angles
  Image format conversion (i.e. "save as)

IMACS Software

- Objective code
- File Directory (file location transparent to user)
- Should incorporate intelligent "pre-fetch" capability (i.e.
  send images to anticipated locations)
- Scaleable
- Fault detecting, fault isolating
- Management statistics to be included (traffic volumes,
  rates)

On-Line Storage

- The local storage devices will be local hard drives,
  appropriately sized to maintain current images for a period
  of at least 2 days.
- The network storage device will consist of a RAID
  (Redundant Array of Independent Discs), appropriately
  sized to maintain images for a period of at least one month.

Archival Storage

- Archival storage will most likely consist of CD-R, MOD, or
  DLT jukebox(es), available on-line. The size of the
  archive, in the first instance, will be sufficient for two years
  current images.
- Future upgrades / additions to archive storage may
  incorporate HDVDs (High Density Video Discs), as this
  technology becomes available, reliable, and cost-effective.

Expectations are for 30 - 90 GB capacity 5.25" discs. A realistic date for this technology is probably 2000.

Network(s)
- Vendor to list range of networks which are compatible with quoted IMACS system:
- (e.g. Switch Based Network which is scaleable, and has fault isolation; FDDI backbone which has designed-in redundancy, designed-in management; 100 Mbit Ethernet which is inexpensive, compatible with many existing systems, and proven).

Network Servers
- Need to be large memory (512 MB RAM), very fast computers (e.g. *Sun Sparc, SGI, HP*).
- Network OS will most likely be *Windows NT* or *UNIX*.
- As configured, the network servers do not include hubs, routers, or bridges.

Equipment Specifications

Vendor to provide data pertinent to the following specifications. In the event of a lengthy response, please provide appropriate reference number in the "Supplementary Information Reference Column" (SIR #) and type response on Supplementary Information Sheets. **SIR's <u>must</u> be typed on separate sheets, and <u>not</u> at bottom of these pages, because they will be deleted when responses are reformatted to create a spreadsheet.**

INSTRUCTIONS: This Specifications section is a WORD 97 (SR-1) document. All questions and responses are in TABLE format. **You must type responses in RESPONSE cells, <u>without inserting or creating</u> additional cells/rows**. The cells will automatically increase in size to accommodate any amount of text in your response.

ITEM	IMAGE MANAGEMENT	RESPONSE	SIR #
1.0	**Database**		
1.1	Is database OEM? - Name.		
1.2	Database relational?		
1.3	Database object oriented?		
1.4	RDMS language		
1.5	What hardware platform does the database reside on?		
1.6	Is the database distributed over the network - elaborate.		
1.7	Directory available at all nodes?		
1.8	Redundancy in network - elaborate.		
1.9	SQL searching allowed?		
1.10	Describe password security levels available.		
1.11	Database must be fully DICOM 3.0 conformant.		
1.12	Vendor to provide detail on all DICOM		

		RESPONSE	SIR #
	3.0 service classes supported relevant to database.		
1.13	Types of fields/keys attributes allowed.		
1.14	Maximum number of fields/attributes allowed per record.		
1.15	Maximum number of records allowed.		
1.16	Elaborate on degree of customizability of database.		
1.17	Vendor to describe database configuration proposed.		
ITEM	**IMAGE MANAGEMENT**	**RESPONSE**	**SIR #**
2.0	**File Management**		
2.1	System management software OEM? - Name.		
2.2	What hardware platform does the file manager reside on?		
2.3	Does the file manager reside on the same platform as the database?		
2.4	Describe capability for pre-fetching of images.		
2.5	Describe capability for auto-routing of images.		
2.6	Can patients be identified by barcode?		
2.7	Describe connectivity of file manager to G.E. Cti scanner patient demographics.		
2.8	Describe connectivity of file manager to G.E. High Speed Advantage scanner patient demographics.		
2.9	Elaborate on connectivity of file manager to RIS and/or HIS.		
2.10	File manager to support distributed storage devices over entire network.		

2.11	File manager must be fully DICOM 3.0 conformant.		
2.12	Vendor to provide detail on all DICOM 3.0 services classes supported relevant to file manager.		
2.13	Elaborate on configurability of file manager with respect to:		
	Workstations		
	Users		
	Storage devices		
	Pre-fetching prior exams		
	Auto-routing of images		
2.14	At any given time, how many minimum copies of an exam will exist on the network?		
2.15	Where will they exist (what storage devices)?		
2.16	Vendor to describe file management configuration proposed.		
ITEM	**DISPLAY / ANALYSIS**	**RESPONSE**	**SIR #**
3.0	**Primary Diagnostic Quality Reporting Stations**		
3.1	Hardware platform used		
3.2	Nominal CPU speed		
3.3	CPU Bus bit size		
3.4	Operating system		
3.5	Standard RAM size proposed (MB)		
3.6	Maximum expandable RAM available as option (MB)		
3.7	Local hard drive size (GB)		

3.8	Programming capabilities: State any high level languages supplied with system.		
3.9	Monitor(s) are OEM? - name		
3.10	Number of monitors proposed		
3.11	Optional number(s) of monitors available		
3.12	Size of monitors (cm diagonal)		
3.13	Actual displayed pixels		
3.14	Luminance of monitors (>65 foot lamberts preferred)		
3.15	Monochrome or color?		
3.16	Image formats available (e.g. 2:1, 4:1, 16:1, etc.)		
3.17	Can image display formats be preset, user-defined, exam specific? Elaborate.		
3.18	Is there a "consultation" or "conferencing" feature (e.g. voice and/or cursor movement recording; messaging)? Elaborate.		
3.19	Is there a "Help" feature? Elaborate.		
3.20	Analysis / Manipulation		
	Vendor to state whether the following features are available:		
	a) Image display matrix sizes. State whether interpolated.		
	b) Window/level/invert		
	c) Zoom (all parts of image). Elaborate.		
	d) Zoom hold (for subsequent images).		
	e) Histogram averaging.		
	f) Slice addition (any slices).		
	g) Slice subtraction (any slices).		

	h) Edge enhancement.		
	i) Noise reduction (smoothing and filtering). Elaborate.		
	j) Text annotation.		
	k) Text deletion.		
	l) Region of interest. Elaborate.		
	m) Geometric measurement (distances, angles, areas).		
	n) Profiling (pixel value vs. pixel position).		
	o) Maximum number of images displayed simultaneously on CRT.		
	p) Cine loop.		
	q) Automatic display of all image acquisition parameters.		
	r) Stacked image display - forward/back.		
	s) Synchronized image display with prior studies.		
	t) Image rotation.		
	u) Printing capabilities.		
	v) File conversion capabilities (e.g. .gif, .tif, .bmp, etc.)		
3.21	Can these workstations display 3-D processed images? Elaborate.		
3.22	Power requirements – list all monitor configurations (Volts, Amps)		
3.23	Heat output – list all monitor configurations (BTUs/hour).		
3.24	Footprint (counter space required)		

ITEM	DISPLAY / ANALYSIS	RESPONSE	SIR
4.0	**Clinical Review Stations**		
4.1	Hardware platform used.		
4.2	Nominal CPU speed.		
4.3	CPU Bus bit size.		
4.4	Operating system.		
4.5	Standard RAM size proposed (MB).		
4.6	Maximum expandable RAM available as option (MB).		
4.7	Local hard drive size (GB).		
4.8	Programming capabilities: State any high level languages supplied with system.		
4.9	Monitor(s) are OEM? - name.		
4.10	Number of monitors proposed.		
4.11	Optional number(s) of monitors available.		
4.12	Size of monitors (cm diagonal).		
4.13	Actual displayed pixels.		
4.14	Luminance of monitors.		
4.15	Monochrome or color?		
4.16	Image formats available (e.g. 2:1, 4:1, 16:1, etc.)		
4.17	Is there a "Help" feature? Elaborate.		
4.18	Analysis / Manipulation		
	Vendor to state whether the following features are available:		
	a) Image display matrix sizes. State whether interpolated.		
	b) Window/level/invert		
	c) Zoom (all parts of image). Elaborate.		

d) Zoom hold (for subsequent images).		
e) Histogram averaging.		
f) Slice addition (any slices).		
g) Slice subtraction (any slices).		
h) Edge enhancement.		
i) Noise reduction (smoothing and filtering). Elaborate.		
j) Text annotation.		
k) Text deletion.		
l) Region of interest. Elaborate.		
m) Geometric measurement (distances, angles, areas).		
n) Profiling (pixel value vs. pixel position).		
o) Maximum number of images displayed simultaneously on CRT.		
p) Cine loop.		
q) Automatic display of all image acquisition parameters.		
r) Stacked image display - forward/back.		
s) Synchronized image display with prior studies.		
t) Image rotation.		
u) Printing capabilities.		
v) File conversion capabilities (e.g. .gif, .tif, .bmp, etc.)		
4.19 Can these workstations display 3-D processed images? Elaborate.		
4.20 Power requirements – list all monitor configurations (Volts, Amps)		

ITEM	DISPLAY / ANALYSIS	RESPONSE	SIR #
4.21	Heat output – list all monitor configurations (BTUs/hour).		
4.22	Footprint (counter space required)		
ITEM	**DISPLAY / ANALYSIS**	**RESPONSE**	**SIR #**
5.0	**PC Review Stations**		
5.1	Hardware platform used.		
5.2	Is hardware platform restricted (i.e., Can it be any PC?)		
5.3	Can hardware platform be purchased by the CHA through their suppliers?		
5.4	Nominal CPU speed proposed.		
5.5	Minimum CPU speed recommended.		
5.6	CPU Bus bit size.		
5.7	Operating system(s).		
5.8	Standard RAM size proposed (MB).		
5.9	Minimum RAM size recommended (MB).		
5.10	Maximum expandable RAM available as option (MB).		
5.11	Local hard drive size proposed (GB).		
5.12	Minimum hard drive size recommended (GB).		
5.13	Programming capabilities: State any high level languages supplied with system.		
5.14	Monitor is OEM? - name.		
5.15	Number of monitors proposed.		
5.16	Optional number(s) of monitors available.		
5.17	Size of monitors (cm diagonal).		

5.18	Actual displayed pixels.		
5.19	Luminance of monitor.		
5.20	Monochrome or color?		
5.21	Image formats available (e.g. 2:1, 4:1, 16:1, etc.)		
5.22	Is there a "Help" feature? Elaborate.		
5.23	Analysis / Manipulation		
	Vendor to state whether the following features are available:		
	a) Image display matrix sizes. State whether interpolated.		
	b) Window/level/invert.		
	c) Zoom (all parts of image). Elaborate.		
	d) Zoom hold (for subsequent images).		
	e) Histogram averaging.		
	f) Slice addition (any slices).		
	g) Slice subtraction (any slices).		
	h) Edge enhancement.		
	i) Noise reduction (smoothing and filtering). Elaborate.		
	j) Text annotation.		
	k) Text deletion.		
	l) Region of interest. Elaborate.		
	m) Geometric measurement (distances, angles, areas).		
	n) Profiling (pixel value vs pixel position).		
	o) Maximum number of images displayed simultaneously on CRT.		

ITEM		RESPONSE	SIR #
	p) Cine loop.		
	q) Automatic display of all image acquisition parameters.		
	r) Stacked image display - forward/back.		
	s) Synchronized image display with prior studies.		
	t) Image rotation.		
	u) Printing capabilities.		
	v) File conversion capabilities (e.g. .gif, .tif, .bmp, etc.).		
5.24	Can these workstations display 3-D processed images? Elaborate.		
5.25	Power requirements – list all monitor configurations (Volts, Amps)		
5.26	Heat output – list all monitor configurations (BTUs/hour).		
5.27	Footprint (counter space required).		
ITEM	**DISPLAY / ANALYSIS**	**RESPONSE**	**SIR #**
6.0	**PC Review - Software Only (for Home review).**		
6.1	Minimum hardware platform required.		
6.2	Is hardware platform restricted (i.e. can it be any PC?)		
6.3	Nominal CPU speed proposed.		
6.4	Minimum CPU speed recommended.		
6.5	Operating system(s) allowed or required.		
6.6	Standard RAM size recommended (MB).		
6.7	Minimum RAM size recommended (MB).		

6.8	Local hard drive size proposed (GB).		
6.9	Minimum hard drive size recommended (GB).		
6.10	Can the software support more than one monitor?		
6.11	Size of monitors (cm diagonal) recommended.		
6.12	Actual displayed pixels.		
6.13	Can the software support a high resolution, high contrast greyscale monitor? Elaborate.		
6.14	Image formats available (e.g. 2:1, 4:1, 16:1, etc.)		
6.15	Is there a "Help" feature? Elaborate.		
6.16	Analysis / Manipulation.		
	Vendor to state whether the following features are available.		
	a) Image display matrix sizes. State whether interpolated.		
	b) Window/level/invert.		
	c) Zoom (all parts of image). Elaborate.		
	d) Zoom hold (for subsequent images).		
	e) Slice addition (any slices).		
	f) Slice subtraction (any slices).		
	g) Edge enhancement.		
	h) Noise reduction (smoothing and filtering). Elaborate.		
	I) Text annotation.		
	j) Text deletion.		
	k) Region of interest. Elaborate.		

	l) Geometric measurement (distances, angles, areas).		
	m) Profiling (pixel value vs pixel position).		
	n) Maximum number of images displayed simultaneously on CRT.		
	o) Cine loop.		
	p) Automatic display of all image acquisition parameters.		
	q) Staked image display - forward/back.		
	r) Synchronized image display with prior studies.		
	s) Image rotation.		
	t) Printing capabilities (to paper copy laser printer).		
	u) File conversion capabilities (e.g. gif, .tif, .bmp, etc.)		
6.17	Can the software display 3-D processed images? Elaborate.		
6.18	Does the software support image compression? Elaborate.		
6.19	What network interface board(s) are supported.		
6.20	Does the software support POTS, ISDN, Cable connectivity?		
6.21	Does the software support push/pull capability?		
6.22	State thoroughly DICOM conformance levels, service classes of software.		

ITEM	STORAGE	RESPONSE	SIR #
7.0	**RAID**		
7.1	Number any type of magnetic disk drives (manufacturer).		
7.2	Storage capacity (GB).		
7.3	Storage capacity (number of images). State matrix size of images.		
7.4	Typical access time (from recall initiation to paint on CRT).		
7.5	RAID "current" storage should have sufficient capacity for one (1) month's worth of CT exams, as well as all prior CT exams for this current list.		
7.6	Vendor to elaborate on configuration of RAID(s) on network.		
7.7	Power requirements (Volts, Amps)		
7.8	Heat output (BTUs/hour).		
7.9	Footprint (space required).		
ITEM	STORAGE	RESPONSE	SIR #
8.0	**On-Line Archive**		
8.1	Jukebox configuration? Elaborate.		
8.2	Number and type of jukeboxes (manufacturer).		
8.3	Magneto-optical or WORM disks.		
8.4	Storage capacity per disk (GB).		
8.5	Optional tape-based system.		
8.6	Fixed or removable discs.		
8.7	Total storage capacity of jukebox proposed (GB).		
8.8	Storage capacity (number of images). State matrix size of images.		

8.9	Typical access time (from recall initiation to paint on CRT).		
8.10	Compression of data for archiving (yes/no).		
8.11	Is compression fully recoverable (yes/no).		
8.12	Elaborate on type and range of compression available.		
8.13	Is archiving automatic?		
8.14	Can archiving be customized?		
8.15	Elaborate on redundancy in archive.		
8.16	Archive "current" storage should have sufficient capacity of one (1) year's worth of CT exams, as well as all prior CT exams for this current list.		
8.17	Power requirements (Volts, Amps)		
8.18	Heat output (BTUs/hour).		
8.19	Footprint (space required).		
ITEM	**NETWORK**	**RESPONSE**	**SIR #**
9.0	Network to be installed by (or under the direction of) CHA Region Information Systems Department.		
9.1	Does vendor offer "turn-key" approach to networking?		
9.2	Network sizing to be sufficient to provide exam transfer between referral hospital sites in a timely manner. Vendor to elaborate on this.		
9.3	Network Protocol:		
9.4	Type of LAN(s):		
	FDDI		

			SIR
	100 MB Ethernet (100 Base-T and/or 100VG).		
9.5	Ethernet?		
9.6	TCP/IP?		
9.7	DICOM conformance:		
	objects.		
	commands.		
	classes.		
9.8	Native image format.		
9.9	Image compression used.		
9.10	Nominal network speed - elaborate.		
9.11	Transmission media:		
	UTP.		
	fibre.		
ITEM	**INTERFACING**	**RESPONSE**	**SIR #**
10.0	Vendor to completely describe DICOM conformance for entire network, including (but not limited to):		
	objects.		
	commands.		
	classes.		
10.1	Vendor to completely describe RIS/HIS interface levels.		
10.2	Network must interface seamlessly to existing CT sanners:		
	G.E. CTi scanner (Vers. x.xx) at Site 1.		
	G.E. CTi scanner (Vers. x.yy) at Site 2.		
	G.E. High Speed Advantage scanner		

	(Vers. y.zz) at Site 1.		
	G.E. High Speed Advantage scanner (Vers. a.bb) at Site 2.		
	G.E. Advantage windows workstation (Vers. d.ff) at Site 1.		
	G.E. Advantage windows workstation (Vers. g.hh) at Site 2.		
10.3	Network must interface seamlessly to existing MRI scanners:		
	Siemens Symphony (Vers. 1.23) at Site 1.		
	Philips Gyroscan 1.5 (Vers. 3.45) at Site 2.		
10.4	Vendor to elaborate on extent of networking possibilities with Site 1 Kodak US network (Vers. 2.2).		
	Vendor to elaborate on extent of networking possibilities with Site 2 A.L.I. US network (Vers. r.cc).		
10.5	Network must interface seamlessly to existing digital angiography and fluoroscopy equipment:		
	Toshiba ADR 1000 R/F system (Vers. x.xx).		
	Philips EasyDiagnost R/F (Vers. y.yy)		
	Philips EasyDiagnost R/F (Vers. y.dd)		
	Siemens Sireskop SX R/F (Vers. x.x)		
	Philips V5000 Angio System (Vers. d.dd)		
	Philips V3000 Angio System (Vers. g.g)		
	Siemens Multistar TOP Angio System (Vers. d.dd)		
10.6	Vendor to elaborate on extent of networking possibilities with Site 1 Picker NM network (Vers. 2.2).		
	Vendor to elaborate on extent of		

ITEM	PRODUCTION OF DIGITAL GENERAL RADIOLOGY IMAGES	RESPONSE	SIR #
	networking possibilities with Site 2 ADAC NM network (Vers. r.cc).		
11.0	**Film Digitizers**		
11.1	Name and Model Number		
11.2	Must have capability to digitize entire range of film sizes: 18 x 24 cm 24 x 30 cm 35 x 35 cm 35 x 43 cm		
11.3	Vendor to elaborate on matrix sizes available for each film size above. User selectable?		
11.4	Bit depth (8,10,12) available for above film sizes and matrix sizes?		
11.5	Vendor to provide list of DICOM compatible fields available for image header, e.g.: Patient Name Patient ID Patient Date of Birth Study ID Other State maximum character length for each of above.		
11.6	Acquisition of above fields by: Keyboard RIS/HIS interface (elaborate) Barcode reader		

	Scan performance:		
11.7	Digitizer spot sizes (microns)		
11.8	Density resolution (OD)		
11.9	Density range (OD)		
11.10	Scan time for full 35 x 43 cm film, 2048^2 x 12 matrix (sec)		
11.11	Total time to scan 35 x 43 cm film at 2048^2 x 12, build, and send image (typical).		
11.12	Multiple film loader/holder available? Elaborate.		
11.13	Sustained, automatic throughput of 35 x 43 cm films, 2048^2 x 12 bits. (Sec/film)		
	Image Manipulation		
11.14	Image preview? Elaborate.		
11.15	Flip image Left / Right capability?		
11.16	Flip image Vertically?		
11.17	Rotate image in 90 degree increments?		
11.18	Histogram adjustment possible?		
11.19	Image Filters available?		
	Computer Station		
11.20	State make and model.		
11.21	State CPU, RAM, Cache, Hard drive, Monitor, OS, and Network interface configuration.		
11.22	DICOM connectivity levels provided?		
11.23	Autocalibration software? Elaborate.		
11.24	Autorouting capabilities? Elaborate.		
11.25	Digitizer and computer power requirements (Volts, Amps).		
11.26	Total heat output (BTUs/hour).		

11.27	Total footprint (space required).		
12.0	**Computed Radiography**		
12.1	Name and model number of reader.		
12.2	System must have capability to read entire range of cassette sizes: 18 x 24 cm 24 x 30 cm 35 x 35 cm 35 x 43 cm		
12.3	Vendor to elaborate on matrix sizes available for each cassette size above. User selectable?		
12.4	Bit depth (8,10,12) available for above cassette sizes and matrix sizes?		
12.5	Vendor to provide list of DICOM compatible fields available for image header, e.g.: Patient Name Patient ID Patient Date of Birth Study ID Other State maximum character length for each of above.		
12.6	Acquisition of above fields by: Keyboard RIS/HIS interface (elaborate) Barcode reader		
	Reader performance:		
12.7	Laser spot sizes at image plane (microns)		

12.8	Processing time for full 35 x 43 cm plate, 2K x 2.5K x 12 bit matrix (sec).		
12.9	Total time to read 35 x 43 cm plate at 2K x 2.5K x 12 bits, build, and send image (typical).		
12.10	Time to completely erase plate after reading?		
12.11	Multiple/Auto cassette loader available? Elaborate.		
12.12	Sustained, automatic throughput of 35 x 43 cm plates, 2K x 2.5K x 12 bits, including erasure (Sec/plate).		
Image Manipulation			
12.13	Image preview? Elaborate.		
12.14	Flip image Left / Right capability?		
12.15	Flip image Vertically?		
12.16	Rotate image in 90 degree increments?		
12.17	Histogram adjustment possible?		
12.18	Image dynamic range adjustment possible? Elaborate.		
12.19	Image Filters available? Elaborate.		
12.20	Artifact suppression/correction features available? Elaborate.		
Computer Station			
12.21	State make and model.		
12.22	State CPU, RAM, Cache, Hard drive, Monitor, OS, and Network interface configuration.		
12.23	DICOM connectivity levels provided?		
12.24	Autocalibration software? Elaborate.		
12.25	Autorouting capabilities? Elaborate.		
12.26	Reader physical dimensions – L x W x H		

	(cm)		
12.27	Reader and computer power requirements (Volts, Amps).		
12.28	Total system heat output (BTUs/hour).		
12.29	System footprints (total space required).		
	Imaging Plates		
12.30	Does reader flex, in any way, the plates as they are read? Elaborate on geometry/mechanics of "read" function inside reader.		
12.31	Sensitivity of plates and screens (relative speed).		
12.32	Useful exposure range on cassette (mR).		
12.33	Does vendor guarantee plate life (exposure number)? Elaborate.		
12.34	Overall performance of the CR system will need to satisfy Acceptance Testing and QC criteria, currently being developed by AAPM Task Group #10.		
13.0	**Direct Radiography**		
13.1	Name and model number of system.		
13.2	System must have capability to record entire range of standard image sizes: 18 x 24 cm 24 x 30 cm 35 x 35 cm 35 x 43 cm		
13.3	Vendor to elaborate on range of matrix sizes available. User selectable?		
13.4	Bit depth (8,10,12) available for above matrix sizes?		
13.5	Vendor to provide list of DICOM		

	compatible fields available for image header, e.g.: Patient Name Patient ID Patient Date of Birth Study ID Other State maximum character length for each of above.		
13.6	Acquisition of above fields by: Keyboard RIS/HIS interface (elaborate) Barcode reader		
	DR performance:		
13.7	TFT pixel size at image plane (microns)		
13.8	Processing time for full 35 x 43 cm image, 2K x 2.5K x 12 bit matrix (sec).		
13.9	Total time to process 35 x 43 cm image at 2K x 2.5K x 12 bits, build, and send (typical).		
13.10	Lapse time between exposures?		
	Image Manipulation		
13.11	Image preview? Elaborate.		
13.12	Flip image Left / Right capability?		
13.13	Flip image Vertically?		
13.14	Rotate image in 90 degree increments?		
13.15	Histogram adjustment possible?		
13.16	Image dynamic range adjustment possible? Elaborate.		
13.17	Image Filters available? Elaborate.		
13.18	Artifact suppression/correction features available? Elaborate.		

13.19	Other software available (e.g. image subtraction)? Elaborate.		
	Computer Station		
13.20	State make and model.		
13.21	State CPU, RAM, Cache, Hard drive, Monitor, OS, and Network interface configuration.		
13.22	DICOM connectivity levels provided?		
13.23	Autocalibration software? Elaborate.		
13.24	Autorouting capabilities? Elaborate.		
13.25	Computer power requirements (Volts, Amps).		
13.26	Computer heat output (BTUs/hour).		
13.27	System footprint (space required).		
13.28	Sensitivity of DR plate (relative speed).		
13.29	Useful exposure range on plate (mR).		
13.30	Overall performance of the DR system will need to satisfy Acceptance Testing and QC criteria similar to that for CR image plates, currently being developed by AAPM Task Group #10.		
14.0	**Dry Laser Film Printer**		
14.1	Hard copy network film device to be a dry film printer with full DICOM print capability.		
14.2	Make and model.		
14.3	Printing done using laser or thermal head? Elaborate.		
14.4	Film sizes available (cm).		

14.5	Vendor to list number and range of views/formats supported.		
14.6	Maximum resolution (matrix size) of printer.		
14.7	Bit depth of images (number of grey shades).		
14.8	Film to be supplied from magazine(s) rather than cassettes.		
14.9	Film capacity of magazines, and film sizes allowed.		
14.10	Printer to be capable of batch mode printing.		
14.11	Minimum time to print 12 (512^2) images on one film (sec).		
14.12	Printer to be capable of either positive or negative image generation.		
14.13	Printer software to include "black matte" feature surrounding images.		

STATEMENT OF SERVICE SUPPORT - IMACS/PACS Network

Vendor must complete this page as service support will be an important consideration in the final selection of successful supplier.

1. Response time (in hours) to a service request:

   Regular week days: _____

   Weekends: _____

   Public (Stat) holidays: _____

   24-Hour Coverage must be available: _____

2. Number of trained service engineers: _____

   Located at: _____

3. The nearest parts depot is located at: _____

   _____

   Percentage of parts (required to service quoted equipment).

   Stored at this location: _____

   Balance of parts stored at: _____

4. Service (labour) rates to be charged:

   Regular time: _____

   After hours: _____

   Weekends: _____

   Holidays: _____

5. Other charges. List and specify (i.e. travel, accommodation, miscellaneous expenses).

   _____

6. Specify cost for a "Comprehensive Service Contract". (Parts, travel and labour) for a one year period.

   _____

7. Specify cost for a "Preventative Maintenance Contract" and describe:

---

8. Describe the required time to be used for scheduled preventative maintenance.

---

9. Vendor's additional comments (service related). _____

A PACS Case Study
PACS Development at
The Medical University of South Carolina

G. Donald Frey
The Department of Radiology
The Medical University of South Carolina
Charleston, SC

Introduction

The purpose of this paper is to describe the history of Picture Archiving and Communication System (PACS) development at the Medical University of South Carolina (MUSC), with the broader intention of showing the roles that the various people involved played, and to emphasize the importance of medical physics involvement. Although specific products and vendors will be mentioned, it is important to note that the products continually evolve, so that factors influencing purchases at a particular time may not be relevant in the current PACS environment.

Early Development

Radiology Information System (RIS)

PACS development at the Medical University of South Carolina began on September 15, 1989 when the Radiology Information System (RIS) DecRad, which subsequently became IDXRad, "address" was installed. The early data from the IDXRad system showed that more than 20% of the studies that were completed were not reported or billed and that for certain orthopaedic and neurosurgens, the rate of unreported and billed studies exceeded 75%. This high loss of studies, and therefore revenue, was a significant concern and while administrative controls and changes in operations within the radiology department reduced this number to the 7 to 8% range fairly quickly, we began investigating ways to reduce film loss and unreported studies within the radiology department.

PACS Rational

The IDXrad experience illustrates one of the more important PACS principles. PACS development should be problem oriented. Most radiology departments are plagued by a variety of problems that PACS call help ameliorate. Existing problems in Radiology have been exacerbated by changes in the present radiology environment. Managed care pressures to reduce costs and staff on the one hand, and the desire for quicker medical decisions and coverage of more locations on the other, are particular examples.

Quicker medical decision-making requires reduction in the time between the order-ing of a radiological procedure and when the data are available for patient care management. This has many elements that include the administrative aspects of sched-uling the study, moving the patient to radiologic equipment, production of the images, transmission of the images to an interpreting physician, dictation of a report and trans-mission of images, and report to the referring physician. In addition, many departments have seen a reduction in the number of radiologists that are available and the desire to provide radiologic services at more than one location. Thus, radiologists may be sta-tioned at locations where the volume of images generated is smaller than desirable for efficient use of radiologists' time, or there may be no radiologists at a location where quick decisions on a particular study are necessary.

These problems associated with staff management also apply to the management of the radiology images on film. These so-called "hard copy images" are usually stored in large file rooms. Because of cost considerations for space in hospitals, older films are often stored off-site. Thus, the time to retrieve old images for comparison is often lengthy and is measured in hours for recently produced images to days for images that were produced more than a year ago. In addition to this, films are frequently lost and/or stolen. In addition, the physical film can only be available at one location so that it is not available for use by several people at one time and cannot be viewed by people in separated locations for purposes of consultation. The large film libraries in hospitals are costly. The film library at the Medical University of South Carolina that occupied 2000 square feet with an approximate cost to the department of $72,000 per year has been eliminated.

PACS can serve as a possible solution to a number of these problems. Images that are generated in the department are available for interpretation by radiologists within five minutes of their production and are simultaneously available for other physicians. A study at Duke University Medical Center showed that in a PACS environment, internists and surgeons in intensive care units were able to view images 20% faster than they could using conventional film technologies (Humphrey et al. 1995, 1993). These images are potentially available simultaneously to physicians throughout the hospital and can be viewed by physicians in more than one location for teleconferencing. In addition, archived images with retrieval times on the order of hours rather than days are available for physicians. While under a PACS there is still some loss of images, the loss rate is much smaller than with conventional film systems.

As environmental regulation increases, the management of wet chemistry systems becomes more difficult. While mandatory reclamation of silver from fixer solutions is required in most locations, some locations require that spent fixer and developer be treated as hazardous waste and be disposed of that way and in rare instances the wash water from film processors must also be recycled.

A second factor which led to our initial efforts in PACS was the interest of the chairman of the department of that time, who was familiar with some early PACS efforts in nuclear medicine and saw the advantages of having studies available on computers. This leads to a second general point, which is—

Common Problems in Radiology Departments

Managed Care
- Cost Reduction Pressures
- Staff Reductions
- Quicker Medical Decisions
- Radiologist Coverage at More Locations

Film Management Problems
- Lost and Stolen Films
- Time to Retrieve Old Studies
- Single Location Availability
- Storage Costs

PACS development goes smoother if there is a champion of the project high within both the hospital administration and the radiology administration.

The third event which increased interest in PACS development was Hurricane Hugo, which struck Charleston on the night of September 19, 1989. This hurricane destroyed approximately 10% of our film library when one of the auxiliary film libraries adjacent to the hospital was flooded. This pointed out an additional problem with film in that it is quite vulnerable to loss and destruction.

Initial Efforts at Implementation of a PACS

In 1990 we had our first opportunity to enter the PACS arena when as part of a large purchase of radiology equipment, we obtained our first PACS (Philips Comview System). The goals of the Philips Comview purchase were to improve the quality of mobile radiography by switching to computed radiography (CR) to provide immediate access to mobile examinations in the intensive care units by electronic distribution to remote viewing terminals, electronically archive the images so that both film and electronic archives exist to reduce the vulnerability to film loss and damage, and to provide high performance viewing stations in adult and pediatric radiology for more rapid review of ICU (Intensive Care Unit) films.

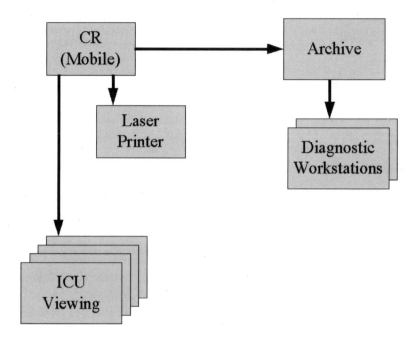

Figure 1. The configuration of the original Philips Comview PACS.

The first two goals were met by this system. Computed radiography improved the consistency of the mobile examinations and reduced, retake rates and the images were transmitted via ethernet to the Philips Comview ICU viewing terminals. There were substantial problems with the electronic archive and the high performance radiologist stations. The electronic archive proved to be so slow in response that it was impractical to use and the radiologist viewing stations were also very slow with image retrieval time, even for images that were stored locally on the units, on the order of 10 to 15 seconds, so that viewing a PA and lateral chest on the units was not practical. Consequently, the electronic archive and the radiologist viewing stations were removed from service, but the computed radiography was retained as were the ICU viewing stations, which were used up until the time they were replaced by a new PACS.

The radiologist viewing stations that were taken out of service had four monitors each. The early radiologist experience with these monitors convinced our radiologists that four monitor stations would not be helpful and that two monitor stations with appropriate software and speed would be more useful. Consequently, all future diagnostic viewing stations have had only two monitors.

The CR part of the initial PACS was very successful so that an additional CR unit was purchased for the trauma center. This second CR reduced the number of lost films from the trauma center since images were held for about 24 hours on the system. If a film was taken to the operating room and not returned, an additional image for interpretation could be printed.

The Philips Comview system had a technical deficiency of slow computer speed and was hampered by trying to use a conventional 10 Mbit/sec Ethernet, even though it was isolated from the rest of the hospital networks. In addition to the technical deficiencies, the Commview system had several operational problems. The first of these was that the images were only distributed to four intensive care units. This limited the utility of the system as an overall PACS. Second, the system did not have a link to our RIS. The lack of a RIS link caused considerable problems in maintaining the integrity of the patient records since the patient name was being entered in different ways by different operators; there were also errors associated with entering the medical record number and the identification number used in the RIS system. Finally, since the system was only set up to use CR data, its utility was limited to a very small section of the total business of the department. At that time, CR was only used for mobile examinations and there was a problem comparing images in that the patient might have two CR images and then a conventional image in the radiology department.

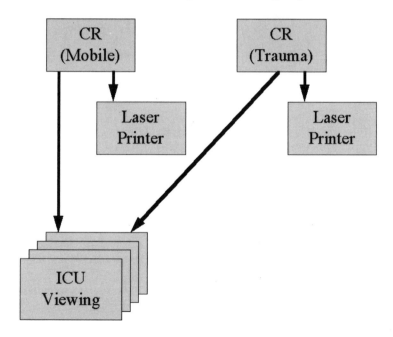

Figure 2. The configuration of the original PACS after the archive and radiologists viewing stations were removed. Because of the initial success of CR for mobile radiography a second CR unit was added in the trauma center.

The Ultrasound Mini-PACS

The next step in PACS development was to obtain a dedicated ultrasound PACS. This was obtained in 1992 and consisted of a file server, a RAID, disk, a small jukebox, and laser printer. The system frame-captured images from four ultrasound scanners. This unit did not have RIS verification of data, but within the limited arena of ultrasound this was not such a large problem. The ultrasound units were equipped with disk drives so that images could be stored when the units were used for mobile studies.

This unit was immediately successful, primarily because images were always available more quickly on this PACS than they were available on film. Radiologists began to use the system to look at images before the films were out of the laser printer, to consult with nonradiology physicians visiting the ultrasound section, and for getting comparison studies. The ultrasound mini-PACS had the advantage for the radiologists of always having comparison studies available. A study that was done showed that images were always available faster on the PACS than they were on film and that the older the images were, the greater the difference was. This was true, even though the jukebox only held about three months of on-line data; for images older than that, the file clerks had to reload old disks. At the same time, images more than a few months old were kept in our remote in-hospital film room and images more than a year old were kept outside the hospital. Sometime during this process, we noted that while films were still being made and archived in the film room, the ultrasound section had spontaneously gone filmless in that the physicians were interpreting soft copy from the PACS workstations and film was not being used within the ultrasound department. Films were still used by the referring physicians but we felt that if electronic copies were available to a few high-use ultrasound physicians (e.g., pediatric nephrology), we could turn off automatic filming and only film studies on demand. In order to achieve this goal we purchased several additional workstations for the areas that were high users of ultrasound images, and automatic filming was turned off in the ultrasound area.

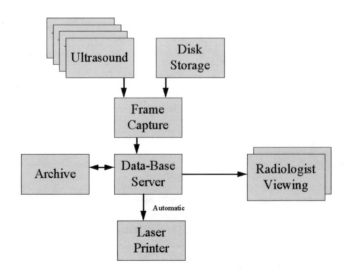

Figure 3. The initial configuration of the ultrasound mini-PACS.

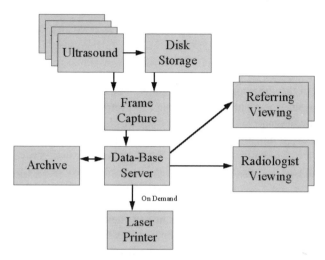

Figure 4. The configuration of the ultrasound mini-PACS showing the addition of workstations outside of radiology. These additional workstations allowed the ultrasound area to go filmless.

Extension to Nuclear Medicine

At the same time we were going filmless in ultrasound, we decided to add a nuclear medicine PACS. This was done by frame capture from six nuclear medicine cameras. Since these cameras all had internal computers, the problem experienced by ultrasound of having to install disk capture systems on the ultrasound units for mobile examinations was avoided. Nuclear medicine went filmless shortly after the ultrasound section.

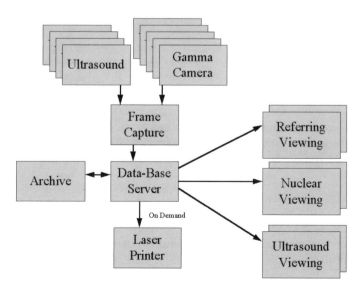

Figure 5. The configuration of the mini-PACS after nuclear medicine was added.

The Full PACS Implementation

Introduction

The success of the ultrasound and nuclear medicine mini-PACS led to the decision to move the hospital to an entirely electronic environment. While there was significant support within the radiology department from the chairman, several key radiologists, and the hospital administrator for radiology, convincing the hospital administration of the importance of moving to an electronic environment was still necessary. This was done by taking the hospital administrator and a representative of the Board of Trustees on a number of site visits where PACS was in use in the CT and MRI area. It was generally felt at the time that these site visits represented a crucial moment in the evolution of PACS at MUSC. The experience of these two individuals seeing PACS working in a clinical environment and of personally being able to use the workstations convinced the hospital administration and the Board of Trustees to allocate a budget of $5 million for the PACS project. While the financial aspect of the PACS is generally beyond the scope of this paper, it is interesting to note that the PACS we have in place has considerably more workstations and one more CR unit than were originally planned even though about $400,000 of the original budget was never spent. We also felt that the project should not be open ended. The budgetary approval occurred in the fall of 1994 and we adopted the goal of going to full soft copy interpretation by the time of the 1996 summer Olympics (July).

The PACS Committee

In order to effect the purchase of the PACS, a PACS purchasing committee was formed consisting of the chairman of the radiology department, an additional radiologist, the radiology department hospital administrator, a representative from hospital purchasing, a representative from the hospital IS (Information Systems) department, a PACS administrator, and a medical physicist. This group was charged with determining what was needed, writing the Request for Proposal (RFP), purchasing the PACS, and implementing it. This group still meets on a regular basis about PACS issues, although presently the representative from IS and the purchasing department do not routinely attend. The committee name has been changed to the Radiology Informatics Committee to stress the importance of the RIS, Dictation, and Office Automation systems as well as the PACS.

Medical Physicist Role

The medical physicist on the committee (GDF) had primary responsibility in six areas. These were: 1) system design, 2) calculation of storage requirements, 3) network traffic analysis, 4) specification writing, 5) acceptance testing, and 6) quality assurance.

Medical physicists have special knowledge about the technical workings of a radiology department. Therefore, medical physics input into the design of a PACS is a key
requirement. Knowledge about where images are used, rates at which images are
moved from one place to another, legal requirements for image retention, technical
requirements, for image retention, image quality requirements, and specifications for
existing equipment are all within the purview of the medical physicist.

Medical physicists are the individuals most knowledgeable about calculation of storage requirements and data transmission requirements for a PACS system. Images are
stored in PACS in many locations: workstations, servers, and short- and long-term
archives. The medical physicist can calculate the expected usage of images and the
requirements for storage at each location. In order to move images from one location
to another, the network that is used must have sufficient capacity. The medical physicist
can calculate the network requirements on different loading and with different degrees
of compression.

The medical physicist should write most of the technical specifications for a PACS.
Specifications should be problem-oriented because different vendors may have different technical solutions to the same radiology problems. The specifications should,
whenever possible, include a testing routine. Common areas that can be tested are workstation performance, image transfer speeds, data integrity, and storage capacity. Since
our system was installed in an existing radiology department, we spent considerable
effort specifying how the proposed PACS would work with the existing PACS equipment, the existing non-DICOM compatible equipment, and the existing RIS system.

When the PACS arrives and is installed, the medical physicist should verify the
technical specifications by acceptance testing.

The medical physicist should also formulate and supervise the quality assurance
protocols that are used for the PACS.

Original Implementation Plan

The initial plan for the full PACS was to install the archive and database server, attach
the existing digital modalities (CT and MRI) to the system, load the database for approximately three months, and begin soft-copy interpretation. At the same time, we were
going to integrate the existing mini-PACS in ultrasound and nuclear medicine into the
system. This was to be followed by the purchase of five CR units (adult, pediatric, OR,
trauma, outpatient) that would also load the database for approximately three months.
Once the CR database loading was complete, the department would go full soft-copy
by July 1996. Site visits were conducted in the spring of 1995 and after visits to a
number of locations we felt that there were perhaps three companies that could provide
a full PACS; but because of state purchasing requirements, many more would likely
submit RFPs if that was the purchasing process used. To reduce the need to evaluate a

large number of RFPs, we initially issued an RFQ (Request for Qualifications). The purpose of the RFP was to eliminate companies that had not installed major PACS. The RFQs requested minimum information from the vendors about PACS they had installed and PACS resources expended by the corporation. After reviewing the qualifications of the companies that proposed to provide a PACS, it was determined that, in fact, only two companies could meet our needs. A detailed RFP was issued in the summer of 1995 and a purchase was placed with Agfa Corporation for the CT and MRI components.

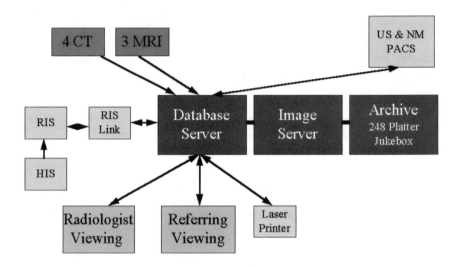

Figure 6. The planned initial installation of the PACS with initial collection of data from the digital modalities (CT & MRI).

Installation

The installation of these components began in late fall 1995. The first components installed were the central archive and database server so that archive loading could begin. A small number of workstations were installed so that faculty interested in using the PACS could do so. A number of problems were quickly discovered. The first of these was that there was no point in starting to load the database until a robust link existed between the PACS and the RIS. It was almost impossible to get accurate patient demographics into the PACS without using the RIS to verify the data. The second was that although it was relatively easy to get the data into the PACS from our digital modalities, there were substantial problems associated with the details of how those data were displayed. For example, one of the MR scanners would send the data very nicely, but would interleave images from early and late echoes, making the data almost impossible to view on a soft-copy terminal. Since we were still printing film at this time, these problems did not affect overall function within the department. In addition, there were some limitations in the soft-copy display stations that made efficient radiologist use of these stations difficult. In the course of early spring 1996 we worked on these problems and by April the properly RIS-verified data were flowing into the PACS. Database loading from that time on was accurate, but it was not until late fall of that year when the CT and MRI section became fully soft-copy.

At the same time, we began installation of a 155 Mbit/sec ATM network for distribution of images. This was ATM over fiber optic cable, the best high speed network available at the time. This network is maintained by MUSC IS staff.

In the meantime, parallel track for CR acquisition was taking place. This included site visits in the fall of 1995. It was our belief that the practical utility of the CR within the radiology department was the single most important factor in the CR purchase. This included RIS verification of the patient data and a smooth, efficient technology interface that included the ability to identify cassettes at more than one location and the ability to use more than one CR reader for an identified cassette. In addition, because of our previous experience, we were very sensitive to the issue of clearing plate jams so we spent some effort in determining which systems allowed easy clearing of plate jams. The CR readers were purchased in January 1996 and installation began shortly thereafter. After approximately three months of database loading, filming was turned off for projection radiography and full soft-copy interpretation began. By the time of the Olympics in July 1996, we were fully soft-copy for projection radiography, nuclear medicine, and ultrasound, but much of CT and MR was still interpreted from film. Following several software upgrades, full CR soft-copy interpretation was implemented later in 1996. The departmental film file library was removed in early 1997. This is the milestone that I used to determine that we had moved into a fully electronic practice. At the same time the film library was removed, we redesigned the adult and neuroradiology reading rooms. The new rooms could be much smaller than the old ones since we needed less diagnostic workstations than for motorized film viewers.

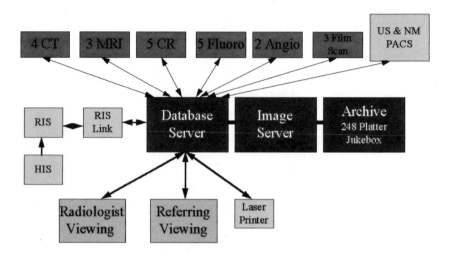

Figure 7. The configuration of the PACS in the summer of 1996. At this time all of the initial installation was complete.

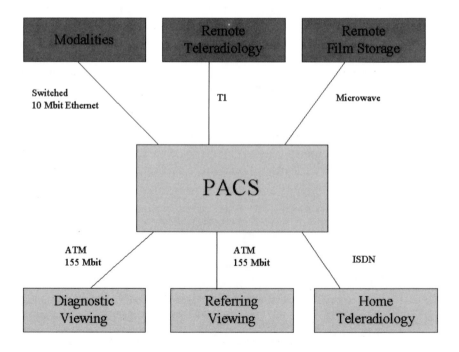

Figure 8. The initial network structure for the PACS.

Description of the Current System

The Current System (Spring 1999)

Presently the PACS accepts images from six ultrasound scanners, seven nuclear medicine cameras, four CT scanners, three MRI scanners, three angiography units, five digital fluoroscopy units, four film scanners, six CR units, two mobile fluoroscopy units (C-arms), and one stereotactic breast biopsy unit. Most of these units have direct DICOM output links to the PACS, but there are some legacy devices. One of these is a CT scanner than captures images by frame-capture, which is not desirable. This scanner is now mainly used for interventional procedures. Although nuclear medicine has been filmless for many years, there are still significant problems in this area. The present system does not adequately handle overlays in the DICOM environment, so some frame capture is still done. Acquisition devices for CT and MRI still have issues in terms of sending sagittal and coronal images, three-dimensional reconstructions, and functional images with color. The heart of the system is the file server database manager. Our PACS is set up as a combination of on-demand auto-routing so that there is a large central database manager and an image server. The database server is a Sun Enterprise 4000 with eight 200 MHz CPUs, 2 Gbyte RAM, and a 30 Gbyte RAID. The system runs an Oracle relational database. The images are managed through a Sun Enterprise 2200 that has dual 200 MHz CPUs, 512 MByte RAM, but 120 Gbyte RAID.

The current system archive holds approximately 24 months of on-line data and consists of two 258 platter jukeboxes using 4.3 Gbyte platters. Data is stored on the system using a full fidelity compression scheme that achieves approximately 3:1 compression.

A variety of networking schemes are used. Most diagnostic and nondiagnostic workstations are connected to the central PACS units using a 150 Mbit/sec ATM network running on fiber optic cables. In our outpatient center images are distributed using switched 100 Mbit/sec Ethernet over copper; 10 Mbit/sec switched Ethernet is used to bring data from the modalities. ISDN phone lines are used for home teleradiology and a T-1 line is used to bring data from a remote site approximately 100 km (62 miles) from Charleston. The remnants of our film archive are stored off-site and can be transmitted or connected to the system using a microwave channel. Diagnostic interpretation by the radiologist is done on eight 2k×2k monitors that are used primarily for projection radiography and by 12 1k×1k systems. These are all dual-monitor systems. Color is provided in nuclear medicine and ultrasound. These units currently run on Sun platforms and while there are some legacy units, most are Sun Ultrasparks that have 196 Mbyte RAM and 9 Gbyte of local storage. The nondiagnostic workstations, approximately 67, are quite various. Certain high-use areas, such as neurosurgery and ENT, employ high performance workstations like the radiologists use. In certain other areas, single monitor film stations are provided, but in most areas, approximately 50, we use PC-based display systems. Initially, these were Pentium PCs, 233 MHz with

32 Mbyte RAM and a 2.6 Gbyte hard disk, using a conventional PC monitor. As the demands for the system increased, these units were upgraded to 400 MHz PCs with 120 Mbyte RAM and a 4 Gbyte hard disk. It was also determined that in many areas, conventional computer monitors were inadequate, so we replaced these with 70 foot-Lambert grayscale monitors. We have also implemented an NT-based server for distributing images in an Internet format.

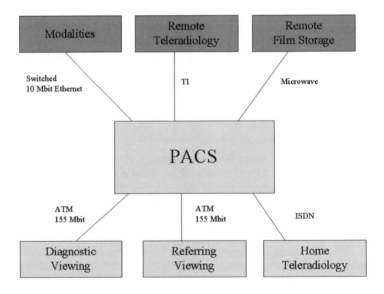

Figure 9. The current PACS configuration.

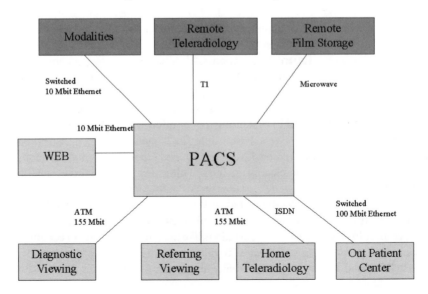

Figure 10. The current PACS network configuration.

Problems

We have had certain ongoing problems with the system. The computers used as the database server and the image server have had to be upgraded or replaced several times. This is due to more use of the system than anticipated and revisions of the software that were more demanding on the system. This was also a problem with the original RIS system that required frequent upgrades in the early years. After several years the system use reached an equilibrium.

The network traffic to the referring physicians viewing stations is much larger than anticipated and continues to be a problem. This is due to our inability to interface with the hospital scheduling system (there isn't one). Thus the clinic staff requests patient images, when the patients arrive in the clinics. Since they believe that they will never get into trouble for having too many images, they frequently request the entire patient record. This slows down the entire PACS system at busy times.

The PACS system does not handle some studies well. Color overlays from Nuclear Medicine, 3D reconstructions from CT and MRI, and functional MRI continue to be problems.

We have not been able to meet the full demand for images outside of radiology. To resolve this problem we are installing a WEB server. This may also solve the problem of physicians outside of radiology who wish a home teleradiology solution.

Future Developments

Future developments for our system will be aimed at solving the problems that remain. We still print more film than we anticipated. This film is mostly used by the operating rooms. The next major PACS project will be to add workstations in all the operating rooms. While CR is very effective, we anticipate increases in productivity from the application of direct capture devices. We are investigating Direct Radiography (DR) devices and expect to install clinical DR in the next fiscal year. Distribution of images to all the hundreds of PCs in our hospital is a challenge we hope to meet by application of Web-based image distribution. The hospital is working on the electronic medical record and we will be integrating the PACS with the EMR. There is considerable demand for the PACS images for nonradiology use. We already send images to surgery for the surgical planning systems and radiation oncology for the 3D treatment planning systems. We expect that the PACS system will accept images from outside of radiology. We presently store the images from endoscopic ultrasound and are working with cardiology to archive the images from the cardiac catheterization labs and cardiac ultrasound. The PACS is already interfaced with the digital dictation system through the RIS. We have installed digital dictation systems but so far they have not been well accepted by the radiologists.

The present archive holds approximately two years of on-line data. After two years, off-line media are managed. This has worked well, but there are a number of areas that we plan to address. The system now uses full fidelity compression. We believe that compressions in the range of 10:1 to 20:1 are practical. If standards for such compression schemes are implemented, we would likely adopt them. In addition we do not have a backup archive. When we installed the PACS we felt that it was so much better than existing film technologies that a backup archive was not necessary. We now feel that a backup archive is necessary and are investigating schemes to copy the existing archive so that we can preserve all of the data in a backup copy.

Effects on Medical Physics' Practice

PACS has had a major effect on the practice of medical physics at the Medical University of South Carolina. The ongoing implementation of PACS takes significant amounts of physics effort. This effort goes into development, problem solving, and quality assurance. Development includes all the problems associated with implementing new systems, including the areas of mentioned above. Second, PACS brings a variety of imaging problems that require physics efforts. These include the appropriate selection of image processing parameters and questions about image quality, radiation safety, and dose issues. However, there are now more questions from physicians from outside of radiology about image quality issues and a significant amount of physics effort is spent with nonradiologist physicians. Finally, the PACS quality assurance takes a considerable effort. We feel that PACS is an important area for medical physicist quality assurance efforts. We routinely find image quality problems in routine quality control (QC) testing that are not seen or reported by users. Thus the QC program is effective because it finds problems at this level. Because of these additional efforts we have added an additional physicist to our group.

The presence of the PACS system has also affected the routine practice of medical physics. Acceptance testing of equipment requires verification of how data is passed to the PACS system. Checks must be done to be sure that image orientation is properly passed to the PACS system. Additional tests verify the accuracy of digital data (e.g., CT numbers), spatial measurements, and image quality.

Routine testing of systems that require image quality testing is done by evaluating the images on the soft-copy displays rather than on film. CR units require significant QC efforts.

Routine QC is made easier by the availability of previous images and the review can be made at the physicist's desk which reduces the required time.

Summary

The total PACS effort at MUSC has taken more than 10 years. While the effort has been lengthy and arduous, the effect has been very positive. We have a system that is more secure, images are much more widely available, and the radiologists have become more efficient. The project has required significant efforts from medical physicists but has also increased the needs for medical physics services. The PACS has also increased the visibility of medical physics to physicians outside of radiology.

References

Humphrey, L.M., Fitzpatric, K., Atallah, N., Ravin, C.E. "Time comparison of intensive care unitswith and without digital viewing." *J Digit Imag* 1995:6:(37-41).

Humphrey, L.M., Fitzpatric, K., Paine, S., Ravin, C.E. "Physician experience with viewing digital radiographs in an intensive care environment." *J Digit Imag* 1993:8:(30-36).

Data Management and Archive Systems

Douglas M. Tucker, Ph.D.
Storage Technology Corporation
Louisville, CO

Introduction/Learning Objective

The purpose of this chapter is to survey data storage systems. Long-term data storage is an important part of any Picture Archiving and Communication System (PACS). In this paper we will discuss the design and implementation of data storage and long-term archives. The discussion will be kept generic, without addressing specific problems associated with the storage and retrieval of medical images. The intent is to provide the reader sufficient information to evaluate commercially available storage product designs and implementations. The author will avoid in-depth discussion of specific technologies or implementation challenges faced in the medical imaging domain.

To achieve this goal, the paper develops the concept of a prototypical storage model. The model is used in the remainder of the paper as the basis for discussion. The model is intended to be a tool for discussion purposes, allowing the reader to compare and contrast the design and implementations of various archive products, and to determine an archive component's functionality in the complete archive. The model should not be interpreted as a "cookbook" recipe for designing and building a medical information data repository.

Storage Model

The execution of a computer software application and the tasks performed by both the hardware and software are abstract and complex. Frequently, these concepts are beyond the mental grasp of the lay person. Humans, by nature, tend to deal with physical realities better than abstract concepts. Computer scientists adopt processing models as formalisms, in large part, to facilitate human communication about the complex abstract concepts that abound in their field.

Processing models provide a uniform methodology to represent programming constructs. Uniform representations beget uniform results. Computational models facilitate the development of software that adheres to common practice standards by defining both data and services. This facilitates the distributed development of high-quality software. Indeed, computational models form the backbone of the explosive growth in Internet-related software. It is possible for multiple programmers, working independently, but upon the same model, to generate a single application that accomplishes a unique task.

In this paper we will define a simple storage model (Figure 1). This model, like many used in computer science, is hierarchical in nature. At the lowest level of the hierarchy is the physical hardware used to provide persistent storage of data. Each successively higher level *encapsulates* or *abstracts* the concepts of the lower level into a logically more complex representation. At the highest level of the model is the application, which embodies the most complex concepts. If one were to start defining the model from the top, abstract concepts familiar to the user's understanding of the application would be represented. In a medical imaging storage application, for example, a high-level concept might include the definition of a medical image as a specialized class of images. At the lowest level, the model would deal with the polarity of an area of a phys-ical storage media.

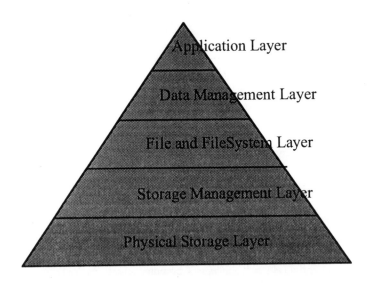

Figure 1: Prototypical application data model

Within the model, steps between each layer are designed to be simple and straight-for-ward to grasp once the concepts associated with the underlying level are understood.

A typical application relies upon many supporting infrastructures to achieve its program goals. Each of the different supporting structures is designed and imple-mented to achieve a specific task relative to the overall goal. Each task, in turn, may be represented by its own processing model. For example, an application may be responsible for user interactions. In today's computing environment, an application is expected to use standard formalism for accepting input and displaying results. If the application is running on a Windows platform, it is expected to support the "look and feel" of the Windows interface, including mouse interactions, tiled windows, etc. It would be an onerous and error prone task for the application developer to develop all of the code necessary to provide this level of user interaction. It would literally take a development force the size of Microsoft's to develop each application. In reality, this is impractical. Therefore, the application developer, and therefore the application, relies upon support infrastructure to accomplish redundant tasks.

Adjacent layers in a computational model access the underlying support infrastructure through a defined *application programming interface,* or *API.* The API is an asymmetric interface between layers. Typically, the upper layer relies upon functionality provided by the lower layer. The lower layer, therefore, provides the API to the upper layer. The API may contain several different functions, or entry-points. Each function is associated with a specific task performed by the supporting infrastructure. For example, waiting for a mouse click may be a specific function provided by the high-level user interface API. The lower level functions that support and implement this function encapsulate specific knowledge of the computer, the pointing device, hardware addresses, and interrupt levels.

APIs can provide interfaces to the computer operating systems, or to libraries of supporting functions. Recursively, supporting functions rely upon standard programming interfaces to lower level functions that ultimately rely upon the operating system. In some cases, APIs may provide (*adhoc* or industry-wide) standard interfaces to hardware components not supported by the operating system.

It is important to understand that the API provides a logical boundary between layers. The interaction between the layers must occur through the API. The API must be flexible enough to accommodate different programming languages and styles, robust enough to provide adequate performance under a variety of different operating conditions, and include all of the lower layer services that the upper layer requires. The upper layer should not manipulate data outside of the context of the lower layer's management API. Doing so will adversely affect the integrity of the functionality provided by the computational model.

Prototypical Storage Model

Application Layer

The application layer represents the highest level in our storage model. Overall, the application performs the task, or set of tasks, achieved. Typically, data management is one of several responsibilities that the application must manage.

As the highest level in our data management hierarchy, the application plays a crucial role. The application is responsible to perform specific tasks. The application:

- *defines* the data objects to be used. For example, a computed radiography (CR) image is defined to have 2180 rows by 1760 columns of pixels. A pixel is defined to be a 10 bit unsigned integer stored in 2 bytes of memory.

- *creates* instances of defined data objects. The chest x-ray image of a specific patient using the data object defined above would require approximately 7.3 megabytes of memory.

- *modifies* instances of existing data. Perhaps it is a function of the application to alter the representation of the image data, with the modified data replacing the existing data.

- *organizes* the data according to a predefined structure. For example, a typical chest examination includes both an AP and a Lateral view that should be associated.

- *manages* data to accomplish predetermined tasks. For example, it may be necessary to store, for extended periods of time, some or all of the data created by an application.

- *destroys* instances of existing data. After seven years, it may no longer be necessary to store the chest examination managed by the system.

The data management hierarchy provides support to the application to accomplish specific tasks in an efficient manner. The choice of whether to use a data hierarchy depends upon the task to be accomplished, the application design, and the resources available to the application. If, for example, the application were to create only one data object that required not to be preserved beyond the execution context of the specific application, long-term data storage would be inappropriate. Similarly, if an application were to create hundreds to thousands of instances of data objects, and needed to manage these objects for years (as in the case of a PACS) , it would be foolish for the application to burden itself with the responsibility of data management.

Data Management Layer

The data management layer resides below the application layer in our data management hierarchy. The data management layer provides a well-defined and standard interface to the application layer to deliver specific services. The data management layer manipulates the data only at the request of the application layer. It expects the application layer to use its services exclusively.

The data management layer handles data in a generic manner. Unlike the application layer, the data management layer does not contain specific knowledge of the data that it manipulates. To the data management layer, the application could be dealing with information related to stock market transactions as well as x-ray images. It is not the responsibility of the data management layer to provide or manipulate application layer contexts.

The data management layer acts at the request of the application layer to associate related data. Associated data is typically referred to as a *record*. For example, the order for a chest exam, the resulting image data and the interpretation of the images by a radiologist may constitute an examination *record*. The individual components of the record (in this case the order, the image, and the interpretation) are referred to as data *fields*. The data management layer provides operations that manipulate records of information. The application manipulates the individual *fields*.

Tasks provided by the data management must be generic in nature. It is not unreasonable to assume that a single data management layer could be used by different applications. In contrast, the services provided must be at a high enough level (i.e., sufficiently abstracted from the underlying system) to be useful to the application layer. Specifically, the data management layer provides services that:

- *Store* data. The data management layer provides functionality to ensure that specific data instances created at the application layer persist beyond the context of the application's execution. For example, if an application referenced in the above section needed to store the chest image for an extended period of time (years, perhaps), it would be unlikely to expect that the application would (a) run forever, or that (b) the same application would be used. In case (a), different application contexts would be created for each execution of the application. Case (b) represents a new (or different) application using data (i.e., data sharing).

- *Retrieve* data. Once the data is stored, it must be reliably retrieved. Reliability is important; the data management layer must ensure that the same data is returned to the application.

- *Manipulate* data. The data management layer has access to all data created by the application layer. Therefore, it should be able to provide certain data manipulation functions such as data sorting and summarizing. Clearly, it is the application's responsibility to instruct how to sort or summarize, and such information must be transferred through the API.

- *Access* specific data. For example, a new chest exam should be viewed with all relevant prior images. It is the application's responsibility to determine what data is relevant, and the data management system's job to find the data.

Improving Data Access—Indexing

To improve access to specific records of data, management systems rely upon shortcuts, or indices. The purpose of the index is to enable the data management system to access a specific record quickly. To improve access, fields with specific interest to the application are identified. These data fields are referred to as *key* fields, and the under-lying records are referred to as *indexed* data. Key fields are managed, often in duplicate to data in the record, in a manner to accelerate access to the original record. To work properly, a key field must uniquely identify the record to which it belongs. Otherwise, ambiguity exists.

Alternatives to the explicit creation of application level indices of data exist. Recent research activities attempt to determine application level patterns of data usage. These so called "meta-data" systems attempt to learn how the application uses data and to provide intelligent access.

Database Management Systems

Database management systems (DBMS) are computer applications that provide com-prehensive data management services. DBMS execute as either stand-alone applications, as integral parts of another application, or both. Examples of common DBMS include Oracle ™, Microsoft's (Redmond, Washington) Access™ and IBM's (Yorktown, NY) DB2™.

DBMS use different models to represent the underlying data. A common representa-tion includes individual records of data as rows within a single large table. Access to a specific record of data is accomplished by searching through the complete table. This type of DBMS is referred to as a sequential access model (SAM), and may rely upon indices (defined above) to improve access (ISAM). The downside to this data repre-sentation is that data common to multiple rows is duplicated within the table.

An alternative model to the SAM mentioned above is the relational databases. Rela-tional databases use multiple tables to remove redundancy from the single table of the SAM model. Original data records are reconstructed by "joining" individual tables, as needed, using relational calculus.

Open Database Connectivity (ODBC) is a standard API for accessing information from different data storage formats. ODBC works with both SAM and relational data for-mats. ODBC is a network-aware industry standard developed, in large part, by Microsoft. ODBC can provide a single application access to data stored in different databases. For example, an ODBC-based application could integrate radiology order information stored in a ISAM database on the Radiology Information System (RIS) with image data stored in a relational database on the PACS.

File Management Layer

The data management layer relies upon services provided by lower levels in the storage hierarchy to achieve it goals. Directly below, and in support of, the data management layer is the file management layer. The file management layer provides standard formalisms to move data to and from physical hardware.

The fundamental construct within the file management layer is the concept of a *file*. A file consists of multiple related *records* (defined above). It is typical for the file management layer to accumulate records of the same type into individual files. For example, a single file may contain all of the records for examination orders, and another file contains all of the records related to the results of the ordered exam. The two files will be related (at a higher level) by the fact that only completed orders will have interpreted results. The file management layer, however, will have no explicit knowledge of this relationship.

The file management layer provides operations related to the manipulation of files. Operations to create, open, close, and delete files must be supported. Once a file is created and open, formalisms to insert data (write) and non-destructively extract (read) data from the file must be supported.

Hierarchical Data Directories

The file management layer typically provides a special type of file, associated only with the functioning of the file management layer. This type of file is referred to as a directory file. The purpose of the directory file is to provide an organizational structure to the separate files that exist within the file management system. A directory file contains information about files that exist within the file system. Related files, as in the example above, can be accumulated and referenced within a single directory structure. The type of data structure that results from this organization is referred to as an inverted tree structure.

File management systems exist at very low levels within the computer application hierarchy. The data structures (files, directories, etc.) are very closely associated with the underlying physical hardware, and the operating system (OS) that creates them. It is unreasonable to assume that a machine running a particular OS would understand a file or filesystem created by the same hardware executing a different OS. To accomplish this level of file and filesystem requires a higher-level application.

There are, however, needs to perform file and filesystem sharing between different operating systems. Certain well-defined file and filesystem formats exists. The most common of these "shareable" filesystems is called Network File System (NFS). NFS was developed by Sun Microsystems (Mountain View, California) in the mid 1980's to support the then expanding needs of client-server applications within academic and commercial computer networks. More recently Microsoft has adopted the Common Internet File System (CIFS) as an alternative to NFS. As expected, differences exist in the underlying data models supported by each filesystem.

Storage Management Layer

One extremely important, and often neglected, service layer exists between the file management layer and the physical hardware layer. The storage management layer attempts to utilize underlying storage hardware as efficiently as possible. Underlying the idea of storage management is that the file management layer should provide fast access to information at the lowest possible cost over time.

If one were to plot a data item's probability of access (ordinate) versus the age of the data (abscissa), a characteristic curve would result. For most data, this curve is monotonically decreases from 100% at creation toward a zero probability of access at infinite time. Within the healthcare industry, like many industries, business-practice, ethical, and legislative requirements dictate that data be kept even when the probability of access approaches zero. Fortunately, most users are willing to tolerate increased time-to-access older data. These two facts are exploited to provide a cost-effective solution to the storage of large amounts of data, while cost-effectively providing rapid access to important data.

Today, storage hardware is distinguished by different performance characteristics (time to first byte, sustained data throughput, cost per unit storage, etc.). Storage management systems, or hierarchical storage management (HSM) systems, attempt to optimize the price-performance curve over the lifetime of data stored within a file. The concept of hierarchy is based on existing hierarchies of cost (and closely related performance) of different storage media. An HSM relies upon high-level information obtained from the application level and the end-user. Different HSM products employ slightly different processing models. Some systems write data to all classes of storage immediately, and remove data from faster, more expensive media as the data ages. Other systems actively move data from more expensive to less expensive media as threshold events occur.

Few archive solutions offered by PACS vendors effectively implement the storage management layer within their products. Many reasons are given for this. Some vendors claim that explicit storage management layer software is expensive, that their application performs these tasks, and that the correct strategy is not to manage storage but to buy only enough storage to accommodate your foreseeable future needs. Unfortunately, none of these arguments are valid. Properly implemented, effective storage management reduces the overall cost of storage and reduces the effects of changes in technology at the physical storage layer. Lastly, by providing storage management as a separate software layer, objective decisions about its use can be made.

Physical Storage Layer

The lowest level of our storage management hierarchy is the physical hardware that provides persistent data storage. Over time, a number of different technologies have been used to provide long-term data storage. Likewise, at any particular time a number of different technologies will be available in the marketplace. It is well beyond the scope of this survey article to explicitly name all, or to definitively survey this broad and fast changing field. Nor will I attempt to associate absolute cost or valuation with any of the technologies discussed. I will attempt only to provide the broadest of categorizations to long-term data storage products currently offered in the marketplace.

Each of these technologies listed below competes at specific price-performance points and some, for brief periods, are able to distinguish themselves from the competition. It is important to realize that each of these technologies will, in time, be succeeded by a newer technology that is able to provide better performance at a lower cost. The prudent purchaser of technology will ensure that his investment is made in the context of specific user requirements, and that the overall application adheres to a well-defined storage model that includes a storage management layer. By doing this, the investment in today's technology addresses a specific business need, and tomorrow can transparently accommodate new technology without the loss of data or diminished performance.

Magnetic Disk

Magnetic disk technology is a pervasive storage technology. The vast majority of online random access storage resides on magnetic disk. Magnetic disks provide fast, reliable access to data. Redundant Arrays of Inexpensive Disk (RAID) technology enhances both reliability and access. Much has been written about magnetic disk and RAID technology. The author suggests that other, more definitive sources be consulted for up-to-date information.

Optical Technology: WORM and MOD

Medical imaging applications have used various optical storage technologies for many years. Optical technologies rely upon the reflective capacity of glass substrate to record information. Laser technology is used to selectively "burn" pits into the glass substrate. Using older Write-Once, Read Many (WORM) technology the substrate could not be alter once information was recorded. New magneto optical disk (MOD) media uses both magnetic and optical properties to both record and erase data.

Several generations of optical storage technology have been used in the medical community. Early PACS implementations used 14" WORM format products from Eastman Kodak (Rochester, NY) or 12" WORM formats from Philips (Best, Netherlands). More recently, 5¼" MOD products have been used. The large format platters provided large storage capacities (up to 14 GB) but suffered high media costs. Newer MOD platter, although storing less data storage per platter (latest technology at 5.2GBs) are significantly less expensive and provide better price per unit storage.

These drives typically use small-computer system interfaces (SCSI) and provide sustained data rates of 3-4 MBs per second.

CD-R, DVD

Performance characteristics of CD-R (Compact Disk—Recordable) and now CD-RW (Compact Disk—Rewritable) technologies have improved enough to be considered as a viable archive medium for small- to medium-sized radiology departments. Media capacity is approximately 600 MBs, and write capabilities are approximately 0.6 MB per second. The drives have become more robust and reliable. Drive and media costs have dropped significantly as the result of commercialization for the home personal computer marketplace.

DICOM (Digital Imaging and Communications in Medicine) has also fully embraced CD technology as a data distribution medium. Protocols exist to create device independent file and file system structures on CD media. DICOM does not endorse CD as an archive media, however. This point is frequently misunderstood.

DVD is an upcoming technology. Video standards and commercial products exist today. Non-video formats are starting to appear. Unfortunately, no single standard dominates, and several competing standards exist. DVD-R, DVD-RAM, DVD+RW, MMVF, and ASMO formats exist. Some of these standards may be appropriate for medical data storage.

DVD has the potential to improve upon shortcomings of CD technology. Most importantly, DVD will significantly improve storage capacity without significant read/write performance degradation. Existing formats offer approximately 5GB media (double sided). Because of the commercial potential of DVD, it is expected that this technology will be significantly less expensive that competing technologies.

Magnetic Tape

Magnetic tape products provided low cost removable storage medium. In the past 30 years, different tape products have been introduced and gone by the wayside. Performance limitations of early products relegated tape to the role of backup-only and disaster recovery purposes. The intent of these backup schemes is to put "dead" data onto the lowest cost media, and hope that you are never forced to read it again (affectionately known as write once, read never). Successive generation of tape products implement newer technology with better price/performance ratios. In the last 5 years, magnetic tape has become a very robust, fast and reliable method of storing "live" data.

Tape media exist as either cartridges or cassettes packages, and several different size packages exist in the marketplace. Cartridges contain a single spool. During the read/write operations, the physical tape is unwound from the cartridge onto a take-up spool that exists within the tape drive mechanism. An example of cartridge technology is the digital linear tape (DLT) products offered by Quantum. Cassette packages, in contrast, include two spools. In a cassette, the tape does not physically leave the package. StorageTek's new 9840 product is an example of a cassette system offered in the physical form-factor as the DLT cartridge. Advantages and disadvantages exist with both packaging technologies. Cartridge systems require pickup and threading mechanisms. Pick-up and threading mechanisms are prone to failure. The tape leader strip, which contains information necessary to initialize and read the tape, is also subject to damage. Cassettes are less prone to handling problems. For a given package, however, cartridges are able to hold more recording media than cassettes.

Three basic tape media type exists, with variations of each basic format. Previous papers have discussed tape formats, and detailed discussion would be inappropriate in the context of this survey article. It is worthwhile to note that three basic formats exist:

1. ½" wide cartridge tape. Examples of this tape format include Storage Technology Corporation's 9840 and Redwood products, IBM's Magstar, and Quantum Corp's Digital Linear Tape (DLT)

2. 8 mm wide cartridge tape. Exabyte and Sony manufacture products using this tape format.

3. 4 mm wide cartridge. Hewlett Packard's Digital Audio Tape (DAT) is an example of this tape format.

Like film and optical media, tape devices have specific price, performance, capacity, and reliability characteristics. Individual products are designed and manufactured to address the needs of specific markets. 4 mm and 8 mm products typically target low price points and are therefore very applicable for desktop and small server or distributed archive applications. ½" tape products are designed for demanding environments such as large server, mainframe, and central archive applications. While more expensive, the ½" products tend to be more robust and reliable.

The following is a quick review of the four major components of retrieval performance for any removable media device:

1. **Initialization:** The media is placed into the throat of the transport made ready for read/write operations.

2. **Search:** For a device that stores data serially, the media must by forwarded to the beginning of data. For tape products this involves some combination of fast forwarding and searching; for optical products this step occurs almost instantaneously. Optical products have traditionally provided a clear performance advantage in this step. Newer tape products, however, are extremely competitive.

3. **Data transfer:** Read data from or write data to the media.

4. **Unload:** Rewind the media and remove the media from the transport.

High-capacity tape media has traditionally meant poor performance. High capacity comes from long tapes combined with high-density data recording. These facts have adversely affected the usability of traditional tape products as "live" data storage products. Tape manufacturers attempt to overcome this limitation in several ways, including the use of novel indexing techniques to facilitate rapid tape positioning. Newer tape products, specifically StorageTek's 9840, combine cassette packaging (reduced tape initialization time), mid-positioning of tape (first byte of data is now _ tape length away), and serpentine written data tracks to significantly improve tape performance. Random retrievals of medical image studies (20 GB of data) can be performed, on average, within 20 seconds.

Robotic Technology

Individual media, whether magnetic disks, optical or tape, have insufficient capacities to address the storage needs of many applications. Tape and optical recording devices, fortunately separate the read/write mechanism from the storage media. This allows for multiple pieces of media to be serviced by one, or a few, readers. A manual procedure for replacing media, adequate for low data demand environments, is inadequate for high-volume, high-performance data archives. Medical imaging applications clearly fall into the high-volume, high-performance arena.

Advances in the robotic technology have been applied to this data storage problem. Automated library systems (ALS or "jukeboxes") consists of one or more readers, multiple shelves for media storage, and a robotic picker arm. The picker arm moves media to and from storage shelves and reader devices. The ALS attaches directly to a computer (usually an NT or UNIX server) via a SCSI interface (Small Computer Systems Interface) or serial port. Control of the ALS is separate from the control and data paths of the drive. These two activities must be coordinated by software on the host computer for the complete system to function properly.

ALSs for optical storage products are available with shelf capacity up to 250 platters. Newer products available from Plasmon hold ~500 platters and from DISC that hold ~1,000 platters. Tape ALSs are available from a number of manufacturers, including StorageTek, ATL, and ADIC. Products range from managing 5-7 tapes to thousands of tapes. High-end products from StorageTek enable multiple ALSs to be physically connected. Tapes can be automatically passed between interconnected libraries. This feature has been shown to be useful in extending the utility of both ALSs and tape transports.

ALS operations require mechanical movement and responses by both the robotics and the drive mechanisms. In multi-user environments, many applications may be simultaneously requesting information from the archive. As more and more people request information from a central archive storage device, queuing delays can affect the performance of the archive. The most common delay with ALS systems occurs when there are an insufficient number of drives to service simultaneously all pending reads or writes operations. Manufacturers have developed sophisticated mathematical queuing models used to design, build, and implement ALS systems. These tools should be consulted during the design and implementation of an archive using ALS technology.

Conclusions

This paper discusses the design and implementation of data storage and long-term archives. The author has attempted to keep the discussion generic, without dealing with specific problems associated with the storage and retrieval of medical images. The intent was to provide a useful summary and overview of storage technology, and not to delve deeply into the specific challenges faced in the medical imaging domain. The reader should be armed with sufficient information to deal intelligently and effectively with the sales and marketing information provided by PACS and information technology (IT) vendors.

The prototypical storage model presented in this paper is not intended to be a "cookbook" recipe for designing and building a medical information data repository. The reader should be aware that there might be no commercially available archive application that faithfully implements this model. The model should be used for its intended purpose, to act as a communication tool and a model against which specific implementations can be judged and evaluated.

Basic Ultrasound Imaging

James A. Zagzebski
Medical Physics Department
University of Wisconsin
Madison, WI

Fundamentals

Ultrasound imaging generally involves transmitting brief pulses of acoustic energy into the body and detecting and displaying echoes from interfaces and scatterers in tissue. Figure 1 illustrates a simple pulse-echo experiment, where echo signals are detected from interfaces and displayed either as amplitude signals or bright-up pulses vs. echo arrival time. The echo return time indicates the distance from the reflector to the transducer. A speed of sound of 1540 m/s is assumed in the computation of reflector distance from echo return time. This is considered the average speed of sound in soft tissue.

The sources of echoes are interfaces formed by tissues that have different acoustic impedances, where the acoustic impedance can be taken as the product of the speed of sound multiplied by the density.

A-MODE AND B-MODE

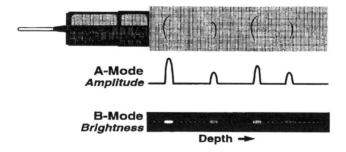

Figure 1. Simple pulse-echo experiment. Echoes follow a transmit pulse by the transducer are displayed as a function of echo arrival time, or reflector depth.

If we have a large, smooth interface formed by two tissues whose impedances are Z_1 and Z_2, the amplitude reflection coefficient,

$$R = \frac{Z_2 - Z_1}{Z_2 + Z_1}$$

describes the ratio of the reflected to incident pressure amplitude for such a "specular" reflector. This equation assumes perpendicular beam incidence. Although specular interfaces are "ideal" conditions that are seldom realized, the equation offers guidance regarding energy partitioning (amount reflected vs. transmitted) at interfaces. Table 1 illustrates the effect of applying this equation to hypothetical interfaces in the body. One can see that several interfaces are fairly reflective, namely bone-to-soft tissue and fat-to-soft tissue. Most interfaces, however, are expected to be fairly weakly reflecting.

Table 1. Approximate reflection coefficients for selected biological interfaces. The dB value is calculated using 20*log(R). (After Wells 1968)

Interface	R, Amplitude Reflection Coeff.	dB re perfect reflector
Skin-to-air	0.99	-0.09
Muscle-to-bone	0.56	-5
Fat-to-muscle	0.112	-19
Fat-to-blood	0.089	-21
Blood-to-muscle	0.025	-32
kidney-to- liver	0.0125	-38

If specular reflections were the only source of echoes from soft tissue, ultrasound images would be rather dull and featureless. In fact, the majority of echo information in an ultrasound scan originates as a result of scattering by small "acoustical inhomogeneities" in the body. Unlike reflection from a specular interface, which can be very directional, scattering is omnidirectional, so there is hardly a dependence on the magnitude of the echo signal on the orientation of the scattering volume. The most notable exceptions are muscle fibers, which exhibit stronger scattering for sound waves perpendicular to the axis than at oblique angles and the renal pyramids, which also exhibit strong dependencies on orientation.

The strength of scattered signals has thus far not been well documented for modern ultrasound equipment operating with high frequency transducers. However, Kossoff (1976) demonstrated the typical echo signal amplitudes produced by their equipment operating using 2 MHz transducers.

This is presented in Fig. 2. Strong echo signals are obtained from specular interfaces, particularly when they are located near the patient skin surface. Weaker signals are produced by scatterers located within organs. The weakest scattering occurs from blood, which appears echo free, except when scanned by high frequency transducers. Figure 2 suggests an overall dynamic range (sometimes referred to as the global dynamic range) of at least 100 dB is necessary to provide an adequate detection of weak scatterers simultaneously with out undue saturation of the amplifiers caused by strong specular interfaces.

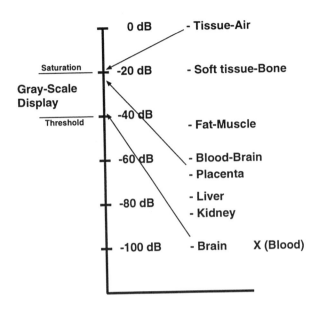

Figure 2. Typically measured echo signal amplitudes
from organ interfaces and from within selected organs.

Part of the echo level variation noted in Fig. 2 is a result of attenuation of the
ultrasound beam in tissue. Attenuation is caused by scattering and reflection at
interfaces and by absorption, that is, conversion of ultrasonic energy into heat. It
usually is specified in decibels/cm or sometimes in nepers/ cm. Table 2 lists typical
attenuation values for several soft tissues. These are for 1 MHz ultrasound waves,
and specify one-way attenuation.

Table 2. Attenuation coefficients at 1 MHz for tissues. (Taken from Bamber 1999;
except * which is from Lu 1999.)

Tissue	dB/cm at 1MHz
Blood	.2
Spleen	.35
Liver	.52*
Skeletal muscle	1.1
Skull bone	1.0

Attenuation of ultrasound is caused both by absorption and scattering. For
parenchyma tissue it is dominated by absorption. This results in attenuation
depending on the ultrasound frequency, with approximately a first power
dependence on frequency. High frequency beams, as a result, cannot penetrate into
tissue as effectively as lower frequency beams.

Ultrasound Imaging Equipment

Producing Images

B-mode (Gray scale) imaging is done almost exclusively using hand-held transducers containing arrays of piezoelectric elements for gray scale imaging. Figure 3 shows a typical scanner used in radiology and obstetrics departments. A block diagram showing principal components of the scanner which pertain to gray scale imaging is presented in Fig. 4. The illustration is for an array transducer that uses 128 channels, where a channel consists of an element in the transducer assemble and its pulser-receiver-digitizer circuit in the scan console. Fewer numbers of channels are common in low-end scanners, as the channel density can significantly add to the cost of a system.

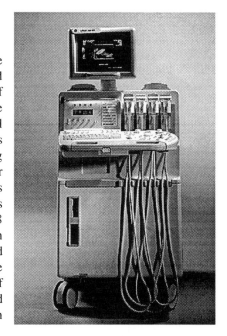

Figure 3. High-end ultrasound scanner, such as used in radiology or obstetrics applications. (Courtesy of General Electric.

The transmitter applies electrical impulses to individual elements in the array. In older generation scanners the transmit pulses were broad-bandwidth electrical impulses, which caused the transducer to "ring" at its resonance frequency. Thus, the frequency of operation was closely dictated by the resonance frequency of the transducer itself, and it was necessary to change transducers to change ultra-sound frequencies.

Modern transducer construction results in probes that have frequency band-widths of 80% or higher. This is broad enough that the transducer can be operated at any one of several frequencies, say 2.5 MHz, 3.5 MHz and 4 MHz for a typical abdominal probe. The transmit signal, then, consists of a sine wave or a square wave burst that has the desired ultrasound frequency. Multi-frequency, or "multi-herz" transducers accept transmit pulses of different frequencies, allowing the operator to select the exact frequency that imaging is done.

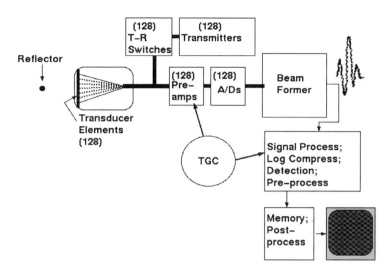

Figure 4. Important components of a 128-channel gray-scale scanner.

Electronically Controlled Transmit Focus

Control of the timing of the transmit pulse applied to each element allows the beam to be focused electronically. This is done by introducing time delays among the transmit pulses sent to individual array elements. Multiple transmit focal zones can also be used, although this sometimes results in the image frame rate decreasing. This is because each transmit pulse can be focused only at a single distance. To allow for several transmit focal depths simultaneously, the scanner transmits with the array focused at the shallowest zone and accepts echoes signals from this depth only. Then another transmit pulse is applied along the same beam line, only this one with the focal distance deeper, and echoes are picked up from near this second zone. This can be done for 5 or more separate transmit focal zones. Multiple transmit focusing has advantages in improved lateral resolution, but the tradeoff is that image frame rate is significantly degraded.

Digital Beam Former

After each transmit pulse, a rapid switch links elements in the array to the receiver chain. Echo signals picked up by individual array elements are amplified, digitized and then applied to the receive beam former. The beam former introduces precisely controlled time delays amongst the echo signals from individual elements, effectively focusing the array as echoes are received. It then sums these signals coherently, creating a single echo signal wave-train for each beam line used to form the image.

Modern systems utilize digital beam formers, where the echo signal in each channel is digitized, followed by digital delays and summation. Thus, prior to the beam former, there are up to 128 echo signals, depending on the number of channels in the scanner. After beam forming there is one echo signal wave train for each beam line.

Imaging is done by systematically transmitting acoustic pulses along well-defined beam lines and receiving echoes from scatterers and reflectors along this each line (Fig 5). Echo signals are displayed on a line that corresponds to the central axis of the active ultrasound beam; the echo delay time enables the depth of origin of the echo signal to be applied. Typically, 100-200 individual transmit-receive pulse-echo sequences are used for an entire image, each one directed into a different direction, or beam line.

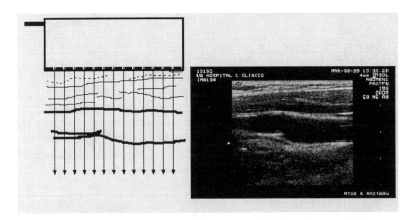

Figure 5. Generating an image of the common carotid artery using a linear array transducer. (Left) Image acquisition using parallel bam lines; (Right) Resultant image.

Transducer Types

Figures 6 and 7 illustrate the types of arrays that are in use. Phased arrays consist of a group of 64-128 individual elements, typically about 1/2 wavelength in width. All elements are used for transmitting and receiving along each beam line. By introducing precisely specified time delays among the transmit pulses sent to individual elements, the transmitted beam can be steered in different directions and can be focused at a given transmit focal depth. Similarly, the receive pattern can also be directed along the same line by applying time delays to echo signals detected by the individual elements, prior to summing in the beam former. The phased array has the advantage of using a fairly small "footprint" yet providing a sector image format. Most echo cardiography scanners use phased arrays because

PHASED ARRAY

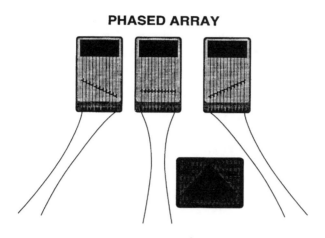

Figure 6. Phased array scanner. Beam steering is done by controlling time delays in the transmit pulses and among the received echoes prior to summation.

scanning must be done from fairly small "windows" within the intercostal spaces or beneath the rib cage. Phased arrays also are used by a few major manufacturers for abdominal scanning.

ELECTRONICALLY SCANNED ARRAYS

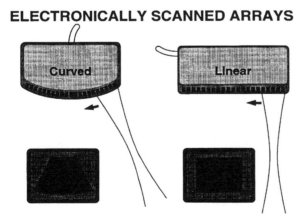

Figure 7. Curvilinear and linear arrays.

The linear array transducer (Fig. 7) consists of an array of piezoelectric elements, 1/2 to 1 wavelength wide, and several millimeters long, arranged side-by-side. Conceptually, a beam is produced by simultaneously transmitting and receiving with a group of, say, 15-20 elements. This beam is centered along the middle of the active element group. After all echoes are detected from along a beam line, element switching shifts the center of the beam one element inward, and the process is repeated. This continues for the entire length of the array, producing a single image. The shape of the array and the fact that beams emerge perpendicular to the array surface dictates that resultant images have a rectangular format, corresponding to the parallel beam lines employed to construct the image.

The curvilinear array operates similarly to the linear array, using groups of elements to transmit and receive for each beam line and applying element switching to define different beam lines. The curved surface of this scan head results in the beam lines fanning out, forming a sector scanned region. Therefore, from a small footprint on the patient surface, a relatively large field of view is visualized for deep structures.

Signal Processing in B-Mode Imaging

There are several important signal processing stages in an ultrasound scanner listed in Fig. 4 above. These include TGC, or time gain compensation, logarithmic compression, frequency filtration, detection and pre and post processing.

TGC compensates for attenuation of the sound pulse by tissues. Echo signals arriving from deeper structures are of lower amplitude than signals from shallow structures because of attenuation losses. By varying the receiver gain with echo arrival time so the amplification is proportional to the reflector depth, the scanner compensates for this attenuation. Both internal TGC, set up by the manufacturer for specific imaging situations and transducers, as well as operator set TGC is applied. Operator controls of this function usually are in the form of a set of perhaps 8 slider gain potentiometers, each controlling the gain at a different depth.

Some phased array echocardiography scanners also provide a "lateral" gain control. Gain slider-potentiometers adjust the receiver gain to different levels for different lateral positions in the phased array image sector. This compensates for different amounts of beam attenuation occurring from side-to-side on the image, which occurs commonly when imaging the heart through the intercostal spaces.

Following TGC the useful echo signal dynamic range at any location on the image (the "local dynamic range") can easily exceed 60 dB; for some scanners it approaches 80-90 dB. Logarithmic amplification is applied to compress the signal amplitude range into a range that can be handled effectively by display monitors. Logarithmic compression generally results in weak echo signals from scattering within organs occupying the major part of the display dynamic range (see Fig. 2). The degree of compression is under user control.

B-mode imaging is done by intensity modulating the display in proportion to the echo signal amplitude (Fig. 1). Bright-up pulses are obtained by rectification of the RF echo signal, followed by low pass filtering, generating the echo signal envelope. Another way to derive the envelope of the echo signal is to compute the "analytic signal" by taking the Hilbert transform of the echo signal, $Q(t)$. Thus, if $I(t)$ is the real part of the signal, the square root of $I(t)^2 + Q(t)^2$ forms the envelope of the signal. The envelope can be used for intensity modulation.

Ultrasound pulses propagating through tissue undergo preferential attenuation of higher frequency components. Thus, for a given center frequency pulse, echoes arriving from deeper structures are effectively of lower frequency content than echoes arriving from very shallow structures. To take advantage of the available frequency content in pulses, some instruments apply a frequency filter that changes dynamically as echo signals arrive from progressively deeper structures. This is done prior to the envelope detection process.

Scanning Speed and Frame Rate

The scanning speed or alternatively, the maximum frame rate, is an important performance characteristic of ultrasound imaging machines. Fundamentally, the frame rate is limited by the speed of sound in tissue, which establishes the delay time needed to acquire echo signal information from the maximum range possible. For a speed of sound of 1540 m/s, the delay time is 13 microseconds for each centimeter of depth imaged. By not allowing overlap of image data from one pulse-echo sequence to the next, this translates into a maximum pulse-repetition frequency of 77,000/D(cm), where D(cm) is the image depth in cm. If this PRF is to be shared by N acoustic lines for each frame, the maximum frame rate is:

$$FR_{max} = \frac{77,000}{ND(cm)}$$

As a simple example, if the depth imaged is 24 cm and 200 beam lines are used per frame, this translates into a maximum frame rate of 16 images per second. As already mentioned, frame rates are lowered by using multiple transmit focal zones, because of the need to apply separate transmit pulses for each focal distance. Higher frame rates are possible by reducing the imaged field width (lowering N) or by reducing the depth setting (D) on the image.

In most of today's high-end scanners, some degree of parallel processing also is used. The transmitted beam is focused but not tightly. Receive beam forming (see below) does focusing during echo reception. By simultaneously processing several look directions, frame rates can be improved over those applied using single channel operation.

"Harmonic Imaging"

When an ultrasound wave propagates through tissue, if the pressure amplitude is high the beam gradually distorts with increasing distance traveled. The distortion is caused by finite amplitude effects, in which the compression part of the sound pulse propagates faster than the rarefaction part (Carstensen 1980). Recently it has been discovered that harmonic echo signals, associated with this nonlinear propagation of ultrasound waves in tissues, are detectable using clinical equipment (Baker 1999). So called "native tissue harmonic imaging" appears to produce better image quality than standard, "linear imaging," particularly in large, difficult-to-scan patients.

It is believed that ultrasound pulses are degraded in patients that have thick body walls, particularly when fat to non-fat interfaces are present. Refraction, scattering and reverberations all play a role in producing these distortions. Distortions lead to acoustic noise on images, reducing contrast of soft tissue structures. Nonlinear propagation results in gradual build-up of higher harmonic components in the ultrasound beam. The actual relationship between the harmonic and fundamental depends on the beam intensity, depth and the attenuation coefficient in the medium. If the harmonic component of the beam is generated beyond the patient body wall, any echoes resulting from reflection of the harmonic beam would be expected to be cleaner and less prone to acoustic noise from propagating through the body wall.

Broad bandwidth transducers and signal processing capitalizes on this behavior. By transmitting, say, 2 MHz pulses into tissue and detecting harmonic frequency echoes that result from the harmonic transmission can be imaged. Differences in image quality at the between standard scanning and harmonic scanning are easily demonstrated in patients.

Harmonic imaging also works effectively with contrast agents. In fact, it was to improve the signal-to-clutter ratio in Doppler, particularly when contrast agents were applied, that harmonic imaging was first introduced. Most ultrasound contrast agents consist of gas-filled spheres stabilized within a thin shell. The spheres are easily compressed under the action of an ultrasound field. In other words, they very easily produce nonlinear wave transitions, accompanied by harmonic echoes. Contrast agent harmonics have been used effectively both in Doppler and color flow imaging as well as with gray scale imaging.

3-D Imaging

Ultrasound has progressed rapidly and continues to evolve as a real-time imaging modality. A good deal of image interpretation occurs during actual examinations, as sonographers optimize scanner settings based on anatomical structures successfully viewed on B-mode images. Image interpretation is done on planar views that are taken of selected anatomical sites during scanning.

Alternative image acquisition methods are now available in which volumetric data sets are acquired and off-line image processing enables image slice selection as well as other 3-D visualization features (Riccabona 1997, Comeau 1998). The majority of 3-D ultrasound imaging systems acquire volumetric data by sweeping the scanning plane over the scanned volume and acquiring large sets of standard 2-D images. With proper registration of the transducer position during acquisition of each plane, the orientation of each image plane can be found and used in volumetric displays.

There are 3 popular ways to acquire the volumetric image data. These are all based on sweeping 2-D imaging probes over the volume. One commercial version uses special array probes housed within a mechanical assembly (Riccabona 1997). The operator locates the region to be imaged, manipulating the transducer on the skin surface as in standard ultrasound imaging. The operator then holds the assembly stationary while a motor within the transducer housing sweeps the scanned plane; images are stored from as many as 200 scanning planes, after which they are available for reformatting and analysis. Mechanical manipulations have also been applied to other regions such as intercavitary scanners and small parts scanners for imaging the carotid artery (Fenster 1998).

Another method for acquisition is to utilize "freehand" manipulation of the scanning probe and record the transducer position corresponding to individual scanning planes. For example, an electromagnetic sensor can be attached to the transducer (Riccabona 1997). The sensor picks up signals from stationary transmitters in the scanning room. The relative locations of each image plane is determined as images are acquired. This approach can cause nonuniform fill-in of the volume, creating missing data.

Another free-hand approach uses no intrinsic tracking mechanisms, but tracks the image plane using image correlations. As the ultrasound scanning plane is translated, speckle caused by randomly positioned scatterers decorrelates (Chen 1997). This would be viewed very easily when you scan a phantom or a large organ such as the liver, and slowly translate the scanning plane by moving the transducer. And observe individual speckle dots on the image as they flush and fade during this translation. The distance required for describing waxing and waning of this stochastic process is the correlation distance. Conversely, the relative correlation in speckle data from one image plane to the next can be used to estimate the distance the transducer scan plane has moved.

Third, a new form of ultrasound imager is being developed that provides volumetric scans by electronic scanning a 2-D transducer array. The transducer consists of a 2-dimensional array. The region imaged is a pyramidal volume. The transducer array shape along with extensive parallel processing during echo reception provides volume data set updates up to 45 times per second.

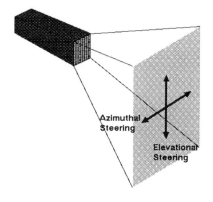

Figure 8. 3-D scanner using a 2-dimensional transducer array (adapted from drawings from Volumetrics, Durham, NC.)

This scanner has been used primarily in echo-cardiography, where the challenge of imaging a volumetric data set of the same volume is great. A popular display approach provides simultaneous images of 2 or 3 "acquisition" planes, that is, planes corresponding closely to those that are viewed using convention-al imaging. Along with these, it has been found useful to display several C-scan ("constant depth scan") views looking at planes perpendicular to the direction the ultrasound beams travel.

The challenge with any 3-D data set is defining effective means to view the data. For higher contrast surfaces, such as the fetal face or contour, surface rendering is very effective. Data segmentation necessary for obtaining the surface can be done on the basis of echo signal strength, especially if echo signals from near by structures can be edited from the 3-D data set.

Speckle noise makes many traditional image segmentation routines difficult to apply to ultrasound. Major borders such as the fetal face or the inside of a blood vessel wall are success-fully displayed using surface rendering. Color flow images of flow within vessels usually are of sufficient contrast to allow volume rendering software to apply here as well. However, the use of cut plane techniques does appear to be useful in ultrasound images. From the volumetric data set, image planes that are inaccessible using standard 2-D imaging have been found very useful.

Resolution Limits

Lateral and Axial Resolution

The spatial resolution available in modern scanners is determined for the most part by the transducer performance. A schematic illustration of the "resolution cell" is presented in Fig 9. We still use terms such as "axial" and "lateral" resolution in describing resolution capabilities in ultrasound. Axial resolution is a measure of the closest that two interfaces can be to one another along the direction of beam propagation and still be distinguished on the display. It is established by the pulse duration and frequency bandwidth of the transducer-pulser system.

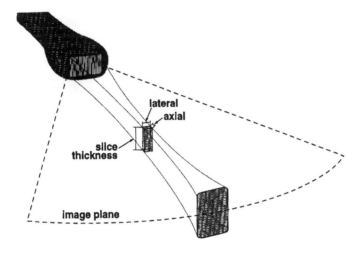

Figure 9. Resolution cell for B-mode imaging.

The lateral resolution refers to the closest that two reflectors or scattering regions can be to one another along a line that is perpendicular to the direction of beam propagation yet in the image plane. This is determined by the effective width of the combined transmit-receive beam pattern, measured in the image plane. Transmit-receive focusing by the beam former attempts to optimize this. At one of the focal distances the lateral resolution goes as

$$L.R. \approx \frac{\lambda F}{D}$$

where λ is the wavelength, F is the focal distance being considered and D is the effective aperture for that focal distance. Array transducer systems vary the aperture with the echo arrival time and with operator settings, so it is difficult to establish values for the lateral resolution.

The strong dependence of resolution on wavelength (and frequency), as well as the capabilities of modern systems, can be illustrated by imaging special resolution targets within a test phantom. These are shown in Figure 10, 13 MHz (left) and 4 MHz (right) images of resolution fibers in a phantom. Horizontal spacing of top row is 2 mm, 1 mm, 0.5 mm and 0.25 mm. The same vertical spacing exist for the oblique set.

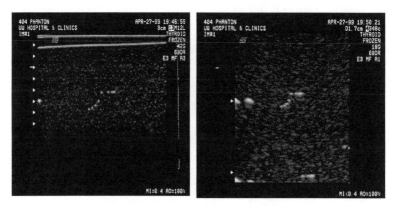

Figure 10, 13 MHz (left) and 4 MHz (right) images of resolution fibers in a phantom; for an abdominal imaging transducer and for a high frequency, small parts transducer.

Slice Thickness

The width of the beam perpendicular to the image plane determines the slice thickness, or the thickness of the section that contributes to echo signals seen on the gray scale image display. For the majority of array systems, slice thickness is the worst of the 3 measures of spatial resolution. These arrays do not use electronic focusing of the beam in the slice thickness, or elevational direction. Instead they employ a fixed focal length mechanical lens for elevational focusing. The lens/aperture is optimized for a single depth. Closer to the transducer the slice thickness approaches the size of the aperture, as measured in the slice thickness direction. Distal to the elevational focal length, the beam again diverges and slice thickness degrades substantially.

Slice thickness is a limiting factor in the ability of an ultrasound system to visualize focal objects (Rownd 1997). For example, with an abdominal imaging transducer, 4-mm cyst-like objects are obliterated within the first 4 cm of the image field as well as beyond about 12 cm, even though the lateral and axial resolutions are usually within 4 mm. Such objects are best viewed when located near the elevational focus of the array.

There is a class of transducers, referred to as 1 1/2-D arrays, that partially overcome this limitation of slice thickness (Wildes 1997). The name stems from the fact that the array itself consists of rows of elements, for example 7 rows with 128 elements in each row. The extra elevational cut in the array elements allows the manufacturer to introduce electronic beam forming methods for the elevational focus as well as for the in-plane, lateral focus. However, these are not fully 2-dimensional arrays, where the element pitch would be sufficient to for beam steering and high definition focusing in the elevational direction. Nevertheless, the improvements in focal structure definition with these devices, particularly in the near field region, is dramatic!

Coded Excitation

The ultrasound industry continues to research methods that will allow use of higher frequency transducers with their inherently superior resolution capabilities. However, to use a very high frequency, say 7 MHz, in an area where significant beam penetration is required, for example, imaging the adult liver, requires a very large amplitude transmit pulse to provide sufficient penetration. In fact, the transmit pulse amplitude often is limited either by technical considerations (power supply limits; limits to the tolerable voltage within the array elements themselves, for example) or by exposure considerations (maximum tolerable "mechanical index," defined as the pressure amplitude in MPa divided by the square root of the center frequency in MHz).

One way around this limit has been introduced by one manufacturer. Rather than transmit a sine wave burst from the transducer, the transmitter takes advantage of the wide latitude in excitation waveforms capable from the broad band-width transducer, and emits a long duration pulse that has a special code governing the exact pulse shape. The long pulse duration provides transmit pulses that are more energetic than a traditional short transmit pulse. The special code allows the axial resolution associated with short duration pulses to be recovered. During the detection process, the instrument must apply special filters that apply the original transmit code to reestablish short pulse conditions (Haider 1997). Thus far, this techniques has been applied successfully to transducers operating as high as 7 MHz.

Doppler Processing and Display

The Doppler effect is a change in the frequency of sound waves when there is relative motion between the source and reflector. Doppler frequency shifts are used in ultrasound devices to detect moving interfaces, especially blood flow. The Doppler frequency, f_D defined as the difference between the transmit frequency and the received frequency, is given by

$$f_D = \frac{2f_0 v \cos\theta}{c}$$

where f_o is the transmitted frequency, $v \cos\theta$ is the component of the reflector velocity along the direction of the ultrasound beam and c is the speed of sound. For typical reflector speeds encountered in blood flow f_D is in the audible frequency range. Very simple Doppler devices operating as continuous wave transmitters and receivers are available for basic flow detection applications, such as detecting fetal heart rates.

Pulsed Doppler (Fig. 11) provides great flexibility for defining precisely the region from which Doppler signals are recorded. It is the most widely used Doppler application in radiology and cardiology departments and is an available operating mode on most ultrasound scanners. In pulsed Doppler sine-wave bursts of acoustic energy are transmitted along a single beam line by the transducer. Echoes picked up by the transducer are applied to the beam former as in gray scale imaging. Doppler processing most commonly applies quadrature, detection, in which the beam-formed echo signal is sent into two branches. In one branch it is multiplied by a signal in phase with the transmit waveform, the other by a signal 90 degrees out of phase. Low pass filtering in each branch yields quadrature base-band signals from which the Doppler signal is derived.

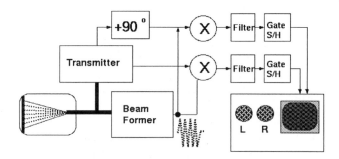

Figure 11. Schematic diagram illustrating portion of diagnostic ultrasound instrument used for pulsed Doppler acquisition and display. A Doppler signal is formed in the sample and hold (S/H) by applying many pulse-echo sequences.

The pulsed Doppler signal is generated from a defined sample volume by electronically gating the quadrature signals at a precise time following the transmit pulse and applying this signal to a sample and hold circuit. Only signals from the sample volume, defined by an operator positioned sample "gate" appear in the sample and hold (S/H in Fig. 11). The pulsed Doppler signal is formed by multiple pulse-echo sequences for transmit pulses sent along the same beam line with the same sample gate location. If reflectors are moving at the location defined by the gated region, there will be phase changes in the echo signal from one pulse-echo sequence to the next. These, of course are detected by Doppler processing, producing a time varying change in the sample and hold output. Signals from stationary reflectors, on the other hand, are identical from one pulse-echo sequence to the next and produce no time varying waveform.

The quadrature Doppler signals contain both reflector speed and directional information. These can be combined in a way that presents Doppler signals on a pair of stereo speakers, with signals for flow towards the transducer applied to one speaker and those for flow away from the transducer applied to the other. In addition, the signals may be sent to a spectral analyzer to display the instantaneous spectrum of the Doppler signals originating from the sample volume. Fundamentally, the spectral display presents Doppler signal frequency along the vertical axis, time along the horizontal axis and the signal power within each frequency component represented as brightness (Fig. 12). An "angle correct" adjustment may be oriented by the operator so that it points in the direction of flow as perceived on an ultrasound image of the vessel. When this is done the scanner computes the Doppler angle (angle between the flow direction and the Doppler beam axis) and converts the vertical axis of the spectral display to reflector velocity.

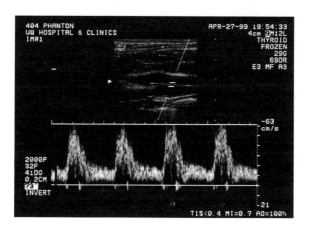

Figure 12. Spectral display of a Doppler signal obtained from the central region of the carotid artery.

The method of forming the pulsed Doppler signal is one of the "sampling", where the sampling frequency equals the pulse repetition frequency (PRF) of the Doppler processor. Aliasing will occur if the PRF is less than 2 times the Doppler frequency. Aliasing is identified easily as a wrapping of the spectral display, with high positive velocities, for example, appearing as negative velocities at the point where aliasing occurs. Apparent flow reversal during aliasing is accompanied by loss of the high frequency components of the Doppler signal. An operator adjusted "spectral scale" (velocity) on the scanner is linked to the PRF. When the spectral scale is increased, the PRF also increases. However, an upper limit to the PRF occurs because of the pulse-echo transit time in tissue. The same limit discussed in the maximum scanning speed section, PRF = 77,000/D'(cm) where D'(cm) is now the sample volume depth in cm, applies. Thus, a sample volume depth of 10 cm imposes a limit of 7.7 kHz on the PRF, or a 3.85 kHz limit on the maximum Doppler signal frequency. Rearranging the Doppler equation, we have

$$v = \frac{f_D c}{2 f_0 \cos \theta},$$

thus, a 3.85 kHz maximum Doppler frequency translates into a maximum reflector velocity of 84.7 cm/s for a 3.5 MHZ transmit frequency in tissue (sound speed is 1540 m/s and θ assumed to be 0 degrees). The maximum detectable velocity increases when lower ultrasound frequencies or larger Doppler angles apply.

Some scanners allow a "high PRF" mode to be selected by the operator. This mode increases the PRF in Doppler, to the point that after an initial transmit pulse, subsequent transmit pulses are applied even before echo signals arrive from the depth corresponding to the range gated sample volume. The range gate still is used to accept signals from the desired depth of interest. However, becasue of the overlaps in the transmit-receive pulse-echo sequences, range ambiguities in the origin of the Doppler signals may occur.

COLOR FLOW IMAGING

Echo data acquisition for color flow imaging can be view as an extension of Doppler signal acquisition, only now velocity data from an extended region of interest are detected and displayed. Recall from previous discussions, Doppler processing is sensitive to the phase of returning echo signals. Typically, the returning echo signals are heterodyned with signals that are in phase coherence with the transmitter. Both in phase (often denoted by ``I") and quadrature channels (denoted ``Q") contain the Doppler processed echo signals.

In conventional, spectral Doppler, the data are acquired from a fixed depth location along the beam axis. In color flow imaging, the processing is extended to the entire echo signal wavetrain following transmission of a each burst of ultrasound. Multiple pulse-echo sequences are necessary to acquire sufficient information to estimate reflector velocities for points along each beam line.

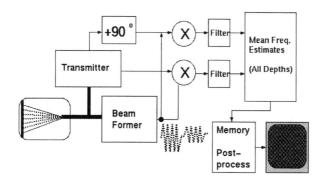

Figure 13. Major components of a scanner involved
with forming color flow images.

An important consideration in this application is Doppler signal acquisition and processing time. In order to have acceptable frame rates, say about 20 images per second, along with a reasonable line density and color flow field size, say 50 lines, only brief glimpses of the Doppler signal from each location are obtained during each image frame. With the parameters just given, there is at best 1 millisecond available for each beam line before moving to the next line. (50 lines × 20 images per second = 1,000 lines per second. Hence, there is 1 msec per line. For high frequency Doppler signals one can get a reasonable estimate of the Doppler signal in this time. For low frequency Doppler signals, say 250 kHz, this acquisition time results in only 1/4 cycle of signal. This signal itself could be contaminated by noise, due for example to statistical fluctuations in the echo signal from incoherent scattering. Thus, estimates of the frequency as well as the flow velocity are on somewhat tenuous grounds.

The majority of ultrasound equipment manufacturers use a processing technique called the phase-shift autocorrelation method for deriving color flow information. This method is used by the majority of the manufacturers. The first real time color flow images were obtained using this technique. (Kasai 1985, Forsberg 1995). The method is called the ``phase shift autocorrelation'' technique, because of the resemblance to the mathematical formalism to calculation of an autocorrelation function. An average frequency is obtained at each depth location by taking the mean for 5 - 10 pulse-echo sequences. After this process, the imager shifts to a new line and the procedure is repeated.

As mentioned above, typically at least 5-10 pulse echo sequences are used along each beam line for each estimate of velocities during a given scan or frame. Thus, it is easy to see that image frame rates can be reduced substantially below those for conventional imaging, especially if comparable field sizes are used. Color flow imaging machines try to solve the image rate problem using one or more of the following:

- Reducing the size of the color field. Often one sees on a combination color and B-mode image that the B-mode image occupies a 100 degree or so sector, while the color image only occupies a small fraction of the B-mode field.

- Reducing the line density in color mode. This method relies upon interpolation to fill in the missing links between actual data spots. Images can appear considerably grainier with higher frame rates if this is applied.

- Reducing the number of pulse-echo sequences per line. In rapidly moving flow situations, such as the chambers of the heart, this often is an acceptable method.

Aliasing

The color flow image is subject to the limitations of aliasing, just as aliasing is possible in pulsed Doppler examinations. When aliasing is present, one sees the effect of a "wrapping around" of the color data, with high aliased velocities jumping to high velocities of the opposite polarity, etc.

It is important to keep in mind that the color flow image depicts motion and flow relative to the ultrasound beam direction. A horizontally moving flow pattern can easily appear as though moving in both directions (i.e., red in one segment of the flow pattern and blue in another) because of this principle. A vessel that courses in a complicated manner through the body can appear differently in different segments, because of different angles it makes with the ultrasound beam direction. Physicians have learned to read into these flow patterns and make appropriate compensation during diagnoses.

Power Mode

The most recent version of color flow imaging which is available with virtually all systems is "Power Mode." This is a processing method that is argued to be much more sensitive to slow flow than conventional color flow imaging. Its basic features are:

- The displayed values on the image are not velocities; rather, they are related to signal power. The signal strength is encoded in image brightness.

- Significant temporal averaging takes place, providing (estimates say) 10-15 dB greater sensitivity.

- Directional information and velocity magnitude information are ignored.

Image Storage Requirements in Ultrasound

Many ultrasound departments have transferred from film recording to film less recording because of the convenience of image store and the need to transfer images effectively from different locations. In spite of the fact that images are stored in a digital format in the scan converter/memory of the ultrasound unit, many image archive units acquire image data using a frame grabber to digitize the video image data as it is reformatted for presentation to image monitors. This is changing as manufacturers move to provide DICOM interfaces to image archival and display, print and retrieval equipment. However, the video frame acquisition model is still a useful one to compare image storage requirements.

A typical single patient case folder in a radiology department often contains 20-30 images per visit, with typically 1/3 of the images being color. Acquisition is currently by way of video frame, operating approximately at television resolution rates and acquiring complete video frames rather than only the ultrasound echo image data. Thus if stored as tiffs, the storage requirement may be up to approximately 400 kbytes/image. Color flow images typically require up to 800 kbytes for storage. A patient study of 30 images, 1/3 of which are color thus requires approximately 12 Mbytes of storage. Thus, a busy ultrasound department scanning 40 patients per day produces easily 480 Mbytes of image and patient data. Image compression schemes are used routinely to reduce the amount of data that would have to be archived, but the uncompressed data size gives an idea of the storage requirements.

If the above number seems small, there is movement on the horizon that would increase storage requirements. For example, very often ultrasonographers use "video clips" particularly for spectral Doppler traces but sometimes for color flow images as well. Currently most PACs storage systems do not make these available for storage, although ultrasound mini-PACS manufacturers are developing the capabilities. Storage of video clips is essential in systems that are used in echocardiography; thus, digital archiving in applications where still images dominate the patient records is much more firmly established than in cardiology.

3-D ultrasound data sets with its 200 or so image base would result in still greater needs for image storage. A single 200 image set might require as many as 300 kbytes/image $\times$ 200 images = 60 Mbytes of storage if uncompressed data were used. It may be possible to reduce this, because an entire video frame only contains ultasound echo data over about 1/2 the useful area. Moreover, when storing 3-D volume sets, it may make more sense to acquire detected image data directly from the scanner rather than concentrate on video formatted data, where interpolation has filled in missing video pixels and significant blank space is provided for displaying scanner settings, patient demographics and time data. Nevertheless, it is likely that future ultrasound storage requirements will greatly surpass those presently used.

Acknowledgments: The author is grateful to Ms. Lisa Humphrey for assisting in the preparation of this manuscript. This work was partially supported by NIH grant R01CA39224.

References

Baker, A. "Nonlinear effects in ultrasound propagation." In *Ultrasound in Medicine*, Edited by F. Duck, A. Baker and H. Starritt. Bristol: Institute of Physics, 1999, pp.23-38.

Bamber, J., "Ultrasonic properties of tissues." *Ultrasound in Medicine*, Edited by F. Duck, A. Baker and H. Starritt. Bristol: Institute of Physics, 1999, pp. 57-88.

Carstensen, E., Law, W., McKay, N. "Demonstration of nonlinear acoustical effects at biomedical frequencies and intensities." *Ultrasound Med Biol* 6: 359-368, 1980.

Chen, J. F., Fowlkes, J., Carson, P., Rubin, J. "Determination of scan plane motion using speckle decorrelation: theoretical consideration and initial test." *Int. J. of Imaging Syst. Technol.* 8: 38-44, 1997.

Comeau, R. M., Fenster, A., Peters, T. M. "Intraoperative US in interactive image-guided neurosurgery." *Radiographics* 18(4): 1019-27, 1998.

Evans, D., McDicken, W., Skidmore, R., Woodcock, J. *Doppler Ultra-sound: Physics, Instrumentation and Clinical Applications*. London: Wiley, 1989.

Fenster A., Lee, D., Sherebrin, S., Rankin, R., Downey, D. "Three-dimensional ultrasound imaging of the vasculature." *Ultrasonics* 36(1-5): 629-33, 1998.

Forsberg, F. *Principles of Doppler Imaging, in Medical CT and Ultrasound: Current Technology and Applications*, American Association of Physicists in Medicine Summer School. Edited by L, Goldman and J, Fowlkes. Madison: Advanced Medical Publishing, 1995.

Haider, B., Lewin, P., Thomenius, K. "Pulse elongation and deconvolution filtering for medical ultrasound imaging." *IEEE Trans Ultrasonics, Ferroelectrics and Freq Control* 45: 98-113, 1997.

Kasai,C., Namekawa, K., Koyano, A., Omoto, R. "Real-time two-dimensional blood flow imaging using an autocorrelation technique." *IEEE Trans on Sonics and Ultrasonics* SU-32: 458-465, 1985.

Kossoff, G., Garrett, W., Carpenter, D., Jelkins, J., Dadd, M. "Principles and classification of soft tissues by grey scale echography." *Ultrasound in Med. and Biol.* 2:89-105, 1976.

Lu, Z., Zagzebski, J., Lee, F. "Ultrasound backscatter and attenuation in human liver with diffuse disease." *Ultrasound Med. and Biol.,* 1999 (in press).

Riccabona M., Pretorius, D. H., Nelson, T. R., Johnson, D., Budorick, N. E., "Three-dimensional ultrasound: display modalities in obstetrics." *Journal of Clinical Ultrasound* 25(4): 157-67, 1997.

Rownd, J, Madsen, E., Zagzebski, J., Frank, G. "An automated system for determining low contrast lesion detectability in ultrasound imaging." *Ultrasound Med Biol* 23: 245-260, 1997.

Thomenius, K. "Instrumentation for B-mode imaging." In *Medical CT and Ultrasound: Current Technology and Applications*, American Association of Physicists in Medicine Summer School. Edited by L, Goldman and J, Fowlkes, Madison: Advanced Medical Publishing, 1995.

Wells, P.N.T. *Biomedical Ultrasonics*. London: Academic Press, 1968.

Wildes, D., Chiao, R., Daft, C., Rigby, K., Smith, L., Thomenius, K. "Elevation Performance of 1.25D and 1.5D transducer arrays." *IEEE Trans Ultrasonics, Ferroelectrics and Freq Control* 44: 1027-1037, 1997.

Vilkomerson, D., Greenleaf, J., Dutt, V. "Towards a resolution metric for medical ultrasonic imaging." 1995 IEEE Ultrasonics Symposium Proceedings, IEEE, 445 Hoes Lane, Piscataway, N.J., 1995.

Zagzebski, J. *Essentials of Ultrasound Physics*. St. Louis: Mosby, 1996.

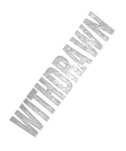
DATE DUE

2/5/01			
6/28/02			
11-20-02			
12/4/02			
MAR 2 2 '04			
DEC 0 8 '04			
MAR 2 9 2007			
APR 1 5 2009			
GAYLORD			PRINTED IN U.S.A.